High Performance Computing for Intelligent Medical Systems

IOP Series in Next Generation Computing

Series editors

About the series

The motive of this series is to develop a trusted library on advanced computational methods, technologies and their applications.

This series focuses on the latest developments in next generation computing, and in particular on the synergy between computer science and other disciplines. Books in the series will explore new developments in various disciplines that are relevant for computational perspective including foundations, systems, innovative applications and other research contributions related to the overall design of computational tools, models and algorithms that are relevant for the respective domain. It encompasses research and development in artificial intelligence, machine learning, block chain technology, quantum cryptography, quantum computing, nanoscience, bioscience-based sensors, IoT applications, nature inspired algorithms, computer vision, bioinformatics etc. and their applications in the areas of science, engineering, business and social sciences. It covers a broad spectrum of applications in the community, from industry, government, and academia.

The aim of the series is to provide an opportunity for prospective researchers and experts to publish works based on next generation computing and its diverse applications. It also provides a data-sharing platform that will bring together international researchers, professionals and academics. This series brings together thought leaders, researchers, industry practitioners, and potential users of different disciplines to develop new trends and opportunities, exchange ideas and practices related to advanced computational methods and promote interdisciplinary knowledge.

High Performance Computing for Intelligent Medical Systems

Edited by
Varun Bajaj and Irshad Ahmad Ansari
Indian Institute of Information Technology Design and Manufacturing, Jabalpur, India

IOP Publishing, Bristol, UK

ISBN 978-0-7503-3815-8 (ebook)
ISBN 978-0-7503-3813-4 (print)
ISBN 978-0-7503-3816-5 (myPrint)
ISBN 978-0-7503-3814-1 (mobi)

DOI 10.1088/978-0-7503-3815-8

Version: 20210701

IOP ebooks

British Library Cataloguing-in-Publication Data: A catalogue record for this book is available from the British Library.

Published by IOP Publishing, wholly owned by The Institute of Physics, London

IOP Publishing, Temple Circus, Temple Way, Bristol, BS1 6HG, UK

US Office: IOP Publishing, Inc., 190 North Independence Mall West, Suite 601, Philadelphia, PA 19106, USA

Dedicated to my father Late Mahendra Bajaj and Family members.

— Varun Bajaj

Dedicated to my family members.

— Irshad Ahmad Ansari

Contents

Preface xvi

Acknowledgements xviii

Editors biographies xix

Contributors biographies xxi

1 Automatic detection of hypertension by flexible analytic wavelet transform using electrocardiogram signals 1-1

Kapil Gupta, Smith K Khare, Varun Bajaj and Irshad Ahmed Ansari

1.1 Introduction 1-1

1.1.1 Various intervals of ECG 1-2

1.1.2 Related work 1-3

1.2 Methodology 1-4

1.2.1 Dataset 1-5

1.2.2 Flexible analytic wavelet transform 1-5

1.2.3 Feature extraction 1-7

1.2.4 Classification techniques 1-9

1.2.5 Performance parameters 1-9

1.3 Results 1-10

1.4 Conclusion 1-15

References 1-15

2 Computational intelligence in surface electromyogram signal classification **2-1**

Turker Tuncer, Sengul Dogan, Fatih Ertam and Abdulhamit Subasi

2.1 Introduction 2-1

2.2 Computational intelligence in biomedical signal processing 2-4

2.3 Background 2-7

2.3.1 Discrete cosine transform 2-7

2.3.2 Fast Fourier transform 2-7

2.3.3 Singular value decomposition 2-7

2.3.4 Ternary pattern 2-7

2.3.5 Support vector machine 2-8

2.3.6 Linear discriminant analysis 2-8

2.3.7 KNN 2-8

2.3.8 Artificial neural network 2-8

2.4 Spider network 2-8
2.4.1 Pre-processing 2-10
2.4.2 Feature extraction 2-10
2.4.3 Feature reduction 2-12
2.4.4 Feature concatenation 2-13
2.4.5 Classification 2-13
2.5 Results and discussions 2-14
2.5.1 Dataset 2-14
2.5.2 Experimental results 2-14
2.5.3 Discussion 2-18
2.6 Conclusions and suggestions 2-19
References 2-19

3 Analysis of IoT interventions to solve voice pathologies challenges 3-1
Wahengbam Kanan Kumar, Mithlesh Prasad Singh, Aheibam Dinamani Singh, Rajesh Kumar and Kishorjit Nongmeikapam

3.1 Introduction 3-1
3.1.1 Pathology assessment 3-2
3.1.2 Internet of things in voice pathology 3-3
3.2 Electroglottography 3-5
3.2.1 Quantitative analysis 3-7
3.3 Voice pathology datasets 3-7
3.3.1 Voice ICar fEDerico II (VOICED) 3-7
3.3.2 Massachusetts eye and ear infirmary 3-8
3.3.3 Saarbruecken Voice Database 3-8
3.3.4 Arabic voice pathology database 3-8
3.4 Acoustic speech features with machine learning for voice pathology classification 3-9
3.4.1 Feature extraction techniques 3-9
3.4.2 Voice pathology analysis and detection techniques 3-11
3.5 Discussion and conclusion 3-22
References 3-24

4 Deep learning for cuffless blood pressure monitoring 4-1
Jamal Esmaelpoor, Zahra Momayez Sanat and Mohammad Hassan Moradi

4.1 Introduction 4-1

4.2 Physiological models 4-2
4.3 Data source 4-4
4.3.1 Preprocessing procedures 4-4
4.4 Deep learning models for blood pressure monitoring 4-6
4.4.1 LSTM model 4-7
4.4.2 PCA-LSTM model 4-9
4.4.3 Convolutional neural network model 4-11
4.4.4 CNN–LSTM model 4-13
4.5 Discussion 4-14
4.5.1 Comparison with other methods 4-16
4.6 Conclusion 4-18
References 4-19

5 Reliability of machine learning methods for diagnosis and prognosis during the COVID-19 pandemic: a comprehensive critical review **5-1**

Hamid Reza Marateb, Mohammad Reza Mohebbian, Mehdi Shirzadi, Arezoo Mirshamsi, Shadi Zamani, Atena Abrisham chi, Fatame Bafande and Miguel Ángel Mañanas

5.1 Introduction 5-1
5.2 Methods 5-2
5.2.1 January–March 5-2
5.2.2 April–June 5-3
5.2.3 July–September 5-5
5.2.4 October 2020 to February 2021 5-8
5.2.5 Machine learning methods 5-12
5.2.6 Critical issues 5-18
5.3 Conclusion and future scope 5-20
References 5-21

6 Forecasting confirmed cases of Corona patients in India using regression and Gaussian analysis **6-1**

Dhyan Chandra Yadav and Saurabh Pal

6.1 Introduction 6-1
6.2 Regression analysis in machine learning 6-4
6.3 Related work 6-9
6.4 Methodology 6-10
6.4.1 Data description 6-10

6.5 Results 6-11
6.6 Discussion 6-13
6.7 Conclusion 6-13
Acknowledgments 6-15
References 6-15

7 A model for advanced patient feedback procedures in diagnostics 7-1
Marjo Rissanen, Antti Rissanen and Kalle Saastamoinen

7.1 Introduction 7-1
7.2 Focus on diagnostics 7-2
7.2.1 Diagnostic error as a concept 7-2
7.2.2 Diagnostic errors in healthcare 7-2
7.2.3 Common reasons for diagnostic failures 7-3
7.2.4 Preventing diagnostic errors in cooperation with patients 7-3
7.3 Diagnostics and safety challenges in healthcare 7-4
7.3.1 Patient safety and equity challenges 7-4
7.3.2 Enhanced patient safety with rational cost control policy 7-5
7.4 Importance of patient feedback in the diagnostics phase 7-5
7.4.1 Need for timely feedback 7-5
7.4.2 The role of timely feedback 7-6
7.5 The challenges of diagnostics-centered clients' feedback 7-6
7.6 Enhancing technology acceptance in system development 7-7
7.7 Phases of diagnostics and the requirements for doctors 7-8
7.7.1 Requirements for competence and compassion 7-8
7.7.2 Diagnostic process from the view of doctors 7-8
7.7.3 Diagnostic process from the view of patients 7-8
7.8 A model for instant patient feedback 7-9
7.8.1 General principles 7-9
7.8.2 Structure of the model 7-9
7.8.3 Patient management with the model 7-10
7.8.4 Meaning of the fixed format phase of the model—phase 1 7-12
7.8.5 Meaning and management of the free format phase—phase 2 7-13
7.8.6 Clients' opinions of the feedback delivery system—phase 3 7-15
7.9 Client feedback as a translational development challenge 7-15
7.9.1 Enhancing process synergy in organizations 7-15
7.9.2 Maturing and validating patient-targeted feedback systems 7-16

7.10 Conclusion 7-16
References 7-17

8 Soft computing techniques for efficient processing of large medical data **8-1**
Hussain Ahmed Choudhury and Nidul Sinha

8.1 Introduction 8-1
8.2 Understanding the concept: video compression 8-3
8.3 Image compression standards 8-4
8.3.1 JPEG 8-4
8.3.2 JPEG2000 8-4
8.3.3 JPEG-LS 8-5
8.3.4 JPEG-XR 8-5
8.3.5 H.265 8-5
8.3.6 Types of coding and frames 8-6
8.4 Motion estimation and the necessity of it in video coding? 8-7
8.4.1 Forward and backward motion estimation 8-7
8.4.2 Block matching concept 8-8
8.5 What is soft computing: techniques and differences 8-9
8.6 Standard techniques for motion estimation 8-10
8.7 Soft computing techniques for motion estimation 8-10
8.8 Conceptual terms used in different SC techniques 8-11
8.8.1 Chromosomes and genes 8-11
8.8.2 Chromosome representation 8-11
8.8.3 Cross-over 8-11
8.8.4 Mutation 8-11
8.8.5 Weighting function and PBME 8-11
8.9 Some well-established soft computing based BMA 8-11
8.9.1 Genetic algorithm-BMA 8-11
8.9.2 Inter-block/inter-frame fuzzy search algorithm 8-13
8.9.3 Basic block-matching using particle swarm optimization 8-13
8.9.4 Harmony search block matching algorithm 8-14
8.9.5 Cat swarm optimization (CSO-BMA) 8-15
8.9.6 CUCKOO search based BMA (CS-BMA) 8-16
8.9.7 The ABC-BM algorithm 8-18
8.9.8 ABC-DE 8-18

8.9.9 HS-DE based BMA 8-18
8.9.10 'Deterministically starting-GA' (GA_{Det}) 8-19
8.9.11 Enhanced Grey-wolf optimizer-BMA (EGWO-BMA) 8-20
8.9.12 Chessboard search pattern strategy 8-21
8.10 Results and discussion 8-22
Acknowledgment 8-25
References 8-25

9 A comparison of Parkinson's disease prediction using ensemble data mining techniques with features selection methods 9-1
Dhyan Chandra Yadav and Saurabh Pal

9.1 Introduction 9-1
9.2 Related work 9-2
9.3 Methodology 9-3
9.3.1 Data description 9-4
9.3.2 Whisker plotting 9-5
9.3.3 Histogram plotting 9-5
9.4 Algorithms description 9-5
9.4.1 Decision tree 9-5
9.4.2 Naïve Bayes 9-6
9.4.3 Random forest 9-6
9.4.4 Extra tree 9-6
9.4.5 Bagging ensemble method 9-7
9.4.6 Features selection method in Parkinson's disease 9-8
9.5 Results 9-8
9.5.1 Evaluation of result after prediction on Parkinson's dataset 9-9
9.5.2 Result of features importance methods 9-9
9.5.3 Chi-square test 9-9
9.5.4 Extra tree 9-9
9.5.5 Heat map 9-10
9.5.6 Evaluation of results after features selection 9-10
9.6 Discussion 9-10
9.7 Conclusion 9-14
Acknowledgments 9-15
References 9-15

10 A comparative analysis of image enhancement techniques for detection of microcalcification in screening mammogram **10-1**
Gaurav Makwana, Ram Narayan Yadav and Lalita Gupta

10.1 Introduction 10-1
10.2 Image enhancement in spatial domain 10-4
10.2.1 Histogram modeling 10-4
10.2.2 Histogram equalization 10-5
10.2.3 Histogram matching 10-5
10.2.4 Averaging filter 10-5
10.2.5 Gaussian filter 10-6
10.2.6 Median filter 10-6
10.3 Image enhancement in frequency domain 10-7
10.3.1 Butterworth filtering 10-8
10.3.2 Gaussian low-pass filter 10-8
10.3.3 Homomorphic filtering 10-8
10.3.4 Discrete wavelet transform 10-9
10.4 Convolutional neural network 10-11
10.5 Evaluation criteria 10-13
10.5.1 Mean square error 10-13
10.5.2 Peak signal-to-noise ratio 10-13
10.5.3 SNR 10-13
10.5.4 Mean 10-14
10.5.5 Variance 10-14
10.6 Results and discussion 10-14
10.7 Conclusion 10-18
References 10-19

11 Computational intelligence for eye disease detection **11-1**
Amit Kumar Verma

11.1 Introduction 11-1
11.2 Anatomy of the eye 11-2
11.2.1 The cornea 11-3
11.2.2 The human retina 11-4
11.3 Retinal diseases 11-5
11.3.1 Retinal tear 11-5
11.3.2 Diabetic retinopathy 11-5
11.3.3 Macula hole 11-5

11.3.4 Degeneration of the macula 11-6
11.3.5 Disorders of the optic nerve 11-6
11.3.6 Glaucoma 11-6
11.3.7 Diabetic macular edema 11-7
11.3.8 Retinopathy of prematurity 11-7
11.4 History of retinal imaging 11-7
11.5 Current status of retinal analysis 11-8
11.5.1 Fundus imaging 11-8
11.5.2 Optical coherence tomography 11-9
11.6 Disease specific analysis of retinal images 11-9
11.6.1 Early detection of retinal disease from fundus photography 11-9
11.6.2 Early detection of systemic disease from fundus photography 11-10
11.6.3 3-Dimensional OCT and retinal diseases—image guided therapy 11-10
11.7 Fundus image analysis 11-10
11.7.1 Glaucoma detection using retinal imaging 11-11
11.7.2 Dementia detection using retinal imaging 11-12
11.7.3 Heart diseases detection using retinal imaging 11-12
11.7.4 Choroidal melanoma detection using retinal imaging 11-13
11.7.5 Advantages of retinal imaging 11-13
11.8 Comparative analysis between various retinal imaging methods 11-13
11.9 Conclusion 11-13
References 11-14

12 Recent trends in medical image segmentation with special focus on brain tumours and retinal images **12-1**

Mithlesh Prasad Singh, Aheibam Dinamani Singh, Rajesh Kumar, Kishorjit Nongmeikapam and Wahengbam Kanan Kumar

12.1 Introduction 12-1
12.1.1 Types of biomedical imaging 12-2
12.1.2 Biomedical image segmentation 12-3
12.1.3 Segmentation evaluation 12-4
12.2 Retinal images segmentation 12-6
12.2.1 Datasets 12-6
12.2.2 Fundus photography 12-8
12.2.3 Challenges in retinal vessel segmentation 12-8
12.2.4 Review of literature 12-9

12.3 Brain tumour segmentation 12-12
12.3.1 Brain tumour segmentation databases 12-13
12.3.2 Classification of brain tumour 12-14
12.3.3 Brain photography 12-14
12.3.4 Challenges 12-15
12.3.5 Image pre-processing 12-16
12.3.6 Image post-processing 12-16
12.3.7 Traditional machine learning in tumor segmentation 12-17
12.3.8 Deep learning 12-18
12.4 Discussion and conclusion 12-20
References 12-21

13 Analysis of AI based PID controller for health care system 13-1
Vandana Dubey, Harsh Goud and Prakash Chandra Sharma

13.1 Introduction 13-1
13.2 Types of chronic disease 13-4
13.2.1 Cancer 13-4
13.2.2 Blood pressure 13-5
13.2.3 Diabetes 13-6
13.2.4 Arthritis 13-9
13.3 Analysis of the biomedical system 13-10
13.3.1 Classical controller in a biomedical system 13-11
13.4 Mathematical modeling of the biomedical system 13-12
13.4.1 MAP control 13-12
13.4.2 Intracranial tumor's temperature control 13-12
13.4.3 Blood glucose 13-13
13.4.4 BP control after surgery in a diabetic patient 13-14
13.4.5 Heart modeling using PM 13-15
13.4.6 Tumor growth control 13-15
13.5 Conclusion 13-16
References 13-16

Preface

The medical and healthcare domain is a cornerstone of society, but modern medicine is highly dependent on engineering. There are machines and systems for analyzing patients, thus making diagnosis possible. X-ray and electrocardiography (ECG) are examples of such systems. X-ray, CT-scan and MRI (medical resonance imaging) provide visual representations, whereas ECG and EEG generate biological signals. Similarly, there are machines for management of patients as well. In the medical and healthcare sector a large amount of data is generated in every step, from the sensing of the ailment, to examination, correlation, classification and its management too.

The present era is witnessing a large-scale development in the field of computational intelligence (CI). High performance computing has emerged as a powerful solution to deal with complex problems. The development happening around the high performance computing and related fields is affecting us in a very positive way. The field of medical science has benefited greatly from the field of the computational intelligence. This has led to the development of intelligent medical systems (IMS). IMS are a result of research collaboration of high performance computing with medical science. The development of IMS requires a large amount of data generation, storage and processing. To apply high performance computing in the medical domain, in depth knowledge and understanding of the medical system is required.

This large amount of data is a necessity for correct analysis and correlation of disease. The generation, collection, storage and labeling of such large data is quite a challenging task. With the advent of wearable devices data generation is increased manyfold. The high performance computing tools seem a powerful option for working on such a large amount of data. They have the ability to perform complex tasks with high speed and accuracy. This knowledge helps researches to apply CI concepts for enhanced performance of medical systems. IMS are able to provide human-like ability and intelligence to existing applications. In this way, IMS can be utilized to get a deep insight into various healthcare and medical problems. It can also aid in controlling, analyzing and management of medical applications. The field of CI makes it possible to address the various issues concerning human health and medical systems. IMS will be fruitful for significant improvement in human life.

The in-depth analysis of large data is the prime requirement for the development of IMS. This can be very helpful in medical and healthcare applications. High performance computing is definitely the answer for computing needs in the medical domain. Deep computational architecture, with capabilities like low-level feature extraction and data augmentation can give a new direction to the present research in medical systems. Considering the future aspects of high performance computing and its involvement in the medical field, IMS is a widely researched area. The idea behind this book is to focus on the advancements in the domain of high performance computing for medical systems. The chapter-wise description of this book as follows.

Chapter 1 presents automatic detection of hypertension and normal electrocardiogram signal by using flexible analytic wavelet transform and different classification techniques. Chapter 2 explores a novel CI approach called spider network classification of basic hand movements. This CI approach provides an effective solution for disabled people based on a man–machine interface employing surface electromyogram signals. Chapter 3 demonstrates dysfunction of speech or voice that leads to a wide range of psychiatric disorders resulting from stigmatization from peers and the community. Different aspects of voice pathology research, applications for the Internet of Things, different datasets, feature extraction, and classification techniques are discussed. Chapter 4 develops several architectures based on deep neural networks (DNNs) and develops more appropriate models to meet the demands of the British Hypertension Society and the Association for the Advancement of Medical Instrumentation Standards.

Chapter 5 provides analysis of critical STARD/TRIPOD issues of more than 45 machine learning methods for the detection of COVID-19 during the pandemic. In addition, various strategies have been recommended to avoid systematic flaws and improve the clinical reliability of such systems. Chapter 6 presents four different functional models for Covid data analysis of Indian Covid patients accessed from Kaggle. Chapter 7 explores a model for improved patient feedback in diagnostics. The work focuses on a model that helps healthcare consumers to formulate and express their opinions quickly and easily about a perceived diagnostic phase in their care. Chapter 8 presents digital radiographs and other computerized methods used for the diagnosis of different diseases. It is required to compress and process the data efficiently with limited hardware resources, hence various soft computing techniques are applied in the field of video compression to make the process faster by accelerating the motion estimation. Chapter 9 describes how the brain manages the control system and blood circulation by nerve cells, so it becomes important to know about the symptoms of initial stage neuron disturbance in the body system. Therefore, to protect the human body, machine learning algorithms are used to analyze Parkinson's disease symptoms. Chapter 10 presents mammogram images enhancement to improve the image quality for better interpretation and detection of breast cancer. In chapter 11 retina imaging helps in the diagnosis of proper eye disease along with complications of diabetes retinopathy, hypertension, myocardial infarction, etc. Therefore, the anatomy of the eye, physiology of the various eye diseases, retinal imaging methods-2D fundus imaging, and 3D optical coherence tomography (OCT) and their comparative analysis are done. Chapter 12 provides a survey on biomedical image segmentation for brain tumors and retina segmentation, abnormality detection, advantages, disadvantages, and automated-learning techniques ranging from traditional machine learning to deep learning are done. Also, it provides a glimpse of key gaps and potential future scope for biomedical image segmentation of retina and brain tumors. Chapter 13 discusses an AI-based proportional integral derivative (PID) controller with various biomedical systems and a comparative study of all primitives and novel control strategies for the AI-based PID controller regarding the health care system is explored.

Acknowledgements

Dr Bajaj expresses his heartfelt appreciation to his mother Prabha, wife Anuja, daughter Avadhi, for their wonderful support and encouragement throughout the completion of this important book on high performance computing for intelligent medical systems. His deepest gratitude goes to his mother-in-law and father-in-law for their constant motivation. This book is the outcome from sincere efforts that could be given to the book only due to great support from the family.

Dr Ansari expresses his gratitude and sincere thanks to his family members and teachers for their constant support and motivation.

We sincerely thank Professor Sanjeev Jain, Director of PDPM IIITDM Jabalpur for his support and encouragement. We would like to thank all our friends, well-wishers and all those who keep us motivated in doing more and more, better and better. We sincerely thank all contributors for writing the relevant theoretical background and applications of this book.

We express our humble thanks to Dr John Navas and all editorial staff of IOP Publishing for great support, necessary help, appreciation and quick responses. We also wish to thank IOP Publishing for giving us this opportunity to contribute on some relevant topic with a reputed publisher. Finally we want to thank everyone, in one way or another, who helped us to edit this book.

Dr Bajaj especially thanks his family who encouraged us throughout the time of editing book. This book is heartily dedicated to his father who took the lead to heaven before the completion of this book.

Last but not least, we would also like to thank God for showering us his blessings and strength to do this type of novel and quality work.

Varun Bajaj
Irshad Ahmad Ansari

Editors biographies

Varun Bajaj

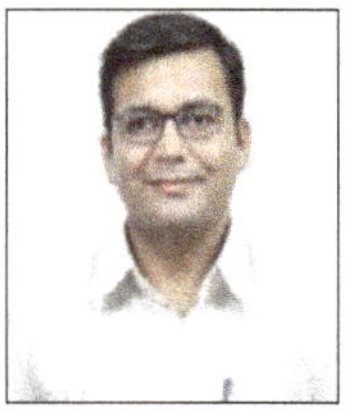

Varun Bajaj PDPM IIITDM Jabalpur, Jabalpur, India

Varun Bajaj (PhD, MIEEE 16 SMIEEE20) has been working as a faculty member in the discipline of Electronics and Communication Engineering, at Indian Institute of Information Technology, Design and Manufacturing (IIITDM) Jabalpur, India since 2014. He worked as a visiting faculty member in IIITDM Jabalpur from September 2013 to March 2014. He worked as Assistant Professor at Department of Electronics and Instrumentation, Shri Vaishnav Institute of Technology and Science, Indore, India during 2009–2010. He received his BE degree in Electronics and Communication Engineering from Rajiv Gandhi Technological University, Bhopal, India in 2006, MTech degree with Honors in Microelectronics and VLSI design from Shri Govindram Seksaria Institute of Technology and Science, Indore, India in 2009. He received his PhD degree in the Discipline of Electrical Engineering, at Indian Institute of Technology Indore, India in 2014.He is an Associate Editor of IEEE Sensor Journal and Subject Editor-in-Chief of *IET Electronics Letters*. He served as a Subject Editor of *IET Electronics Letters* from November 2018 to June 2020. He was made a Senior Member IEEE in June 2020, MIEEE 16–20, and also contributing as active technical reviewer of leading International journals of IEEE, IET, and Elsevier, etc. He has authored more than 110 research papers in various reputed international journals/conferences such as IEEE Transactions, Elsevier, Springer, IOP Publishing etc. He has edited books with IOP Publishing and CRC Press (Taylor & Francis Group). The citation impact of his publications is around 2470 citations, h index of 24, and i10 index of 60 (Google Scholar, March 2021). He has guided six (three completed and three in process) PhD scholars and six MTech scholars. He is a recipient of various reputed national and international awards. His research interests include biomedical signal processing, image processing, time–frequency analysis, and computer-aided medical diagnosis.

Irshad Ahmad Ansari

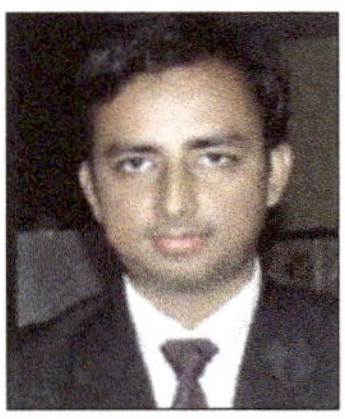

Irshad Ahmad Ansari PDPM IIITDM Jabalpur, Jabalpur, India

Irshad Ahmad Ansari has been working as a faculty member in the discipline of Electronics and Communication Engineering, at PDPM Indian Institute of Information Technology, Design and Manufacturing (IIITDM) Jabalpur, India since 2017. He received his BTech degree in Electronics and Communication Engineering from Gautam Buddha Technical University, Lucknow, India in 2010, MTech degree in Control and Instrumentation from Dr B R Ambedkar National Institute of Technology Jalandhar, Punjab, India in 2012. He completed his PhD from IIT Roorkee with MHRD teaching assistantship, and subsequently joined Gwangju Institute of Science and Technology, South Korea as a postdoctoral fellow. His major research interest includes image processing, signal processing, soft computing, brain computer interface and machine learning. He is a Senior IEEE member. He is presently guiding three PhD scholars. He has authored more than 32 research papers in various reputed international journals/conferences of publishers like IEEE, Elsevier, Springer etc. He is also serving as an active and potential technical reviewer for various journals of repute.

Contributors biographies

Ms Athena Abrishamchi

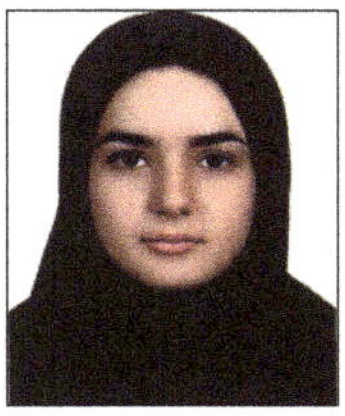

Athena Abrishamchi Faculty of Engineering, University of Isfahan, Isfahan, Iran

Ms Athena Abrishamchi is a Biomedical Engineering MSc student at the University of Isfahan. She finished her BSc degree in biomedical engineering at the University of Isfahan in 2019. In 2018 summer, she joined the AI research group at the Medical University of Isfahan and worked on detecting lung cancer through deep learning methods. Also, her research interests include machine learning, deep learning, machine vision, and data mining.

Fatame Bafande

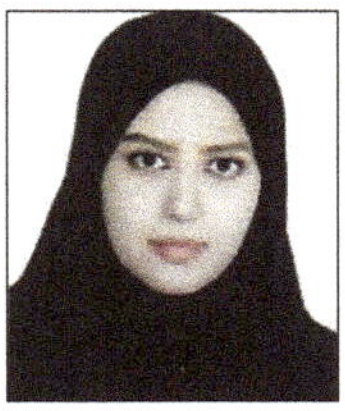

Fatame Bafande Faculty of Engineering, University of Isfahan, Isfahan, Iran

Fatemeh Bafande, has been studying for an MSc in Biomedical engineering in the University of Isfahan since 2019. She took a BSc degree in Electronic and Electrical Engineering from Hamadan University of Technology in 2018. Her research interests include pattern recognition, machine learning, data mining, and signal/image processing.

Hussain Ahmed Choudhury

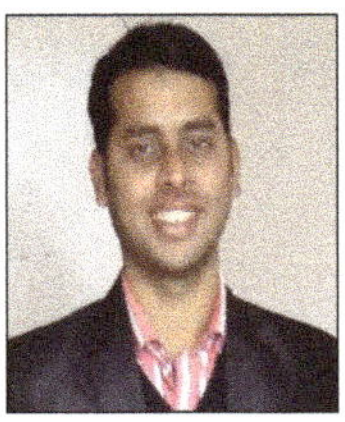

Hussain Ahmed Choudhury CVR College of Engineering, Ibrahimpattanam, Hyderabad, India

Dr Hussain Ahmed Choudhury, PhD received his BTech degree from Assam University silchar, MTech from NERIST-AR and PhD degrees in Computer Science and Engineering from National Institute of Technology, Silchar, Assam, India in 2010, 2014 and 2020, respectively. He joined Jain University Bangalore as Assistant Professor in CSE-Specialization from 2018 to 2020. Since December 2021, he has been working as an Associate Professor with the Department of Computer Science-IT department of CVR College of Engineering, Hyderabad under JNTU, India. Dr Hussain has authored/co-authored 16 publications in various high impact factor, peer-reviewed, journals. He has written one book chapter and he presented about six papers in international conferences. His area of research includes image processing, data visualization, computer networks and soft computing techniques.

Sengul Dogan

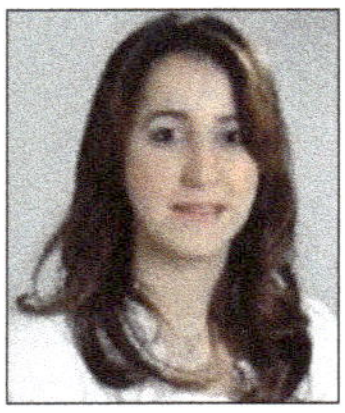

Sengul Dogan Digital Forensics Engineering, Technology Faculty, Firat University, Elazig, Turkey

Sengul Dogan received a master's degree in bioengineering and a PhD in electrical and electronics engineering from Firat University, Elazig, Turkey, in 2007 and 2011, respectively. She is currently an Associate Professor with the Digital Forensics Engineering, Technology Faculty, Firat University. Her main research interests include computer forensics, mobile forensics, image processing, and signal processing. She has been working actively on developing algorithms in machine learning for biomedical data.

Vandana Dubey

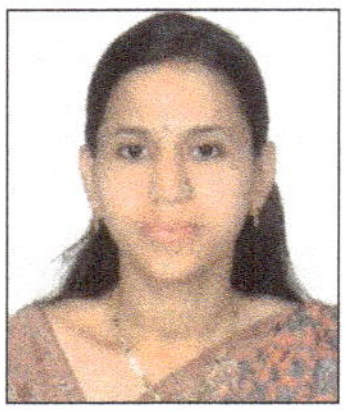

Vandana Dubey Department of Electronics, Manipal University Jaipur, India

Ms Vandana Dubey, PhD (pursuing) from Manipal University Jaipur-Rajsthan, in Information and Technology Engineering. Received ME (72.8%) from IET-DAVV Indore-M.P., BE (73.13%) from BANSAL R.G.P.V. Bhopal-M.P., Diploma (67.01%) from S.R.G.W.P. R.G.P.V. Sagar-M.P., degrees in Electronics and Communication Engineering, in 2010, 2006 and 2003, respectively. She received a 'Best student award' in Diploma. She started her academic carrier in 2007. Since January 2015, she has been with the IPS Academy, an autonomous institute, Indore, where she is currently an Assistant Professor. Her research interests include physical layer security, PID controller, reinforcement learning, machine learning and artificial intelligence. She has published 13 research papers in national/ international conferences and journals. She is a lifetime member of the IETE (Institution of Electronics and Telecommunication Engineers).

Fatih Ertam

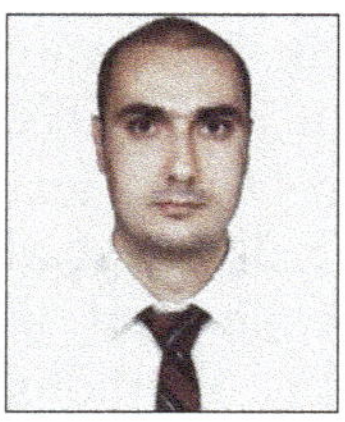

Fatih Ertam Digital Forensics Engineering, Technology Faculty, Firat University, Elazig, Turkey

Fatih Ertam received a PhD degree in software engineering from Firat University, Elazig, Turkey, in 2016. He is currently an Associate Professor with the Digital Forensics Engineering, Technology Faculty, Firat University. His current research interests include artificial intelligence, deep learning, digital forensics, and network security.

Jamal Esmaelpoor

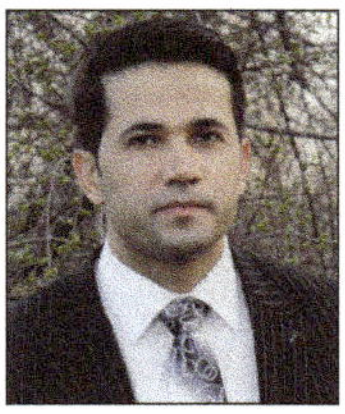

Jamal Esmaelpoor Islamic Azad University Boukan Branch, Boukan, Iran

Mr Jamal Esmaelpoor is a lecturer at Azad University, Boukan Branch and also continues his studies at Amirkabir University of Technology, Tehran, Iran. His research interests include biomedical signal processing, artificial intelligence in biomedicine, and medical instrumentation.

Harsh Goud

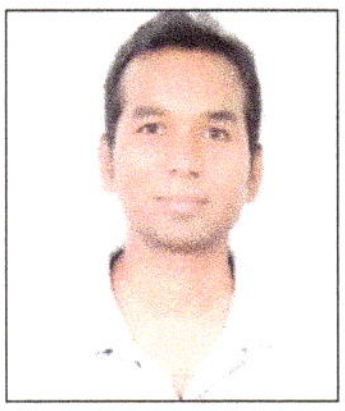

Harsh Goud Department of Electronics, Indian Institute of Information Technology Nagpur, India

Dr Harsh Goud, PhD received his BE degree in Electronics and Instrumentation Engineering from Shri Govindram Seksaria Institute of Technology and Science, Indore in 2005, and ME degree in Digital Techniques and Instrumentation from Shri Govindram Seksaria Institute of Technology and Science, Indore in 2008. His PhD is in Electrical Engineering from Maulana Azad National Institute of Technology, Bhopal in 2019. He joined Institute of Engineering and Science IPS Academy Indore as an Assistant Professor in 2010. Since January 2021, he has been with the Faculty of Electronics and Communication Engineering Department, Indian Institute of Information Technology, Nagpur, where he is currently an Assistant Professor. His research interests include instrumentation, control system and robotics. Dr Harsh has authored/co-authored 11 publications in various high impact factor, peer-reviewed, journals. He has presented three papers in international conferences.

Kapil Gupta

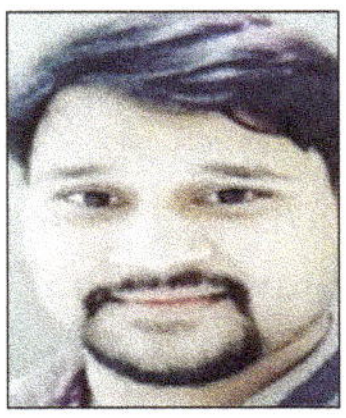

Kapil Gupta PDPM IIITDM Jabalpur, Jabalpur, India

Mr Kapil Gupta is a research scholar in Indian Institute of Information Technology, Design and Manufacturing Jabalpur, India. He received a BE degree with Honors in Electronics and Communication Engineering from Oriental Institute of Science and Technology, Bhopal, India in 2011, and an MTech degree in Nano Technology, from School of Nano Technology, Rajiv Gandhi Technical University, Bhopal, India in 2013. His research interests include non-stationary signal processing, biomedical signal processing, nano materials.

Lalita Gupta

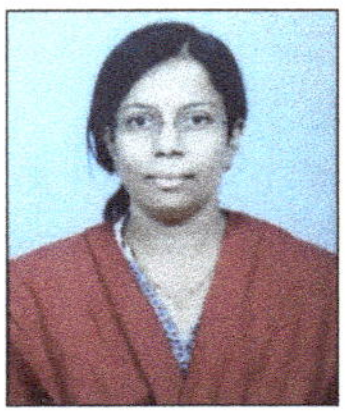

Lalita Gupta Department of Electronics and Communication Engineering, Maulana Azad National Institute of Technology, Bhopal, India

Lalita Gupta is Associate Professor at the Department of Electronics and Communication Engineering, Maulana Azad National Institute of Technology, Bhopal, India. She received her BE degree in Electronics and Telecommunication Engineering from Pt. Ravi Shankar Shukla University Raipur in 2003, MTech degree in Digital Communication from Maulana Azad National Institute of Technology, Bhopal, India in 2007 and PhD in Electronics and Communications Engineering from Maulana Azad National Institute of Technology, Bhopal, India in 2012. Since July 2004 she has been associated as a faculty member with the Maulana Azad National Institute of Technology, Bhopal. She is a member of IEEE, IETE, ICEIT. Dr Gupta has 30 research publications in various international journals and conferences of repute. Her research interests are signal and image processing.

Smith K Khare

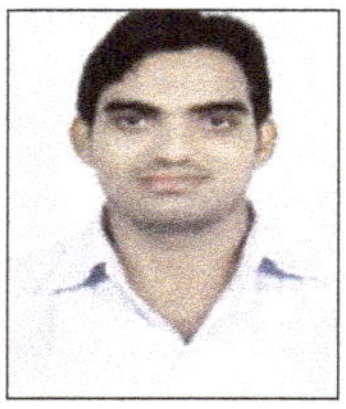

Smith K Khare PDPM IIITDM Jabalpur, Jabalpur, India

Mr Smith K Khare is a research scholar in Indian Institute of Information Technology, Design and Manufacturing, Jabalpur, India. Mr Smith has authored/co-authored 13 publications in various high impact factor, peer-reviewed journals for publishers like IEEE Transactions, Elsevier, etc. He has published two papers in international conference proceedings. He is serving as a journal reviewer for IEEE, Elsevier and several other reputed publishers. His research interests include biomedical signal processing, pattern recognition, machine learning and deep neural networks.

Rajesh Kumar

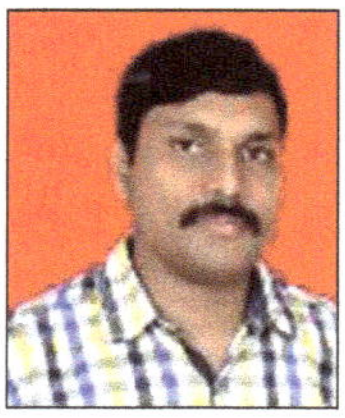

Rajesh Kumar Department of ECE, NERIST, Nirjuli, India

Rajesh Kumar PhD was born in India. He received his Bachelor of Engineering in ECE from Bangalore University in 2001, Master of Engineering Science in Control Systems from NIT, Patna in 2007 and PhD in the field of sensors from Jamia Millia Islamia, New Delhi (A Central University) in 2012. He has 18+ years of teaching experience in various capacities at RPSIT, Patna (Bihar), AKGEC, Ghaziabad (UP) and ABESEC, Ghaziabad (UP) at an undergraduate and post-graduate level of engineering education. He is presently working as Associate Professor in the Department of Electronics and Communication Engineering at North Eastern Regional Institute of Science and Technology (Under MHRD, Gov. of India), Nirjuli, Itanagar, India. He has published numerous research articles in journals and conferences at national and international level. His area of research is in the field of sensing technology using MEMS, RF MEMS, biosensors, WSN and mobile communication.

Wahengbam Kanan Kumar

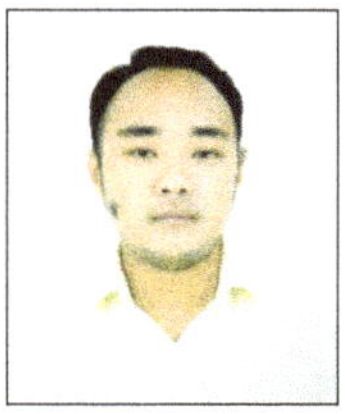

Wahengbam Kanan Kumar Department of ECE, NERIST, Nirjuli, India

Wahengbam Kanan Kumar, PhD received his BE degree in Electronics and Communication Engineering from Manipur University, India in 2012, and MTech degree from M.M.U. Mullana in 2015. He is currently working as a JRF and nearing PhD completion at NERIST. He has published eight SCI journal papers during his PhD tenure with reputed publishers like IEEE, Elsevier, Springer Nature, Wiley, ACM and IOS Press. He has also published numerous research articles in conference and book series. His current research interests include image processing, computer vision, pattern recognition, medical image processing, biomedical signal processing, and speech.

Gaurav Makwana

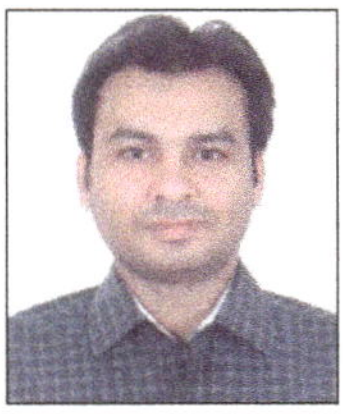

Gaurav Makwana Department of Electronics and Communication Engineering, Maulana Azad National Institute of Technology, Bhopal, India

Gaurav Makwana is a doctorate researcher in Department of Electronics and Communication Engineering, Maulana Azad National Institute of Technology, Bhopal, India. He received his BE degree in Biomedical Engineering in 2006 from Shri Govindram Seksaria Institute of Technology and Science, Indore, India and ME in Digital Techniques and Instrumentation in 2010 from Shri Govindram Seksaria Institute of Technology and Science, Indore, India. He was lecturer in Department of Biomedical Engineering, Shri Govindram Seksaria Institute of Technology and Science, Indore, India from December 2006 to August 2008. Since March 2011, he has been associated as a faculty member with the Department of Electrical and Electronics Engineering, Shri Vaishnav Institute of Technology and Science, Indore, India. His research interests are medical instrumentation and image processing.

Miguel Ángel Mañanas

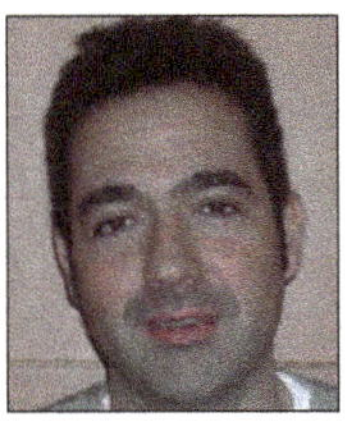

Miguel Ángel Mañanas Escola Tècnica Superior d'Enginyeria Industrial de Barcelona (ETSEIB), Universitat Politècnica de Catalunya-Barcelona Tech, Barcelona, Spain

Miguel Ángel Mañanas, PhD, received his Telecommunications Engineering degree and PhD in Biomedical Engineering (BME) from Universitat Politècnica de Catalunya (UPC) in 1993 and 1999, respectively. He is currently an Associate Professor at the Department of Automatic Control (ESAII) at the same university, member of the Biomedical Engineering Research Center (CREB) at the UPC and member of the CIBER-BBN. He is the founder and leader of the multidisciplinary BIOsignal Analysis for Rehabilitation and Therapy Group (BIOART, UPC) composed of engineers and physicians. His research is focused on applying engineering techniques in health areas. His career has been particularly focused on biomedical signal processing and biological system modeling, in three fields: (1) neuromuscular: evaluating neuromuscular disorders and motor rehabilitation by high-density electromyography; (2) neurological: evaluating brain activity by electroencephalography and magnetoencephalography; (3) respiratory: modeling the respiratory control system and simulating pulmonary diseases and mechanical ventilation. He is the co-author of 65 JCR articles (31 in Q1 and 23 in Q2), has more than 100 peer-reviewed scientific communications, and co-invented two patents. He has co-supervised eight PhD theses. He has also been PI of 30 national/international projects. He received the Leonardo Award from BBVA Foundation as a career recognition in 2016.

Hamid Reza Marateb

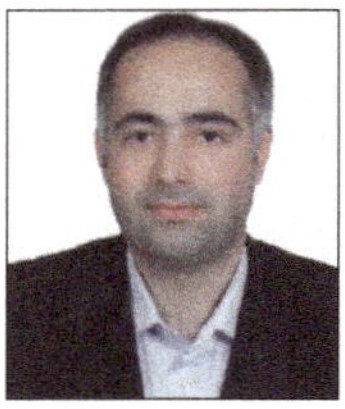

Hamid Reza Marateb Faculty of Engineering, University of Isfahan, Isfahan, Iran

Hamid Reza Marateb, PhD received BS and MS degrees from the Shahid Beheshti University of Medical Science and Amirkabir University of Technology, Tehran, Iran, in 2000 and 2003, respectively. He received his PhD and the post-doctoral fellowship from the Laboratory of Engineering of Neuromuscular Systems, Politecnico di Torino, Turin, Italy in 2011 and 2012, respectively. He was a visiting researcher at Stanford University in 2009 and Aalborg University in 2010. He was a visiting professor in UPC, Barcelona, in 2012 and 2017. His research line is cognitive informatics in health and biomedicine, mainly focusing on clinical neurophysiology, computational neurosciences, and medical data mining. Dr Marateb is a reviewer in more than 30 international ISI journals and is now on the editorial board of international journals including *Frontiers in Integrative Physiology*, and *Frontiers in Cognitive Neuroscience*. He also received European Union/Spanish grants (e.g., Marie Curie fellowship and MYOSLEEVE). He is currently with the Department of Biomedical Engineering, Faculty of Engineering, the University of Isfahan, Iran, and also BIOsignal Analysis for Rehabilitation and Therapy Research Group (BIOART), Department of Automatic Control, Biomedical Engineering Research Center, Universitat Politècnica de Catalunya, BarcelonaTech (UPC), Barcelona, Spain.

Arezoo Mirshamsi

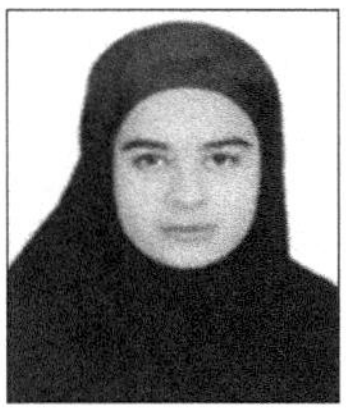

Arezoo Mirshamsi Faculty of Engineering, University of Isfahan, Isfahan, Iran

Arezoo Mirshamsi has been an MS student of Biomedical Engineering of the University of Isfahan since 2019. She graduated from Hamedan University of technology in 2018 with a BS Degree in Biomedical Engineering. The subject of her BS project was stress reduction with biofeedback by investigating heart rate variation while playing an Android game. She was also a member of the Editorial Board of the *Student Journal of Medical Engineering* (2015–2017). Her research interests include EEG and EMG signal processing, artificial intelligence, machine learning, and deep learning.

Mohammad Reza Mohebbian

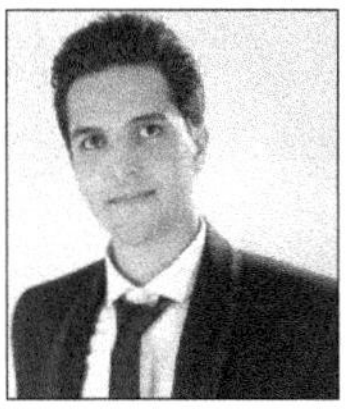

Mohammad Reza Mohebbian Department of Electrical and Computer Engineering, University of Saskatchewan, Saskatoon, Canada

Mohammad Reza Mohebbian studied biomedical engineering at the University of Isfahan for BSc and MSc degrees. He ranked in the top two of the BSc and MSc students. Presently, he is studying electrical and computer engineering at the University of Saskatchewan, Canada. He won a devolved scholarship from the University of Saskatchewan in 2019 and conducted research for Philips Canada during his PhD program. His career is mainly focused on machine learning, deep learning, pattern recognition, and image processing in biomedical fields.

Mohammad Hassan Moradi

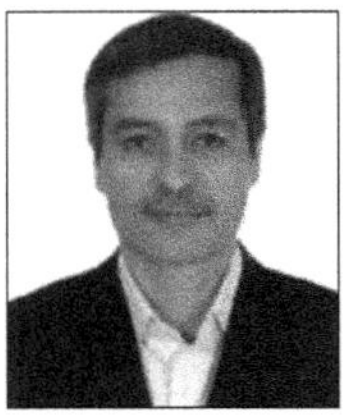

Mohammad Hassan Moradi Amirkabir University of Technology, Tehran, Iran

Dr Mohammad Hassan Moradi is Professor at Biomedical Engineering Department of Amirkabir University of Technology, Tehran, Iran. His research interests include medical instrumentation, biomedical signal processing.

Kishorjit Nongmeikapam

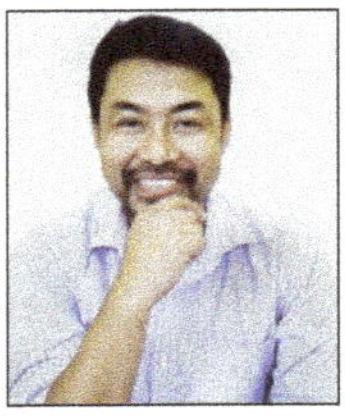

Kishorjit Nongmeikapam Department of CSE, Indian Institute of Technology, Manipur, India

Kishorjit Nongmeikapam, PhD received his BE degree in Computer Science and Engineering from PSG College of Technology, Coimbatore, India in 2003. He completed his ME and PhD in Computer Science and Engineering from Jadavpur University, Kolkata, India in 2010 and 2016, respectively. He worked as a faculty member in Manipur University for 13 years from 2003, and has also currently been a faculty member in Indian Institute of Information Technology (IIIT) Manipur since 2016. His research interests are in the area of image processing, computer vision, pattern recognition, natural language processing, and programming. He has published over 40 scientific papers in many research journals, international and national conferences of repute.

Saurabh Pal

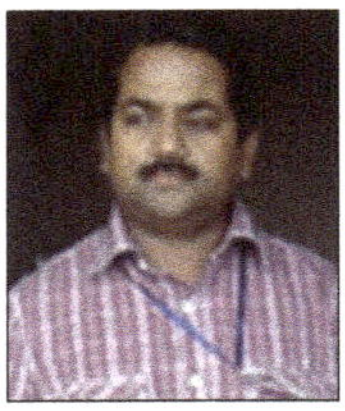

Saurabh Pal Department of Computer Applications, VBS Purvanchal University, Jaunpur, India

Dr Saurabh Pal is Head of the Department of Computer Applications at Jaunpur's Veer Bahadur Singh Purvanchal University. Machine learning, pattern recognition, software engineering, cloud computing, and other topics are among his research interests. Dr Pal has authored or co-authored 80 publications in peer-reviewed journals with high impact factors. Dr Pal has 25 book chapters to his credit and has given about 30 papers at international conferences. Dr Saurabh Pal has been a reviewer for a number of conferences and journals.

Antti Rissanen

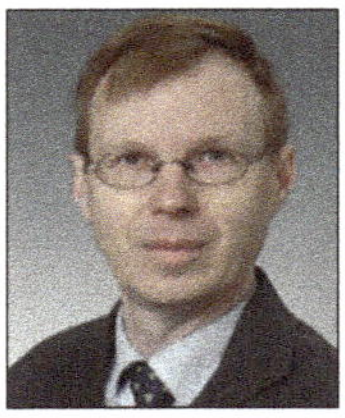

Antti Rissanen Department of Miltary Technology, National Defence University, Helsinki, Finland

Dr Antti Rissanen, PhD received his BSc, MA and PhD degrees in Physics from Helsinki University, Finland in 1981, 1984 and 2011, respectively. He obtained licentiate in technology degree (electric engineering) in 1992 in University of Technology in Tampere. In 1997 he joined the National Defence University (Finland) as a Senior Lecturer for General Technology where he currently works as a researcher. He is also the leader of the Educational Research Group at the Military Technology Department. His research interests include science education, e-learning, and simulations or artificial intelligence in an educational context. Previous research interests are biomedical engineering, signal analysis, technology transfer and thin film technology. Dr Rissanen has authored/co-authored 37 publications in peer-reviewed, journals. Dr Rissanen has written three book chapters and presented about 50 papers at international conferences.

Marjo Rissanen

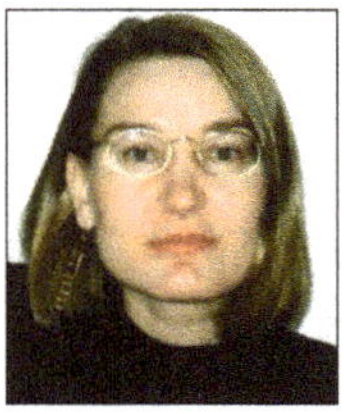

Marjo Rissanen Prime Multimedia Ltd, Helsinki, Finland

Mrs Marjo Rissanen is a senior consultant, focusing on the health informatics design area. She received her master's degree from Helsinki University, Faculty of Medicine, Finland. She has worked in Helsinki University, in the Ministry of Social Affairs and Health, and in consultancy companies in research and design activities. She has worked also in international projects, e.g., in Sri Lanka in a cost-control information system project for an orthopaedic hospital. She has lectured for the academia, health organizations, and industry also in international contexts. Her research interests cover topics connected to translational health technology and design, consumer-targeted health informatics, related quality and design challenges. She has written 16 peer-reviewed articles about timely topics.

Kalle Saastamoinen

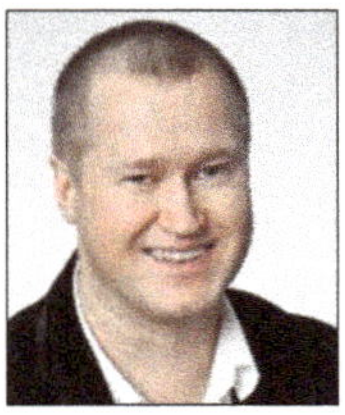

Kalle Saastamoinen Department of Miltary Technology, National Defence University, Helsinki, Finland

Dr Kalle Saastamoinen, PhD received his MSc degree in Mathematics from University of Helsinki in 1999 and PhD degree in Applied Mathematics from Lappeenranta University of Technology in 2008. He worked as a researcher and as a part time lecturer in Lappeenranta University of Technology and South Karelia University of Applied Sciences during 1999–2008. In 2009, he joined the National Defence University (Finland) as a Senior Lecturer for applied mathematics, where he is currently working as a researcher and research coordinator in the Department of Military Technology. His research interests are computational logic and its applications, AI based expert systems, data classification, military technology research, teaching technology and its usage. Dr Saastamoinen has authored/co-authored 71 peer-reviewed publications.

Zahra Momayez Sanat

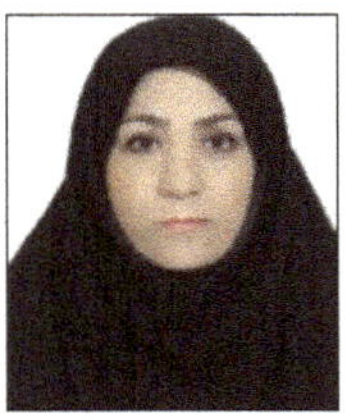

Zahra Momayez Sanat Tehran University of Medical Sciences, Tehran, Iran

Dr Zahra Momayez Sanat received her Specialty Board of internal Medicine, Shahid Beheshti University of Medical Sciences in 2004. She is Assistant Professor at Tehran University of Medical Science, Tehran, Iran.

Prakash Chandra Sharma

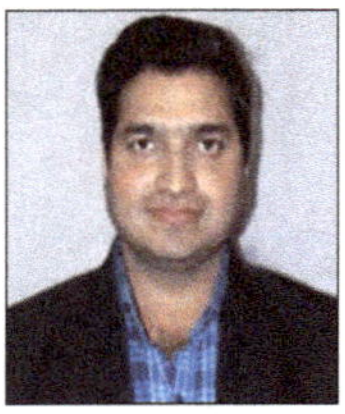

Prakash Chandra Sharma Manipal University Jaipur, Santoshi Nagar, Khamatarai, Raipur, India

Dr Prakash Chandra Sharma is currently working as Senior Assistant Professor in School of Computing & Information Technology at Manipal University Jaipur, India. He has received his honored degree of PhD from Indian Institute of Technology Indore in discipline of Computer Science & Engineering. He completed his Master of Engineering from SGSITS Indore. He has teaching and research experience of 16 years in various areas of Computer Science & Engineering. His research interest includes graph theory, theoretical computer science, artificial intelligence, image processing and wireless network. He has published a number of research papers in various international/national journals (including IEEE, Springer, Elsevier etc.) and in proceedings of reputed international/national conferences as well. He has also published number of book chapters in various edited books with reputed publishers like Elsevier, Springer, CRC Press etc. He is an active reviewer and editorial member of various reputed international journals in his research areas. He has filed and published 10 copyrights and patents. He has chaired many technical sessions in international conferences. He is a member of various professional international societies (including IEEE, CSI, IAENG, Institute of Engineers India). He is a recipient of many awards and recognitions at national level.

Mehdi Shirzadi

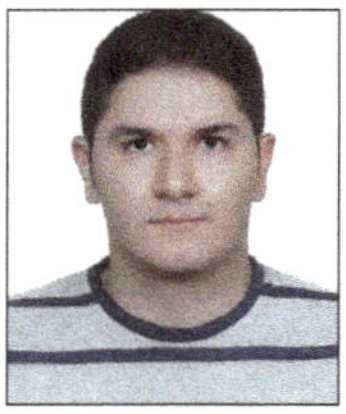

Mehdi Shirzadi Escola Tècnica Superior d'Enginyeria Industrial de Barcelona (ETSEIB), Universitat Politècnica de Catalunya-Barcelona Tech, Barcelona, Spain

Mehdi Shirzadi received BS and MS degrees in Biomedical Engineering from Islamic Azad University of Najaf Abad, Najaf Abad, Isfahan, Iran and the University of Isfahan, Isfahan, Iran, in 2015 and 2018, respectively (raked in the top two students). He is a PhD candidate of Biomedical Engineering at the Universitat Politècnica de Catalunya-Barcelona Tech (UPC), Barcelona, Spain. He won a four-year scholarship from the Ministry of Economy and Competitiveness (MINECO) in Spain in 2019. His research interests include electromyographic signal processing, optimization, medical data mining, and machine learning.

Aheibam Dinamani Singh

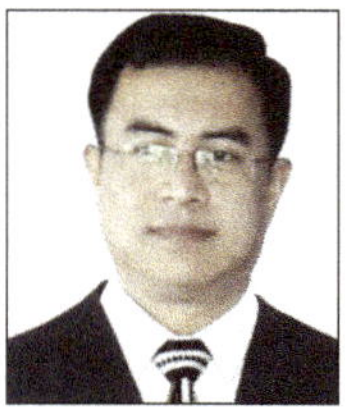

Aheibam Dinamani Singh Department of ECE, NIT Manipur, India

Aheibam Dinamani Singh, PhD received BTech in Electronics and Communication Engineering from North Eastern Hills University, Shillong, India in 2004. He completed his MTech and PhD in Electronics and Communication Engineering from the North Eastern Regional Institute of Science and Technology (NERIST), Nirjuli, Arunachal Pradesh, India, in 2010 and 2015, respectively. He was a teaching faculty member in the Department of Electronics and Communication Engineering, NERIST from 2006 to 2019. He is currently working as Associate Professor in the Department of Electronics and Communication Engineering at National Institute of Technology, Manipur. His research interests are in the area of wireless communication, fading channels, image processing, computer vision, bio-medical image processing, signal processing, antennas array, and millimeterwave antennas. He has published over 60 scientific papers in research journals, international and national conferences of repute.

Mithlesh Prasad Singh

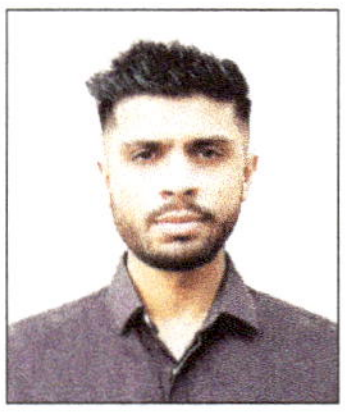

Mithlesh Prasad Singh Department of CSE, Amity University, Gurugram, India

Mithlesh Prasad Singh, MTech received his BE degree in Computer Science and Engineering from Manipur University, India in 2016, and is currently pursuing a master's degree in Artificial Intelligence and Machine learning from Amity University Gurugram. His current research interest includes deep learning optimization, Nature-inspired algorithms, computer vision, medical image and signal processing, natural language processing and e-learning.

Nidul Sinha

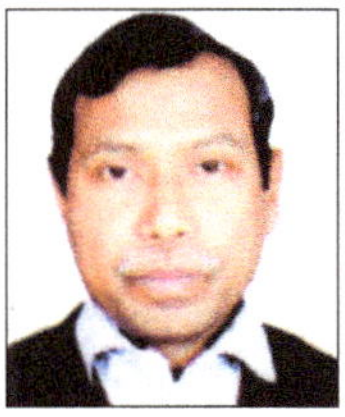

Nidul Sinha NIT Silchar, Cachar, Assam, India

Dr Nidul Sinha was born in Tripura, India, in 1962. He received the BE degree in Electrical Engineering from Calcutta University, Calcutta, India, in 1984, and the MTech degree in Power Apparatus and Systems from Indian Institute of Technology, New Delhi, in 1989. He received a PhD in Electrical Engineering from Jadavpur University, Kolkata, India. His PhD thesis was on 'Application of Intelligent Techniques in Optimal Operation of Power System'. Since then he has been engaged in active research in different areas like automatic generation control, optimal operation of power system under a conventional as well as non-conventional environment, control of renewable energy sources and micro-grid, image de-noising, video motion estimation, EEG based emotion detection, silent speech reading. He has more 100 national and international publications in diverse fields. He was conferred with the senior membership of IEEE in 2008. He has successfully completed four sponsored R&D projects. Further, he has been the reviewer of number of international journals; IEEE, IET, Elsevier, Taylor & Francis, and Springer etc.

Abdulhamit Subasi

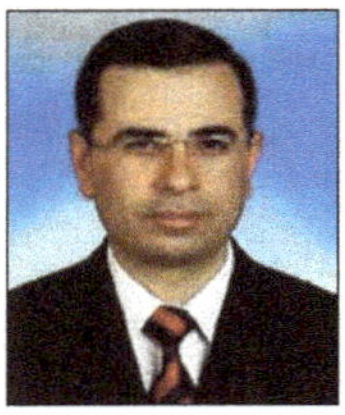

Abdulhamit Subasi Institute of Biomedicine, Faculty of Medicine, University of Turku, Turku, Finland

Abdulhamit Subasi is specialized in artificial intelligence, machine learning, biomedical signal and image processing. Concerning application of machine learning to different fields, he has written more than ten book chapters and more than 190 published journal and conference papers. He is also author of the books, 'Practical Guide for Biomedical Signals Analysis Using Machine Learning Techniques' and 'Practical Machine Learning for Data Analysis Using Python'. He worked at many institutions as an academician and Georgia Institute of Technology, Georgia, USA, as a researcher. He has been awarded with the Queen Effat Award for Excellence in Research, May 2018. He worked as a Professor of computer science at Effat University, Jeddah, Saudi Arabia between 2015 and 2020. Since 2020, he has been working as a Professor of medical physics at Faculty of Medicine, University of Turku, Turku, Finland and visiting researcher at Effat University, Jeddah, Saudi Arabia. He has worked on several projects related to biomedical signal processing and data analysis.

Turker Tuncer

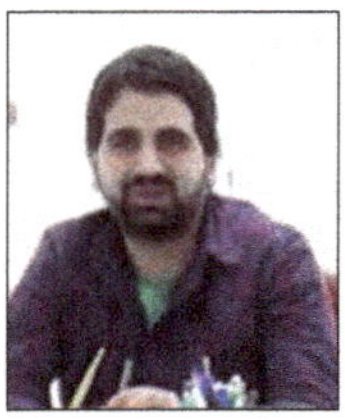

Turker Tuncer Digital Forensics Engineering, Technology Faculty, Firat University, Turkey

Turker Tuncer received a master's degree in electronics and computer sciences and a PhD in software engineering from Firat University, Elazig, Turkey, in 2011 and 2016, respectively. He is currently an Associate Professor with the Digital Forensics Engineering, Technology Faculty, Firat University. His main research interests include feature engineering, image processing, signal processing, information security, and pattern recognition. He has been working actively on developing algorithms in machine learning applied to visual surveillance and biomedical data.

Amit Kumar Verma

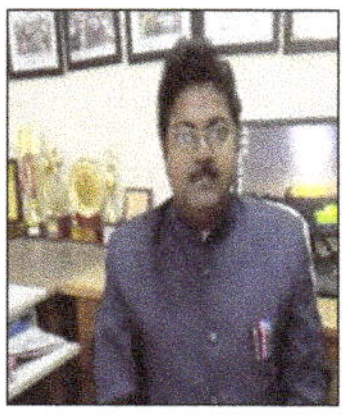

Amit Kumar Verma Department of Pharmacy, MJP Rohilkhand University Bareilly, Biharpur, UP, India

Amit Kumar Verma (Academician and Researcher, Gold medalist, Shikshak Shree Awardee). A renowned Academician working in the Department of Pharmacy MJP Rohilkhand University, UP Govt State University, District Bareilly, Uttar Pradesh. He was the merit holder in his BPharm. He did his postgraduation in pharmaceutical chemistry (MPharm) from Manipal College of pharmaceutical sciences (MCOPS) Manipal, Karnataka India. He took PG project training at Central Drug Research Institute (CDRI) Lucknow. The research topic of his PhD was polymer chemistry and drug delivery. He has wide experience of academic, research and administration. He has published 12 research papers in high-impact publications of SCI, Scopus, UGC etc, with 5 books and more than 12 book chapters to his credit. He is the editor of a book series on COVID-19. He is presently working on a research project on COVID-19. His interest areas include application of artificial intelligence in the disease management and herbal formulation development. He has four patent publications and copyrights to his credit. He has supervised 15 postgraduate students. In the interdisciplinary contribution, he is the research supervisor of the dissertation work of MSC microbiology and chemical engineering students of the University. He is a member of Institutional Ethical Committee supervising 600 Colleges and also the science representative member of the intellectual property right IPR cell of the University, covering around 600 Colleges. In an administrative capacity, he is working as Assistant Dean Student Welfare ADSW, Training placement coordinator, career counsellor and mental counsellor to students during COVID-19. Through the use of electronic and print media Doordarshan, Akashwani radio, newspapers etc, he has enriched the knowledge of Indian citizens. Delivering more than 20 expert invited lectures in renowned institutions of the Army, ITBP Police, educational and in villages indicates his capability of percolating knowledge through society. In corporate life he is discharging the duties of advisor (non-remunerative basis) in the Alobhin Herbal Pharmaceutical private limited, his innovation led to the development of product 'Daisy care' which is available in the commercial market, now working as Brand Ambassador of innovation cell, Ministry of Education. His social contribution creation of ZERO TB Digital platform, an innovative initiative enabling digital caring of tuberculosis patients to help achieve the goal of a TB-free India, is the first in the world. He also runs a self-financed malaria and COVID-19 eradication awareness program in District Bareilly.

Dhyan Chandra Yadav

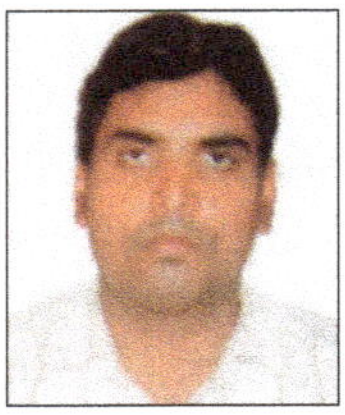

Dhyan Chandra Yadav Department of Computer Applications, VBS Purvanchal University, Jaunpur, India

Dr Dhyan Chandra Yadav, Post-Doc., received his MCA from Veer Bahadur Singh Purvanchal University, Jaunpur in 2008, and his PhD in Computer Applications from SV University Gajraulla, Amroha JapiNagar, U.P. in 2016. He is currently employed as a Post-Doctoral Fellow at Veer Bahadur Singh Purvanchal University, Jaunpur. Pattern recognition, statistical image processing, and knowledge discovery are among his research interests. Dr Yadav has authored/co-authored 25 publications in peer-reviewed journals with high impact factors. Dr Yadav has published two book chapters and has given four presentations at international conferences. Dr Dhyan Chandra Yadav has served as a conference reviewer and a journal reviewer.

Ram Narayan Yadav

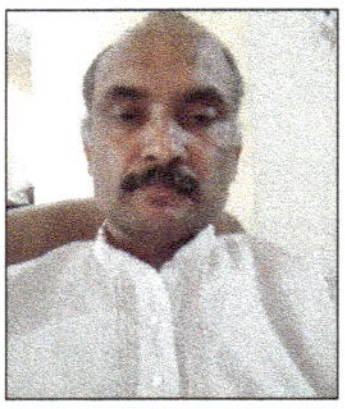

Ram Narayan Yadav Department of Electronics and Communication Engineering, Maulana Azad National Institute of Technology, Bhopal, India

Ram Narayan Yadav received the BTech degree in Electronics from Motilal Nehru National Institute of Technology, Allahabad, India in 1993, MTech degree in Digital Communications from Maulana Azad National Institute of Technology Bhopal, India in 1997 and PhD in Electrical Engineering from Indian Institute of Technology, Kanpur, India in 2005. He joined the department of Electronics and Communication Engineering, Maulana Azad National Institute of Technology Bhopal, India in 1997 where he is currently a professor. He has published more than 70 papers in various international journal and conference including journals of IEEE, IET, Elsevier and Springer. He has supervised 25 masters and 10 doctoral students. He is a reviewer of several IEEE and Elsevier journals. His current research interests are communication systems, image processing, neural networks and applications.

Shadi Zamani

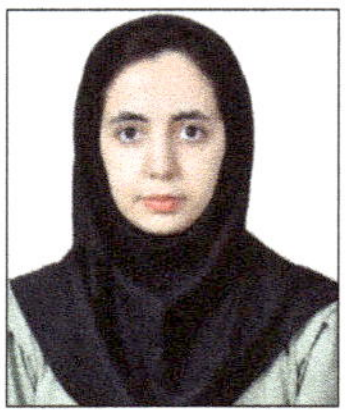

Shadi Zamani Faculty of Engineering, University of Isfahan, Isfahan, Iran

Shadi Zamani received the BS degree in Biomedical Engineering from University of Isfahan, Isfahan, Iran in 2019. She is currently pursuing an MSc degree in Biomedical Engineering in the University of Isfahan since 2019. Her current research interests include machine learning, pattern recognition, data mining and medical image processing.

IOP Publishing

Chapter 1

Automatic detection of hypertension by flexible analytic wavelet transform using electrocardiogram signals

Kapil Gupta, Smith K Khare, Varun Bajaj and Irshad Ahmed Ansari

Hypertension (HPT) is a critical health problem that comes from the higher blood pressure force on the walls of arteries. HPT occurs when systolic blood pressure (SBP) and diastolic blood pressure (DBP) are more than 140 mmHg and 90 mmHg, respectively. It becomes more severe when SBP is greater than 180 mmHg and DBP is more than 120 mmHg. HPT has no direct symptoms but continuous higher blood pressure can urge heart muscles enlargement which will be reflected in the electrocardiography (ECG) report. Due to the non-stationary nature of ECG signals it is difficult to detect HPT manually. Hence, an automatic detection of HPT is proposed using flexible analytic wavelet transform (FAWT) in this chapter. The input signal is decomposed into sub-bands using FAWT and features are extracted from these sub-bands. A set of highly discriminatory features are identified using the Kruskal–Wallis test. These features are fed into the input of different classifiers to classify the HPT and normal ECG signals. The effectiveness of the proposed system is checked by applying tenfold cross-validation and obtained specificity, sensitivity, accuracy, negative predicted value, false positive rate, and false negative rate of 96.74%, 96.95%, 96.60%, 99.69%, 3.04%, and 3.24%, respectively, using ensemble bagged tree classifier.

1.1 Introduction

Hypertension (HPT) is defined as higher pressure of blood, and it is a severe health condition that comes from the large blood pressure force acting on the walls of the arteries [1]. It creates higher blood pressure around the arteries, as the heart works hard to pump oxygenated blood through the rest of the body [1]. According to statistics of the World Health Organization, HPT is the third most common cause of global fatality and responsible for more than eleven million deaths annually [2]. HPT, if not treated in a timely manner may induce various diseases related to kidney, brain and heart [3, 4].

Timely diagnosis and proper medication of HPT may help in reducing the risk of various cardiovascular diseases [5, 6]. From clinical epidemiological observations, optimal systolic blood pressure (SBP) and diastolic blood pressure (DBP) are less than 140 mmHg and 90 mmHg, repectively, in a healthy person [7]. HPT becomes severe when SBP and DBP are more than 180 mmHg and 120 mmHg, respectively [8]. A sphygmomanometer is commonly used to measure blood pressure [8]. Due to various environmental limitations it is being replaced by computerized measurement devices such as aneroid sphygmomanometers and digital electronic pressure transducers [9]. But these meters may provide inaccurate results due to the tendency of error in estimating SBP and DBP in adults [10].

As the pressure of blood can vary, 24-h, monitoring of blood pressure has emerged as a useful tool for diagnosing HPT [11]. Continuous HPT will sharpen heart, nerve, and kidney diseases which will be deliberated in the electrocardiography (ECG) report. Varying electrical activity of the heart is measured by using an ECG report [12]. The isoelectric line is calculated from the baseline voltage of ECG, which is the portion of tracing following the T-wave and preceding the next P-wave [13, 14]. ECG analysis helps the cardiologist to diagnose the symptoms of the various diseases [15].

Segmentation of ECG signal plays a vital role in the analysis of coronary artery disease, blockage in the heart, hypertrophy of heart chambers, etc [16]. ECG signal is the combination of P-wave, QRS complex, and T-wave. P-wave is also known as atria complex, and occurs when the senatorial node produces an action that depolarizes the atria. The P-wave is the first and positive wave of the ECG [17]. The height and width of a normal P-wave is less than 2.5 small squares. Taller P-wave occurs due to the enlargement of the right atria, which is greater than 2.5 mV and causes a pulmonary chronic respiratory disease called pulmonary HPT. A wider P-wave occurs due to the enlargement of the left atria having a duration of 2.5 s. Q-wave is the negative wave due to the depolarization of the basal portion of the interventricular septum. R-wave is the positive tallest wave due to depolarization of the apical portion in the ventricular septum and muscle. S-wave is the smallest negative wave due to depolarization of the basal portion in the ventricular muscle near the atria ventricular ring. The association of Q-, R- and S-wave is called QRS complex or initial ventricular complex. T-wave is the positive wave that occurs due to repolarization of ventricular musculature; with the help of ECG a segment cardiologist can identify the various types of heart activity [18].

1.1.1 Various intervals of ECG

P–R interval: is the time difference between starting of P-wave and starting of Q-wave. A normal P–R interval lies in the range 120–200 ms. Greater P–R interval (value more than 200 ms) indicates first-degree heart block, and if the P–R interval is less than 120 ms it indicates Wolff–Parkinson–White syndrome.

Q–T interval: is the time difference between starting of Q-wave and ending of T-wave. A normal Q–T interval lies in the range of 360–440 ms. A long QT interval ($QT > 440$ ms) indicates hypocalcemia. A short Q–T interval ($QT < 360$ ms) indicates hypercalcemia.

QRS interval: is defined as the time difference between endings of P-wave and starting of T-wave. Normal QRS interval is less than 100 ms, if it is greater than 100 ms it indicates a bundle branch block.

R–R interval: is the time difference in between two consecutive R-waves. A normal R–R interval is 60–120 ms.

Long-lasting HPT affects all these intervals, which is reflected in the ECG test. However, there may be no clinically visible ECG disturbances in the early stage of HPT, and it is difficult to diagnose manually with ECG [11]. Automatic detection of HPT using ECG signal is an emerging research topic in the field of biomedical engineering. Since the recorded ECG signal is contaminated with various types of noise it may cause variation in the width and height of these intervals and error occurs in the prediction of disease [19]. So, preprocessing of ECG is required before feeding the classifier. Preprocessing can be divided into two phases: the noise removal phase suppresses noise present in the signal and the feature extraction phase extracts information from the signal [20]. Jain *et al* developed the ECG denoising method based on empirical mode decomposition using Riemann–Liouville fractional integral [21]. The severity of HPT can be detected automatically using noise-free and segmented ECG signals [22].

1.1.2 Related work

To date, researchers have proposed various methods for detection and classification of HPT using ECG signals. Tripathi *et al* classified the features extracted by using filtering to detect fast and slow heart rhythms [23]. Rajput *et al* determined the HPT diagnosis index which has been used to differentiate in between HPT and normal subject using wavelet filter bank [11]. Chuang *et al* applied empirical mode decomposition to extract different linear and non-linear features [24]. Kiat Soh *et al* used discrete wavelet transform and extract different subbands to diagnose the HPT [10]. Ni *et al* developed multi-scale HRV analysis for calculating the severity of HPT by using wavelet transform to detect R peaks [11]. Melillo *et al* designed a tool for prognosis of cardiovascular and cerebrovascular events using HRV analysis through the series of beat intervals [25]. Zhang *et al* have done analysis of the autonomic nervous pattern in HPT based on short-term HRV by using the RR interval. Different features are extracted to distinguish between hypertensive heartbeat rhythms and normal ones [26]. Kale *et al* extracted the R–R interval for prediction of sensitivity and specificity of a cardiovascular event, random forest classifier has been used for classification of the event [27]. Ortiz-Martin *et al* analyzed the entropy of the LSB values and the Pan–Tompkins algorithm has been used to extract the R-peaks and extracted inter pulse interval [28]. Alkhodari *et al* implemented a machine learning model that handles imbalance data and predicts vascular events in hypertensive patients [29]. Agliari *et al* applied statistical mechanics tools and maximum entropy principle to analyzed temporal correlation in heart rate variability (HRV) against various complexes and chaotic cardiac dynamics [30]. Taye *et al* predicted the occurrence of ventricular tachyarrhythmia which arises from improper electrical heart activity and causes fast heart rate [31]. Agnihotri *et al* predicted present and future cardiac health of an individual based on fast and slow heart rhythms [32]. Koichubekov *et al* analyzed nonlinear indices of HRV signal in HPT using the Pan–Tompkins algorithm to detect the QRS complex and calculate R–R intervals. The spectral of R–R interval samples have been determined by using Welch's method [33]. Bossone *et al* studied the association of features in primary pulmonary hypertension patients [34]. Melillo *et al* designed a cloud-based intelligent health monitoring system to automatically collect and analyze biomedical signals for the identification of HPT patients [35]. Dami *et al* predicted cardiovascular events using a deep belief neural network to reduce the dimension of the features, and used long short-term memory for classification of features [36]. Zhao *et al* identified the association of nervous system functions with minor stroke, using an ECG signal [37]. Thomas *et al* applied automated ECG-derived sleep spectrogram technique to prevent stroke and HPT in the sleeping stage [38]. Paragliola *et al* used a time series-based approach for identification of increases in HPT to discriminate between cardiovascular high-risk and low-risk HPT patients [39]. Schillaci *et al* reviewed the role of ECG signal in the diagnosis of left ventricular hypertrophy to forecast many risk factor adjusted cardiovascular morbidity and mortality in the asymptomatic patients of HPT [40]. Afkami *et al* developed a method for detection of left ventricular hypertrophy by using discrete wavelet transform to find the statistical features and fed it to a support vector machine (SVM) classifier with RBF kernel function [41]. Jothiramalingam *et al* used continuous wavelet transform for detection of R-wave and S-wave to obtain the features of left ventricular hypertrophy. SVM, K-nearest neighbour (KNN), ensember tree (ET) classifier have been used for classification [42]. Kublanov *et al* compared various machine learning methods for the diagnosis of arterial HPT by using short-term HRV signals [43].

Various methods have been proposed for detection and classification of HPT in the literature. The filtering method requires selection of filter coefficients which are difficult to select, whereas in wavelet based methods selection of mother wavelet and decomposition level is difficult. The main contribution of this chapter is to design an automatic ECG detection system to discriminate between normal and HPT patients using flexible analytic wavelet transform (FAWT) and different machine learning algorithms to identify the most discriminant features and most suitable classification technique.

The rest of the chapter is organized as follows. Methodology is presented in section 1.2. The results are discussed in section 1.3, and the conclusion of this chapter is presented in section 1.4.

1.2 Methodology

This section consists of information about the dataset, FAWT, features, and classification techniques. The ECG signals are decomposed into subbands using FAWT. Various time domain features such as mean, mean absolute value (MAV), root mean square (RMS), standard deviation (STD), variance (VAR) and simple square integral (SSI) are extracted from these subbands. Highly distinguishable features are selected using the Kruskal–Wallis test and classified using different classifiers. Figure 1.1 represents a pictorial view of the proposed methodology.

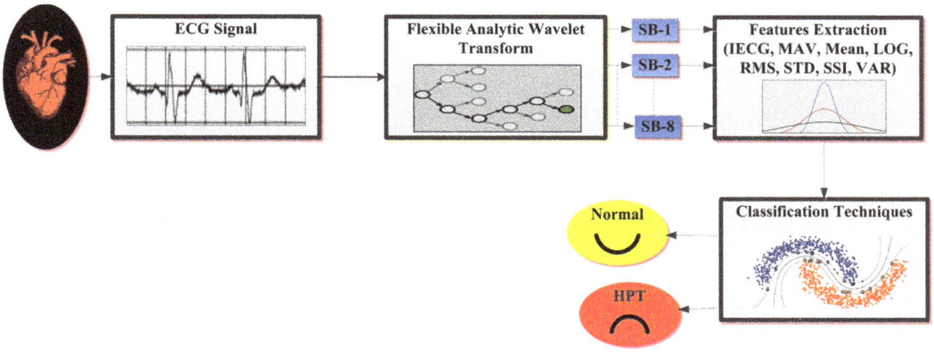

Figure 1.1. Flowchart of the proposed methodology.

1.2.1 Dataset

The ECG dataset downloaded from smart health for assessing the risk of events from the physionet website (https://physionet.org/content/shareedb/1.0.0/). It contains nominal 24-h ECG holter recording of 139 subjects, and available length of ECG recording of each subject is approximately 2 h 10 min: 12 s. ECG signal of each subject is recorded from three channels III, V3, and V5, and sampled at a sampling frequency of 128 Hz, with 8-bit resolution. It contains 49 females of average age 55 ± 5 years and 90 males having average age 72 ± 7 years, respectively. Out of 139 subjects, 17 were identified as high-risk HPT and 122 were identified as normal [9]. In this chapter, ECG recordings are segmented into 2-min epochs. Figure 1.2 represents the three lead ECG recordings of normal and HPT subject.

1.2.2 Flexible analytic wavelet transform

The nature of ECG signal is nonlinear and nonstationary due to which many difficulties are faced in the time-frequency analysis of a signal. Hence this study considered FAWT to decompose the ECG signal into sub-bands. FAWT is the well-structured technique for decomposition of non-stationary and non-linear signal. FAWT contains Hilbert transform pairs of atoms for analyzing positive and negative structure, therefore, it is most suitable for nonstationary signal processing. It uses a bank of filters to decompose a signal into sub bands. An iterative filter bank is used for signal decomposition. It is a combination of two high pass filters and one low pass filter. FAWT low pass and high pass channels are allowed arbitrary sampling rate. In FAWT dilation factor, quality factor and the redundancy can be easily specified by the user, due to this flexibility it allows fast implementation with perfect reconstruction of a finite length signal [44].

The following variables are used in FAWT: low pass up-sampling (s_1), low pass down-sampling (s_2), high pass up-sampling (s_3), high pass down-sampling (s_4), controlling parameter β, quality factor and redundancy rate (R).

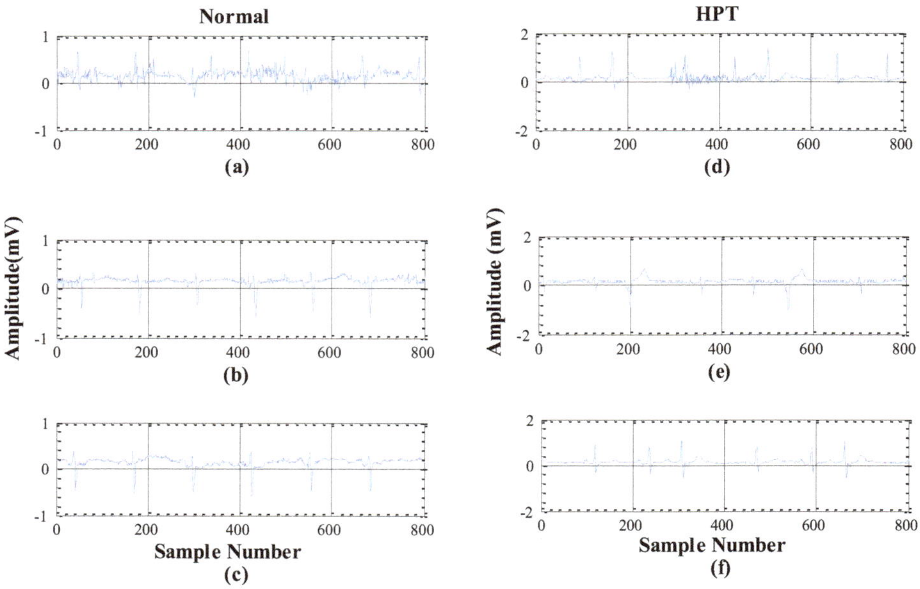

Figure 1.2. (a) Channel-III ECG signal of normal, (b) Channel-V3 ECG signal of normal, (c) Channel-V5 ECG signal of normal, (d) Channel-III ECG signal of HPT, (e) Channel-V3 ECG signal of HPT (f) Channel-V5 ECG signal of HPT.

The frequency response of LPF ($K(\omega')$) is given as

$$K(\omega') = \begin{cases} (s_1 s_2)^2, \ |\omega'| < \omega_{ph} \\ (s_1 s_2)^{\frac{1}{2}}\theta. \ \dfrac{\omega' - \omega_{ph}}{\omega_s - \omega_{ph}}, \ \omega_{ph} \leqslant \omega' \\ (s_1 s_2)^{\frac{1}{2}}\theta. \ \dfrac{\pi - \omega' + \omega_{ph}}{\omega_s - \omega_{ph}}, \ -\omega_s \leqslant \omega' \leqslant -\omega_{ph} \\ 0, \ |\omega'| \geqslant \omega_s \end{cases} \tag{1.1}$$

The frequency response of HPF ($H(\omega')$) is given as,

$$H(\omega') = \begin{cases} (2s_3 s_4)^{1/4}\theta. \ \dfrac{\pi - \omega' - \omega_0}{\omega_s - \omega_{ph}}, \ \omega_0 \leqslant \omega' < \omega_1 \\ (2s_3 s_4)^{\frac{1}{2}}, \ \omega_1 \leqslant \omega' < \omega_2 \\ (2s_3 s_4)^{\frac{1}{2}}\theta. \ \dfrac{\omega' - \omega_2}{\omega_3 - \omega_2}, \ \omega_2 \leqslant \omega' \leqslant \omega_3 \\ 0, \ \omega' \epsilon [0, \omega_0) \bigcup (\omega_3, 2\pi) \end{cases} \tag{1.2}$$

where, phase frequency (ω_{ph}) is given as,

$$\omega_{ph} = \frac{(1 - \beta)\pi}{s_1} + \frac{\epsilon}{s_1} \tag{1.3}$$

$$\omega_s = \frac{\pi}{s_2},\ \omega_0 = \frac{(1-\beta)\pi + e}{s_2},\ \omega_1 = \frac{s_1\pi}{s_2 s_3},\ \omega_2 = \frac{\pi - \epsilon}{s_2},\ \omega_3 = \frac{\pi + \epsilon}{s_3}$$

Quality factor (Q) is used to control the frequency resolution. It is the proportion of focal recurrence and the band width, it can be computed as,

$$Q = \frac{(2-\beta)}{\beta} \tag{1.4}$$

For proper and smoothed reconstruction of the signal β is always less than 1.

Dilation factor (R) is used to control the size of the wavelet and can be expressed as,

$$R = \frac{s_3}{s_4} \times \frac{1}{1 - \left(\frac{s_1}{s_2}\right)} \tag{1.5}$$

For proper recovery of the information and to reduce the losses, R should be greater than 1.

FAWT is time invariant and it provides a covering of flexible time frequency and tunable oscillatory bases.

The subbands obtained from ECG signal using FAWT are shown in figure 1.3.

1.2.3 Feature extraction

In this chapter, features are extracted from the subbands of decomposed ECG signal using the FAWT method.

Eight features are extracted from sub bands which are represented as [45]:

1. **Variance (VAR):** Variance is defined as the expectation of the squared deviation from its mean. It can be given as,

$$\text{VAR} = \frac{1}{N-1}\sum_{i=1}^{N}(x_i - \mu)^2 \tag{1.6}$$

2. **Integrated ECG (IECG):** It is used in the onset detection index in the sub band and the sum of absolute value of these sub bands is defined as *IECG*, it can be expressed as,

$$IECG = \sum\nolimits_{i=1}^{N}|x_i| \tag{1.7}$$

3. **Mean absolute value (MAV):** It is an average of absolute value of a subband and it can be computed as,

$$MAV = \frac{1}{N}\sum\nolimits_{i=1}^{N}|x_i| \tag{1.8}$$

4. **Mean (μ):** It is an average value of a subband extracted from FAWT, it can be expressed as,

$$\mu = \frac{1}{N}\sum\nolimits_{i=1}^{N}x_i \tag{1.9}$$

5. **Simple square integral (SSI):** It expresses the energy contained by sub band and it can be computed as,

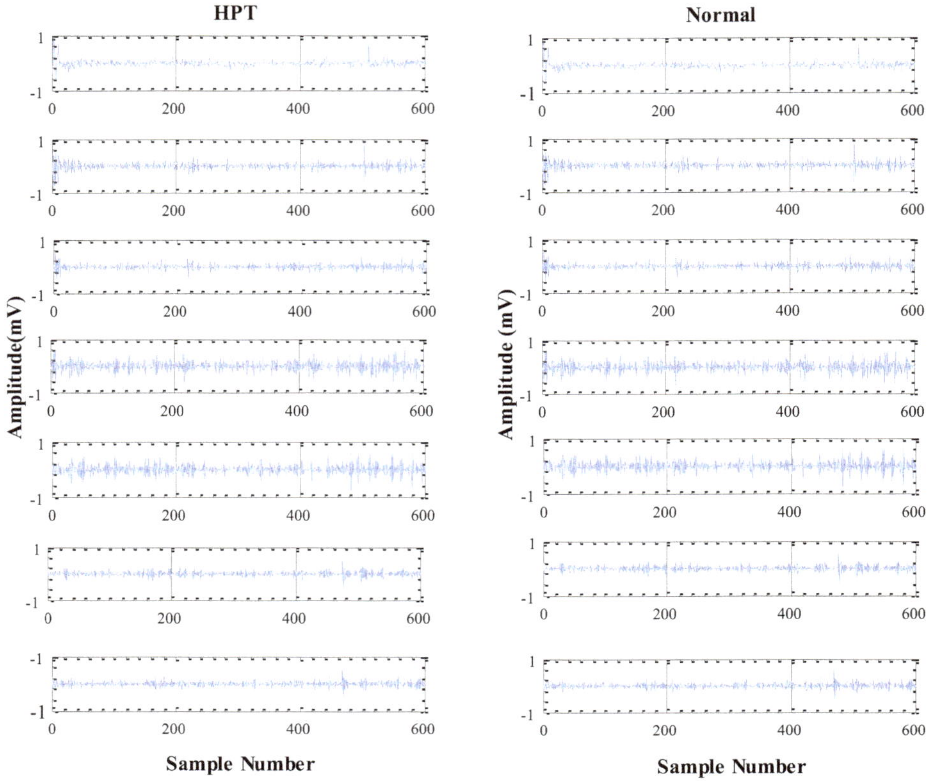

Figure 1.3. Sub bands for normal and HPT class ECG signal.

$$\text{SSI} = \sum_{i=1}^{N} |x_i{}^2| \tag{1.10}$$

6. **Root mean square (RMS):** It is defined as squared mean of sub band and can be given as,

$$\text{RMS} = \sqrt{\frac{1}{N} \sum_{i=1}^{N} x_i^2} \tag{1.11}$$

7. **Standard deviation (STD):** It is the dispersion of signal with respect to the mean, it can be formulated as,

$$\text{STD} = \frac{1}{N-1} \sum_{i=1}^{N-1} (x'_{i+1} - x'_i)^2 \tag{1.12}$$

8. **Log detector (LOG):** It provides an estimate of blood force exerted on the walls of arteries, logarithmic change of nonlinear detector is defined as LOG detector. It can be computed as,

$$\text{LOG} = e^{\frac{1}{N}\sum_{i=1}^{N} x^2{}_i} \tag{1.13}$$

where, x_i is the ith subband with N number of samples.

1.2.4 Classification techniques

Classifiers are used to categorize input data into two or more classes. The feature matrix is provided as an input for classifiers. In this chapter, four different classifiers are used to classify HPT and normal signals. In the case of decision tree classifiers, three kernel functions are used, namely simple tree, complex tree and medium tree. An ensemble tree classifier is used following kernel namely bagged tree, boosted tree, subspace discriminant, and subspace k-NN. Linear, medium Gaussian and coarse Gaussian types of kernel functions are used in SVM. In k-NN, six kernel functions are used, namely the cosine, fine, coarse, medium, cubic and weighted kernels. Details of these classifiers can be found in [46–49].

1. **Decision tree classifiers (DTC):** It is a tree-structured supervised machine learning classifier where internal nodes represent the characteristics of a given input feature, branches represent decision rules and each leaf node represents the output. DTC is used to separate a complicated decision-making process into a set of simpler decisions. The performance of the DTC is based on the type of given input features.
2. **Ensemble tree (ET):** ET classifier is based on the principle of ensemble, that is, the stronger learner is always generated from the group of various weak learners. In this classifier multiple decisions are combined together for producing better classification results.
3. **Support vector machine (SVM):** In SVM two classes can be separated using linear and hyper plane. SVM is the robust prediction method and it depends upon the statistical learning framework. Two types of kernel functions are used in SVM, namely Gaussian and linear.
4. **K-nearest neighbor (K-NN):** It is a nonparametric, supervised machine learning classification technique. K-NN algorithm stores all the given input features and classifies a new feature point based on the similarity. It can be more effective for large input data.

1.2.5 Performance parameters

The performance of the proposed method is analyzed by computing quality parameters, namely specificity (SPE), sensitivity (SEN) and accuracy (ACC), false-negative rate (FNR), negative predicted value (NPV) and false positive rate (FPR) [50].

Accuracy: It is the ratio of the total number of true identified events to the total number of events. It can be computed as,

$$\mathrm{ACC}(\%) = \frac{\mathrm{TP} + \mathrm{TN}}{\mathrm{TP} + \mathrm{FP} + \mathrm{FN} + \mathrm{TN}} \times 100\% \tag{1.14}$$

Sensitivity: Sensitivity belongs to positive class, and it is defined as the percentage of the correctly identified actual positive events. It can be given as

$$\mathrm{SEN}(\%) = \frac{\mathrm{TP}}{\mathrm{TP} + \mathrm{FN}} \times 100\% \tag{1.15}$$

Specificity: Specificity belongs to negative class, and it is defined as the percentage of the correctly identified actual negative events. It can expressed as,

$$\mathrm{SPE}(\%) = \frac{\mathrm{TN}}{\mathrm{TP} + \mathrm{FP}} \times 100\% \tag{1.16}$$

Negative predicted value: It is defined as the ratio of the total number of real negative events to the total number of negative events. It can be computed as

$$\mathrm{NPV}(\%) = \frac{\mathrm{TN}}{\mathrm{TN} + \mathrm{FN}} \times 100\% \tag{1.17}$$

False negative rate: It is defined as when an actual is positive and how often the classifier predicted negative. It can be computed as

$$\mathrm{FNR}(\%) = \frac{\mathrm{FN}}{\mathrm{TP} + \mathrm{FN}} \times 100\% \tag{1.18}$$

False positive rate: It is defined as when an actual event is negative and how often the classifier predicted positive. It can be given as

$$\mathrm{FPR}(\%) = \frac{\mathrm{FP}}{\mathrm{FP} + \mathrm{TN}} \times 100\% \tag{1.19}$$

True positive (TP): It is the number of correctly identified HPT subjects by the proposed model.

False positive (FP): It is the number of normal samples classified incorrectly by the proposed model.

False negative (FN): It is the number of incorrectly identified HPT subjects by the proposed model.

True negative (TN): It is the number of correctly identified normal subject by the proposed model.

1.3 Results

This methodology uses the FAWT and different classification techniques to distinguish between HPT patients and normal patients. There are a total of 139 subjects present, out of which 122 belong to normal class and 17 belong to HPT class, each signal is reshaped into the size of 15 360 samples, there are a total of 65 chunks of each signal, each chunk is given as an input to the FAWT. The FAWT is tuned with the following values of parameters, $J = 7$, sampling parameters $s_1 = 275$, $s_2 = 279$, $s_3 = 1$, $s_4 = 10$, which are kept the same for both normal and HPT classes. All these parameters are selected empirically. Various statistical features are evaluated from detailed coefficient and highly distinguishable features are selected by applying the KW test. The KW test is a ranked based nonparametric investigation of variance. It is used to identify the difference between two or more groups of independent variables on a continuous dependent variable. A feature is considered significant if the probability of *chi* is less than 0.05. Tables 1.1–1.3 represent the KW test results for

Table 1.1. KW test results for channel-III.

	SB-1	SB-2	SB-3	SB-4	SB-5	SB-6	SB-7	SB-8
IECG	6.88×10^{-16}	1.53×10^{-15}	0.9243	2.18×10^{-11}	0.5633	0.4505	0.0071	1.92×10^{-81}
LOG	1.08×10^{-107}	2.95×10^{-101}	4.65×10^{-99}	2.20×10^{-85}	5.40×10^{-65}	5.11×10^{-50}	1.04×10^{-39}	4.38×10^{-100}
MAV	6.88×10^{-16}	1.53×10^{-15}	0.9243	2.18×10^{-11}	0.5633	0.4505	0.0071	1.93×10^{-81}
Mean	6.88×10^{-16}	1.53×10^{-15}	0.9243	2.18×10^{-11}	0.5633	0.4505	0.0071	1.93×10^{-81}
RMS	4.25×10^{-31}	6.08×10^{-6}	1.23×10^{-4}	0.0036	0.2665	0.0002	1.86×10^{-7}	1.41×10^{-16}
SSI	4.25×10^{-31}	6.08×10^{-6}	1.23×10^{-4}	0.0036	0.2665	0.0002	1.85×10^{-7}	1.41×10^{-16}
STD	3.94×10^{-31}	6.08×10^{-6}	1.23×10^{-4}	0.0036	0.2665	0.0002	1.85×10^{-7}	1.41×10^{-16}
VAR	4.25×10^{-31}	6.08×10^{-6}	1.23×10^{-4}	0.0036	0.2665	0.0002	1.85×10^{-7}	1.41×10^{-16}

Table 1.2. KW test results for channel-V3.

	SB-1	SB-2	SB-3	SB-4	SB-5	SB-6	SB-7	SB-8
IECG	0.2156	0.8279	0.1616	1.42×10^{-6}	0.1575	0.7115	6.97×10^{-19}	1.60×10^{-19}
LOG	6.11×10^{-8}	5×10^{-4}	0.012	0.6377	0.3994	0.2171	0.1399	9.56×10^{-6}
MAV	0.2155	0.8279	0.1616	1.42×10^{-6}	0.1575	0.7115	6.97×10^{-19}	1.60×10^{-19}
Mean	0.2155	0.8279	0.1616	1.42×10^{-6}	0.1575	0.7115	6.97×10^{-19}	1.60×10^{-19}
RMS	0.0014	0.0049	0.0748	0.8570	0.1821	0.2162	0.1740	7.22×10^{-34}
SSI	0.0014	0.0049	0.0748	0.8570	0.1821	0.2162	0.1740	7.22×10^{-34}
STD	0.0017	0.0049	0.0748	0.8570	0.1821	0.2162	0.1740	3.85×10^{-14}
VAR	0.0014	0.0049	0.0748	0.8570	0.1821	0.2162	0.1740	7.22×10^{-34}

channels III, V-3 and V-5, respectively. It is seen from these tables that all the selected features are highly distinguishable.

All features are fed as input for the different classifiers and default parameters are used for classification. All three channels of all features are faded into the classifier for each sub band and the size of the obtained feature matrix is 1105×3 for HPT and 7930×3 for normal. Tenfold cross-validation is applied for evaluating the effectiveness of the proposed system, in tenfold cross-validation, input data is divided randomly into ten parts, one is for testing and the remainder are for training. Each part is trained ten times, similarly each part is tested ten times.

Table 1.4 represents the classification accuracy of ensemble classifier using four kernels. The classification accuracy obtained by using Boosted Tree, Bagged Tree, Subspace Discriminate and Subspace k-NN. The maximum accuracy is obtained by using EBT classifier for SB-1, which is 96.6%.

Table 1.5 represents the classification accuracy for three different classifiers, namely SVM, decision tree (DT) and K-NN. Fine tree (FT) kernel in DT gives the highest classification accuracy for SB-1 as 96.4%. Medium tree (MT) kernel in DT gives the highest classification accuracy for SB-7 as 92.5%. Coarse tree (CT) kernel in DT gives the highest classification accuracy is for SB-1 is 89.4%

Fine Gaussian (FG) kernel in SVM gives the highest classification accuracy for SB-8 as 94.2. Medium Gaussian (MG) kernel in SVM gives the highest classification accuracy for SB-4 as 91.1%. Coarse Gaussian (CG) kernel in SVM gives the highest classification accuracy for SB-6 as 88.5. Four types of kernels are used in the k-NN classifier, namely fine (F), medium (M), coarse (C) and weighted (W). The W kernel gives the highest classification accuracy of 94.8% for SB-8.

Highest classification accuracy is achieved using EBT classifier so performance parameters are evaluated for EBT which are summarized in table 1.6.

Highest SEN of 96.95% is achieved for SB-8, highest SPE of 96.74% is obtained for SB-1, highest NPV of 99.69% is achieved for SB-8, and lowest FNR of 3.04% is obtained for SB-8, lowest FPR of 3.24% is achieved for SB-8 using EBT classifier. Figure 1.4 represents the receiver operator characteristics of SB-1 area under the curve as 98%, percentage change in classifier characteristics is obtained by using true positive rate of 99.5% and false-positive rate of 3.97%.

Table 1.3. KW test results for channel-3.

	SB-1	SB-2	SB-3	SB-4	SB-5	SB-6	SB-7	SB-8
IECG	2.38×10^{-13}	4×10^{-4}	0.57	1.24×10^{-11}	0.40	0.641	0.322	9.25×10^{-77}
LOG	4.47×10^{-88}	6.94×10^{-110}	1.08×10^{-114}	1.96×10^{-93}	2.89×10^{-79}	1.94×10^{-61}	2.77×10^{-57}	1.02×10^{-11}
MAV	2.38×10^{-13}	4×10^{-4}	0.57	1.24×10^{-11}	0.40	0.64	0.32	9.25×10^{-77}
Mean	2.38×10^{-13}	0.0004	0.57	1.24×10^{-11}	0.40	0.64	0.32	9.25×10^{-77}
RMS	2.26×10^{-100}	2.56×10^{-78}	2.16×10^{-78}	5.08×10^{-55}	3.38×10^{-39}	7.21×10^{-22}	2.56×10^{-20}	9.48×10^{-74}
SSI	2.26×10^{-100}	2.56×10^{-78}	2.16×10^{-78}	5.08×10^{-55}	3.38×10^{-39}	7.21×10^{-22}	2.56×10^{-20}	9.48×10^{-74}
STD	2.50×10^{-100}	2.56×10^{-78}	2.16×10^{-78}	5.08×10^{-55}	3.38×10^{-39}	7.21×10^{-22}	2.56×10^{-20}	9.48×10^{-74}
VAR	2.26×10^{-100}	2.56×10^{-78}	2.15×10^{-78}	5.08×10^{-55}	1.90×10^{-39}	5.38×10^{-22}	2.56×10^{-20}	9.48×10^{-74}

Table 1.4. Accuracy of ensemble classifier.

SB	Boosted Tree	Bagged Tree	Subspace Discriminate	Subspace k-NN
SB-1	93.8	96.6	87.8	93.3
SB-2	92.6	94.5	87.8	91.8
SB-3	92.3	94.7	87.7	92.1
SB-4	93.1	95	87.7	93
SB-5	93.5	95.2	88	92.6
SB-6	93.9	95.6	88.2	93.2
SB-7	94.7	96	87.9	93.6
SB-8	92	96.2	87.7	87.7

Table 1.5. Classification accuracy of decision tree, SVM, k-NN classifier.

	DT			SVM				k-NN			
					Gaussian						
	FT	MT	CT	L	FG	MG	CG	F	M	C	W
SB-1	96.4	91	89.4	87.6	91.2	88.3	87.8	91.4	88.3	88	92.1
SB-2	95	91	88.8	87.8	89.5	89.4	87.8	87.8	89.4	87.9	89.8
SB-3	93.7	91.4	89.3	87.8	90.2	90.2	87.8	88.9	90.2	88.2	90.9
SB-4	94.4	91	89.9	87.8	90.5	91.1	88.1	90.5	91.1	88.1	91.8
SB-5	95.2	92.3	89.5	87.8	90	90.7	88.2	88.9	90.7	87.9	91.1
SB-6	95.9	92.3	89	87.8	90.3	90.6	88.5	89.4	90.6	87.9	91.3
SB-7	95.5	92.5	89.6	87.8	91.6	91	88.3	90.9	91	88.1	92
SB-8	94.1	91.9	89.7	87.8	94.2	90.5	87.8	94.2	90.5	89.2	94.8

Table 1.6. Performance parameters for EBT.

SB	SEN	SPE	NPV	FNR	FPR
SB-1	95.02	96.74	99.40	4.97	3.24
SB-2	91.11	94.83	99.16	8.88	5.16
SB-3	93.37	94.67	99.40	6.62	5.32
SB-4	91.48	95.07	99.18	8.51	4.92
SB-5	92.67	95.20	99.29	7.32	4.79
SB-6	95.21	95.76	99.52	4.78	4.23
SB-7	94.96	95.97	99.48	5.03	4.02
SB-8	96.95	95.87	99.69	3.04	4.12

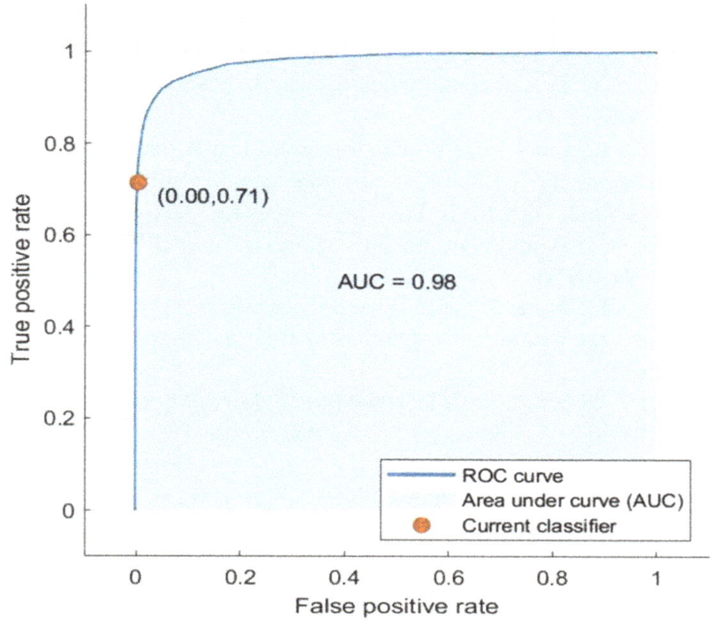

Figure 1.4. Receiver operator characteristics for EBT of SB-1.

1.4 Conclusion

Our busy, unhealthy, hectic lifestyle and a pollution-filled environment can cause fluctuations in the blood force on the walls of arteries, resulting in HPT. Large and sudden change in blood force may damage organs and can cause various disease related to kidney, heart and brain. In this chapter FAWT and EBT-based decomposition and classification technique has been proposed for automatic detection of HPT. Highly discriminatory features are identified using KW test and get the highest classification accuracy of 96.6% using an ensemble-based classifier. The proposed method provides the way for implementing a new approach for automated detection of HPT using ECG which are presently difficult to classify due to the non-stationary and non-linear characteristics of the ECG signal. The FAWT-EBT-based method may help in the automated detection of HPT so that patients can take early medication. The developed system can help the experts in early prediction of HPT. In future, a 24-h blood pressure monitoring system will be implemented for the real-time automatic detection of HPT.

References

[1] Tabassum N and Ahmad F 2011 Role of natural herbs in the treatment of HPT *Pharm. Rev.* **5** 30–40

[2] Ni H, Cho S, Mankoff J, Yang J and Dey A.k. 2018 Automated recognition of HPT through overnight continuous HRV monitoring *J. Ambient Intell. Hum. Comput.* **9** 2011–23

[3] Drozdz D and Kawecka-Jaszcz K 2014 Cardiovascular changes during chronic hypertensive states *Pediatr. Nephrol.* **29** 1507–16

[4] Hall J E 2003 The kidney, hypertension, and obesity *Hypertension* **41** 625–33

[5] Shirole U, Joshi M and Bagul P 2019 Cardiac diabetic and normal subjects classification using decision tree and result confirmation through orthostatic stress index,' *Inform. Med. Unlocked* **17** 100252

[6] Zhu C, Idemudia C U and Feng W 2019 Improved logistic regression model for diabetes prediction by integrating PCA and K-means techniques,' *Inform. Med. Unlocked* **17** 100179

[7] Jain P, Gajbhiye and Tripathy R K 2020 A two-stage deep CNN architecture for the classification of low-risk and high-risk HPT classes using multi-lead ECG signals *Inform. Med. Unlocked* **21** 100479

[8] Schwartz C L and McManus R J 2015 What is the evidence base for diagnosing HPT and for subsequent blood pressure treatment targets in the prevention of cardiovascular disease? *BMC Med* **13** 6437

[9] Melillo P, Izzo R, Orrico A, Scala P, Attanasio M, Mirra M, Luca N and Pecchia L 2015 Automatic prediction of cardiovascular and cerebrovascular events using HRV analysis *PLoS One* **10** e0118504

[10] Kiat Soh D C, Ng E Y K, Jahmunah V, Oh S L, Tan R S and Rajendra Acharya U 2020 Automated diagnostic tool for HPT using convolutional neural network *Comput. Biol. Med.* **126** 103999

[11] Ni H, Wang Y, Xu G, Shao Z, Zhang W and Zhou X 2019 Multiscale fine-grained heart rate variability analysis for recognizing the severity of HPT *Compute. Math. Methods Med.* **2019** 4936179

[12] Rajput J S, Sharma M, Tan R S and Rajendra Acharya U 2020 Automated detection of severity of HPT ECG signals using an optimal bi-orthogonal wavelet filter bank *Comput. Biol. Med.* **123** 103924

[13] Sharma M, Tan R S and Acharya U R 2020 Detection of shockable ventricular arrhythmia using optimal orthogonal wavelet filters *Neural Comput. Appl.* **32** 15869–84

[14] Kwon S, Kang S, Lee Y, Yoo C and Park K 2014 Unobtrusive monitoring of ECG-derived features during daily smartphone use *Proc. 2014 36th Annual Int. Conf. IEEE Engineering in Medicine and Biology Society (Chicago, IL, USA),* 26–30

[15] Islam M K, Haque A N M M, Tangim G, Ahammad T and Khondokar M R H 2012 Study and analysis of ECG signal using MATLAB and LABVIEW as effective tools *Int. J. Comput. Electr. Eng.* **4** 404–8

[16] Haque A K M F, Alil H, Kiber M A and Hasan M T 2009 Detection of small variations of ECG features using wavelet *ARPN J. Eng. Appl. Sci.* **4** 27–30

[17] Lepeschkin E and Surawicz B 2004 The measurement of the Q-T interval of the electrocardiogram *Circulation* **6** 378–8

[18] Rajendra Acharya U, Paul Joseph K, Kannathal N, Lim C M and Suri J S 2006 Heart rate variability: a review , *Med. Biol. Eng. Comput.* **44** 1031–51

[19] Basten B L, Sherman R L, Lametschwandtner A and Spieler R E 2011 Development of embryonic gill vasculature in the yellow stingray, *Urobatis Jamaicensis Respir. Biol.* **294** 1423–32

[20] Kai Li H R and Ziemssen T 2019 Spectral analysis of heart rate variability: time window matters, perspective article *Front. Neurol.* **10** 545

[21] Roy S and Chandra A 2018 A new method for denoising ECG signal using sharp cut-off FIR filter *International Symposium on Devices, Circuits and Systems (ISDCS)* pp 1–6

[22] Jain S, Bajaj V and Kumar A 2018 Riemann–Liouvelle fractional integral based empirical mode decomposition for ECG denoising *IEEE J. Biomed. Health Inform.* **22** 1133–9

[23] Tripath K, Sohal H and Jain S 2020 Computer-aided diagnostic system for feature-based classification using heart rate variability *Biomed. Eng.: App. Basis Commun.* **32** 205009

[24] Soh D C K, Ng E Y K, Jahmunah V, Oh S L, San T R and Acharya U R , 2020 A computational intelligence tool for the detection of HPT using empirical mode decomposition *Comput. Biol. Med.* **118** 103630

[25] Melillo P, Izzo R, Orrico A, Scala P, Attanasio M, Mirra M, Luca N D and Pecchia L 2015 Automatic prediction of cardiovascular and cerebrovascular events using heart rate variability analysis *PLoS One* **10** e0118504

[26] Ruiqi Zhang Z H, Chen Chen G L and Wanhui Wen A 2020 Analysis of autonomic nervous pattern in HPT based on short-term heart rate variability *Biomed. Tech. (Berl)* **66** 71–9

[27] Kale N, Thomas J, Agrawal R, Benjamin B and Thomas J P Predicting cardiovascular events: sensitivity and specificity *Int. Conf. Health Informatics and Medical Systems HIMS'17*

[28] Ortiz-Martin L, Picazo-Sanchez P and Peris-Lopez P 2020 Are the interpulse intervals of an ECG signal a good source of entropy? An in-depth entropy analysis based on NIST 800-90B recommendation. *Future Gener. Comput. Syst.* **105** 346–60

[29] Alkhodari M, Islayem D K, Alskafi F A and Ahsan H K 2020 Predicting hypertensive patients with higher risk of developing vascular events using heart rate variability and machine learning *IEEE Access* **8** 19272–39

[30] Agliari E, Alemanno F, Barra A, Barra O A, Fachechi A, Vento L F and Moretti L 2020 Analysis of temporal correlation in heart rate variability through maximum entropy principle in a minimal pairwise glassy model *Sci. Rep.* **10** 15353

[31] Taye G T, Hwang H-J and Lim K M , 2020 Application of a convolutional neural network for predicting the occurrence of ventricular tachyarrhythmia using heart rate variability features *Sci. Rep.* **10** 6769

[32] Agnihotri P and Jain M , 2019 Cardiac health prediction using electrocardiography Pratishtha Agnihotri *Int. J. Recent Technol. Eng. (IJRTE)* **8** 33–9

[33] Koichubekov B K, Sorokina M A, Laryushina Y M, Turgunova L G and Korshukova I V 2018 Nonlinear analyses of heart rate variability in hypertension *Ann. Card. d'Ang.* 67 174

[34] Bossone E, Paciocco G, Iarussi D, Agretto A, Iacono A, Gillespie B W and Rubenfire M 2002 MelvynRubenfire, the prognostic role of the ECG in primary pulmonary hypertension *Chest J.* **121** 513–18

[35] Melillo P, Orrico A, Scala P, Crispino F and Pecchia L 2015 Cloud-based smart health monitoring system for automatic cardiovascular and fall risk assessment in hypertensive ratients *J. Med. Syst.* **39** 109

[36] Dami S and Yahaghizadeh M 2021 Predicting cardiovascular events with deep learning approach in the context of the internet of things *Neur. Comput. Appl.* **43** 1–18

[37] Zhao M, Guan L and Wang Y 2020 The association of autonomic nervous system function with ischemic stroke, and treatment strategies *Front. Neurol.* **10** 1141

[38] Thomas R J, Peng C-K, Goldberger A L and Gottlieb D J 2009 Prevalent HPT and stroke in the sleep heart health study: association with an ECG-derived spectrographic marker of cardiopulmonary coupling *Sleep* **32** 897–S2

[39] Paragliola G and Coronato A 2020 An hybrid ECG-based deep network for the early identification of high-risk to major cardiovascular events for HPT patients *J. Biomed. Inform.* **113** 10648

[40] Schillaci G, Battista F and Pucci G 2012 A review of the role of electrocardiography in the diagnosis of left ventricular hypertrophy in HPT *J. Electrocardiol.* **45** 617–23
[41] Afkami R G and ali Tinati M 2015 ECG based detection of left ventricular hypertrophy using higher order statistics *23rd Iranian Conf. Electrical Engineering*
[42] Jothiramalingam R, Jude A, Patan R, Ramachandran M, Duraisamy J H and Gandomi A H 2020 Machine learning-based left ventricular hypertrophy detection using multi-lead ECG signal *Neur. Comput. Appl.* **33** 4445–55
[43] Kublanov V S, Dolganov A Y, Belo D and Gamboa H 2017 Comparison of machine learning methods for the arterial HPT diagnostics *Appl. Bion. Biomech.* **2017** 5985479
[44] Safavian S R and Landgrebe D 1991 A survey of decision Wee classifier methodology *IEEE Trans. Syst. Man Cybernet.* **21** 660–74
[45] Sarvani C, Bajaj V, Taran S and Sengur A 2020 Flexible analytic wavelet transform based features for physical action identification using EMG signals *IRBM* **41** 18–22
[46] Khare S K and Bajaj V 2021 Entropy-based drowsiness detection using adaptive variational mode decomposition *IEEE Sens. J.* **21** 6421–8
[47] Siuly S, Khare S K, Bajaj V, Wang H and Yanchun Zhang A 2020 Computerized method for automatic detection of schizophrenia using EEG signals *IEEE Trans. Neural Syst. Rehabil. Eng.* **28** 2390–400
[48] Ullo S L, Khare S K, Bajaj V and Sinha G R 2020 Hybrid computerized method for environmental sound classification *IEEE Access* **8** 124055–65
[49] Khare S K, Bajaj V, Siuly S and Sinha G R 2020 *Classification of Schizophrenia Patients through Empirical Wavelet Transformation Using Electroencephalogram Signals* (Bristol: IOP Publishing Ltd)
[50] Bajaj V and Pachori R B 2012 Classification of seizure and nonseizure EEG signals using empirical mode decomposition *IEEE Trans. Inf. Technol. Biomed.* **16** 1135–42

Chapter 2

Computational intelligence in surface electromyogram signal classification

Turker Tuncer, Sengul Dogan, Fatih Ertam and Abdulhamit Subasi

The objective of this book chapter is to introduce a solution for disabled people based on a man–machine interface, which can work on data processed by computational intelligence techniques. The model utilizes computational intelligence techniques for hand movement classification. On this basis, a novel computational intelligence approach, which is called a spider network for the recognition of basic hand movements employing surface electromyogram signals is presented. The main components of the spider network are pre-processing, feature extraction, feature reduction, and classification. In the preprocessing phase, the surface electromyogram signals from two different channels are concatenated. In the feature extraction phase, Discrete Cosine Transform (DCT) and Fast Fourier Transform (FFT) are applied to concatenated signals to obtain frequency coefficients of the surface electromyogram signal. Besides, Singular Value Decomposition and Ternary Pattern are utilized. The extracted features are divided into two groups according to feature extractors. To select distinctive features, Neighborhood Component Analysis is employed as a weight generator. By using these weights and tangent sigmoid activation function, the features are reduced. In the classification phase, Linear Discriminant Analysis, Artificial Neural Network, k-nearest neighbor, and Support Vector Machine are employed for the classification task. The proposed model is optimized and validated based on the accomplishment of the built framework, which can produce accurate, and consistent solutions for the surface electromyogram based prosthetic device control, intending to help amputees or congenitally deficient limbs. The proposed model achieved 100% classification accuracy in hand movement classification.

2.1 Introduction

As demonstrated by the various applications in wellness, biomedicine, and biomedical engineering, there has been increased attention in computational intelligence (CI) over

doi:10.1088/978-0-7503-3815-8ch2

recent years. The usage of CI in surface electromyogram (sEMG) signal classification is presented in this book chapter. The usage of engineering principles and methods to problems in medicine and healthcare is biomedical engineering. Typical applications include prosthesis and medical instrument design/development, health monitoring with imaging equipment, and diagnostic software. Computational algorithms, involving artificial intelligence, and machine learning are CI approaches. Many CI methods require the establishment of nonlinear mapping between a model's inputs and outputs reflecting the operation of a biomedical system in the real world. Computational intelligence (CI) for diagnostic systems is a new concept in the medical field. CI is a mixture of machine learning algorithms and artificial learning. For the analysis of massive amounts of data, these techniques are extremely useful and have been effectively implemented to problems of pattern recognition and signal classification. In short, CI methods are a potential solution to the rising demand for automatic diagnostic and control systems [1]. In this chapter, we will discuss the basics of automatic hand movement recognition schemes and focus on the fields where CI methods were effectively used for sEMG signal classification.

Surface electromyography (sEMG) signals have been widely employed for myoelectric control as it includes important information on muscular action. The hands play a crucial role in manipulating and grasping several items. The defeat of even a single hand can expressively disturb the human activity. Hence, a prosthetic hand is an attractive solution to furnish the armless person [2–4]. The usage of sEMG differs from rehabilitation apparatus to a man–machine interaction scheme. Several intelligent methods were developed to classify the neuromuscular actions in prosthetic hand control. In this chapter, the sEMG signals based prosthetic hand movement control framework is presented. The hand prosthesis based on the myoelectric control employs the sEMG signals that are taken from the skin surface during the contraction of muscles. Most muscles that control the finger motion are positioned on the left side of a stump. Thus, the action of these muscles can be employed for the prosthesis control after a hand amputation. In order to control prosthesis motion with muscle activity features extracted from the myoelectric signals can be utilized. The feature extraction from sEMG can be achieved by employing numerous techniques involving signal characteristics in time and frequency domain, autoregressive model coefficients, and time-frequency characteristics [5]. On the other hand, a robust hand movements recognition by employing the sEMG signals present diverse challenges. To enhance the classification performance and get rid of those problems, a proper arrangement of the feature extraction and selection methods should be employed. Additionally, an appropriate model to improve the classification performance should be utilized.

Noce *et al* [6] proposed an approach for nerve control in hand prostheses. In the proposed method, a comparative analysis was performed with a pattern recognition technique used for muscle signals and adapted Spike Sorting Algorithms (SSA) for nerve signals. Through the SSA, the peak points of the nerve signals were determined, and the movement was transferred. EMG and ENG signals are used as input parameters. Accuracy is chosen as the performance parameter and the results are presented. The results showed that ENG signals were more effective decision makers. Nishad *et al* [7] proposed tunable Q wavelet transform based sEMG recognition technique. The main goal of the developed approach is to classify electromyogram signals in accordance with the basic six hand movements. The developed approach includes preprocessing, feature extraction, feature selection and classification. The accuracy of this approach was chosen as the success criterion and the results were compared with the existing and widely used techniques in the literature. Yabuki *et al* [8] designed a glove made of silicone rubber with a detection feature. The designed glove has a structure including appearance (shape, texture, color), material (strength, flexibility), mechanical (fingertip shape, joint movements) and detection. In their study, a structure was created for real hand movements through sensors and control units. Shi *et al* [9] proposed a study on the evaluation of electromyogram signals for a bionic glove design. The main objective of this work is to present a methodology, which can mimic the movements of the human hand. Servo motors controlled by Arduino have enabled the movement of bionic fingers. In their study, k-nearest neighbor algorithm is used in the classification phase. Accuracy is selected as the performance parameter. Enoka [10] provides a different perspective for the measurement and analysis of electromyographic signals. According to the results obtained, it is emphasized that EMG signals need to elaborate signal waveforms with various algorithms and detection systems and defined waveforms should be evaluated effectively. Ryu and Kim [11] proposed an approach EMG Signal Graph Matching (ESGM) algorithm based method. They evaluated the physiological muscle activity using their methods. They used conventional feature extraction and classification methods. Junior and de Seixas [12] investigated noise reduction performances on the EMG signals. In their study, the aim is to clear ECG interference from EMG signals as a noise signal. In the proposed method, unlike high-pass filtering, it was observed that most of the EMG spectral content was maintained at low frequencies. Jochumsen *et al* [13] introduced a Bayes based sEMG classification technique to recognize main movements of the arms. Chowdhury *et al* [14] suggested an approach that relies on the correlation of EMG and EEG signals. The key objective of the research was to design a neuro-rehabilitation system. The proposed approach consists of the phases of pre-processing, feature extraction and classification. Accuracy was employed as the evaluation parameter in the study. Tavakoli *et al* [15] developed a prosthetic glove using EMG signals. In the study, basic hand movements are defined, and hand movements are aimed to be transformed into a flexible structure. The accuracy and error matrix parameters have been utilized to test the performance of the study. Tavakoli *et al* [16] designed a wearable glove from EMG signals. This designed glove basically recognizes four movements. The major goal of their research was to provide high mobility with four basic movements defined. To accomplish this objective, an original glove hardware was designed and they constructed their dataset using the glove constructed. In the second stage, the statistical features were extracted from the data obtained. In the third stage, LDA and SVM classifiers were used to obtain performance.

In this work, a novel feature extraction network, which is called a spider network (SN), is proposed. SN includes preprocessing, feature extraction and feature reduction stages. In the preprocessing stage, firstly, the sEMG signals are concatenated. In the feature extraction stage, DCT and FFT are applied to concatenated signals to obtain frequency coefficients of the signal. Then SVD and TP are used together. Neighborhood Component Analysis (NCA) and tangent sigmoid function are used for dimension reduction. In the classification stage, ANN, k-NN, SVM and LDA are employed for hand movement recognition. The principal motivation of the developed SN is to combine several effective methods for signal processing and create an efficient framework for sEMG signal classification with high performance and short execution time. The key objective of the SN is to extract variable features utilizing effective methods and select discriminative features using feature selection methods. Therefore, it uses many transformations for sEMG signal processing. The main contributions of the developed approach are as follows:

- In this chapter, we developed a novel scheme, which utilizes the DCT and FFT for signal processing. Moreover, SVD and TP are utilized as feature extractors. These methods clearly illustrate that the proposed network is a cognitive network. Efficient and optimum methods are used in the proposed SN.
- Moreover, a novel feature reduction method is presented, and this method is used for the first time in the literature. A novel NCA and tangent sigmoid based feature reduction method (Algorithm 2) is presented, and the results prove the success of this method.
- Besides, the average classification accuracy of the developed SN is very high as compared to the literature. The developed model is also compared to the state-of-the-art and these results clearly demonstrate that the proposed SN solves classification of sEMG signals with high classification accuracy. A multi methods-based learning approach is presented and called a deep method since it uses several methods for feature extraction.

2.2 Computational intelligence in biomedical signal processing

A successor of Artificial Intelligence (AI) is Computational Intelligence (CI). CI depends on heuristic algorithms such as neural networks, evolutionary computation, fuzzy systems and deep learning. CI also involves methods which utilize swarm intelligence, etc. CI is a mixture of learning, adaptation, and creation utilized for innovative and intelligent applications. Study in computer intelligence does not exclude statistical approaches, but instead provides a complementary viewpoint of how these techniques are applied. A mixture of fuzzy logic, artificial neural networks, genetic algorithms, connectionist systems such as cybernetics and AI are closely related to CI. Subordinate cognitive functions are concerned with the exploration of CI: visual perception, recognition of artifacts, signal processing, breakthrough of data structures, simple associations and control. In different areas, such as biomedical signal/image analysis, pattern recognition, and robotics, these approaches are utilized to solve the same sort of challenges [17].

At present, these tasks are puzzled by the community of AI utilizing approaches focused on searching, symbolic representation of cognition, logical thinking with machine learning, expert systems, and lingual approaches. AI is a component of CI that focuses on issues, which involve higher cognition to solve these problems employing the symbolic interpretation of knowledge. Other CI strategies in the future may also find solutions for these issues. Reinforcement learning, sequence learning, machine learning, and distributed multi-agent systems are the major areas of overlap between high and low-level cognitive functions. All activities, which need rule-based reasoning built on perceptions, such as machine-driven vehicles, robotics and automation need techniques to solve both high- and low-level cognitive problems, and are therefore a raw meeting ground with the rest of the CI community for AI experts. AI models are symbolically interpreted on the basis of multi-dimensional approach patterns containing brain functions. Instead of symbolic variables, representative brain model functions give no accurate approximation of any problem defined by continuous variables. In order to achieve identical functions, calculations of cognitive processing should be carried out at the correct level. Symbolic dynamics can provide valuable information on complex structures and can be beneficial for modelling the change between processes at low and high levels. The distinction between cognitive functions at low and high levels is just a rough estimation of the brain activities. In the last decade, symbolized cognition was extensively investigated, and robotics adopted developmental estimates. Neural networks are inspired at the lowest level brain processes and structures, whereas symbolic AI approaches are motivated at the highest-level processes. In an unambitious way, individual neurons coherently function on the processing of brain information. CI is a study of intelligent agent design and involves learning all non-algorithmic processes, which can be solved with varying degrees of competence by humans. The main CI techniques should be complemented by information and search-based methods in issues involving intelligence. It is even more necessary for CI to overcome and welcome all strategies that can be used in such solutions, regardless of their inspiration. CI is essentially comprised of those paradigms in AI, which refer to a biological or natural mechanism of some kind [17].

Healthcare is one of the most important problems in contemporary societies, as the life quality of individuals depends directly on it [18]. Nevertheless, the healthcare area is extremely varied, extensively distributed and decentralized. Access to accurate patient records is needed to provide appropriate medical care from a clinical point of view, which is rarely accessible where and when required [19]. There are inherently different statistical properties of medical results. Researchers and practitioners face two difficulties when analyzing those results: the curse of dimensionality and the heterogeneity of feature origins and statistical properties [20]. These triggers lead to biomedical signal analysis problems and factual errors. The fields of statistics, computing and medicine are now facing the challenge of exploring new approaches for biomedical signal modeling. This need is highly related to advancements in other fields, such as machine learning (ML), AI and CI. As the volume of digitally captured and processed medical data is vast and exponentially increasing, data storage and analysis are also emerging to turn this huge data into information and expertise, which helps them achieve their goals [21].

Advanced approaches need to be used to describe these systemic differences in data. For any intellectual behavior, learning is one of the basic requirements. It is known that there is no knowledge without experience. CI provides several major approaches for intelligent retrieval of information today. In addition, its methodology is presently suitable for the study of medical data and, particularly, a broad range of medical diagnostic work on small-specialized diagnostic issues has been carried out [22], where initial CI applications have been identified. CI algorithms that are useful methods for clinical diagnosis have been successfully utilized for the diagnosis and treatment of diseases [23–26]. Evidently, on a wide variety of crucial problems, many CI approaches work very well. Nonetheless, since they are extremely complex and the curse of dimensionality in the data is strong, they have failed to solve the main CI problems [21].

sEMG signals were extensively utilized for the rehabilitation and control of prosthetic devices, aimed for amputees or congenitally disabled limbs, and improving the interaction between machines and people [27]. In order to distinguish various types of myoelectric signals, improved sEMG signals may be used. Due to the various forms of contraction, the variance of EMG signals impacts the classification efficiency of algorithms. Different biomedical signal processing methods are used to remove those differences [23, 28–31]. Those inventions from everyday life could be encountered by people with disabilities with attitudes that vary from people without disabilities. Door-knobs, kitchen appliances, or shirt buttons that may not bother a significant number of people may end up being a challenge for those with a disability. In turn, a lever door handle modified to a door-knob may give that person tremendous help and significance, and be supported and respected by others in addition. A basic buttonhook system may support someone who is struggling to control keys, but it is not practical for most individuals. Therefore, despite some advances posing challenges to disabled peoples' independence, some inventions are intended to suit impairments and some of these are designed for general usage [32]. By improving the skills of individuals through the advancement of all environments, these supporting technologies may work [33].

The hand is one of the most essential aspects of a person and, in the sense of thought, is seen as a fundamental element. The hand is used to sense movements and patterns of real-life encounters and execute simple lifting functions. For instance, with coordinated muscle activity, the basic role of the arm is to grab, raise, wave and conduct other arm rotating movements. The prosthesis hand is an electronic mechanism employed to replace a damaged component in the case of amputees. The hand prosthesis is an augmented yet practical hand, which is designed to perform multiple tasks and can be controlled. For example, to move and consolidate the control center, the myoelectric arm utilizes a regulated muscle contraction produced by an electrical charge. In this way, an amputee can do routine arm tasks, such as grasping, sensing, waving, and other hand-related gestures, through a controlled gesture. In gripping and handling diverse objects, the hands of humans play a vital role. Even the lack of a single hand impacts human operation, and a cure for equipping the armless subject is the prosthetic hand [34]. The upper limb prosthesis is mainly dependent on the use of myoelectric control to identify sEMG signals realized during the contraction of the muscle. Because most of the muscles generating finger motion are left in the stump after hand amputation, they can be utilized for myoelectric control and the operation of these muscles can be used for prosthesis control. Any useful characteristics can be derived from the EMG signals that provide prosthesis control information about muscle function [35]. Because EMG-controlled assistive devices aid disabled people who have trouble navigating user interfaces, such as joysticks and keyboards, more sophisticated hands-free human–machine interfaces are required. In a control system, sEMG signals can be used to trigger robotics and recovery equipment [36, 33].

2.3 Background

In this study, DCT, FFT, SVD, TP, and different machine learning techniques are used to create an SN. Brief explanations about these methods are given in this section.

2.3.1 Discrete cosine transform

The DCT is one of the widely used transformations for signals and images. It helps to obtain transformation coefficients of the signals using cosine based equations. The JPEG algorithm, as the mostly known image compression method, uses DCT. In this study we used 1D-DCT because sEMG signals are used for hand movement recognition [37].

2.3.2 Fast Fourier transform

Coley and Tukey proposed FFT in 1965 to decrease processes of the Discrete Fourier Transform (DFT). This process led to a rapid rise in DFT applications in digital signal processing and other fields. It has also led to the development of other algorithms. All these algorithms are known as FFT algorithms. The number of operations required for the DFT account has been greatly reduced and ease of operation is provided with FFT. FFT is an effective and economical algorithm for calculating DFT. It is one of the phenomena of signal processing. Hence, we used it in the proposed SN [38].

2.3.3 Singular value decomposition

SVD is a matrix factorization method and it generates three components from a matrix. Generally, the singular values have been utilized to construct feature vectors. It is a widely used method in signal processing, image processing, face recognition, perceptual hashing and Google page rank algorithms [39, 40].

2.3.4 Ternary pattern

Texture recognition and analysis are a major problem for image processing and several methods have been presented to solve this problem [41]. One practical solution of the texture analysis is textural descriptors.

2.3.5 Support vector machine

The SVM has various versions and it is a commonly used classifier in the literature. It is a conventional and parametric classifier. The widely used activation functions of the SVM are linear, quadratic, cubic, radial basis and Gaussian [42, 43].

2.3.6 Linear discriminant analysis

LDA is a linear dimension reduction and supervised machine learning technique, which seeks to find vectors in the space in which classes are best separated using class information of data objects. It is a nonparametric classifier. It is simple, fast and effective. Hence, many methods have been used [44].

2.3.7 KNN

KNN is a distance-based classifier. Variable distances are utilized in KNN such as Euclidean, city block, Minkowski, Spearman, Chi-square. It is one of the simplest classification methods. However, it is a lazy classifier because it is not efficient for big data. It is suitable for small datasets. However, KNN proves success of the methods for large datasets using a small dataset [45].

2.3.8 Artificial neural network

Artificial neural network (ANN) is inspired by bio-neurological systems and it is utilized as a classifier and regressor in the literature. ANN is one of the phenomena of machine learning and it has many variations. It uses input, weights and actual output for prediction. Basic mathematical notation of it was shown in equation (2.1) [46].

$$Y = \varphi(X_{*}w^{T} + \text{bias}) \tag{2.1}$$

where $\varphi(.)$ is activation function, X defines input vector, w is weights, Y is output.

2.4 Spider network

The key objective of the developed model is to obtain a cognitive model for basic hand movement recognition. We want to extract low, middle, and high level features using a cognitive method. As we know from the literature, DCT and FFT are effective methods for signal processing. Hence, these are used in a preprocessing step to obtain frequency coefficients of the sEMG signals. Also, TP and SVD are effective feature extraction methods and are used as such. After these processes, large feature sets are obtained. To select distinctive of them, an NCA-based feature reduction method is utilized. The proposed SN uses several classifiers for comparison purposes. These classifiers are chosen to validate the feature extraction power of the proposed SN because these are conventional classifiers. The key objectives of the proposed SN are given below.

- Obtain high classification accuracy.
- Propose a lightweight signal recognition network

The SN includes preprocessing, feature extraction, feature reduction, feature concatenation and classification stages. The pictorial description of the SN is shown in figure 2.1.

As shown in figure 2.1, signal concatenation, DCT and FFT are used in preprocessing to generate secondary signals. SVD and TP are chosen as feature extractors. The extracted SVD-based and TP-based features are concatenated and two types of features are obtained. These are SVD-based and TP-based features. Finally, 2560 TP-based and 80 SVD-based features are extracted from an sEMG signal. In the feature reduction phase, firstly NCA generates weights then these weights and a tangent sigmoid-based feature reduction method are applied onto TP- and SVD- based features. 10-fold cross-validation is employed to obtain results. The milestones of the SN are explained in the subsection.

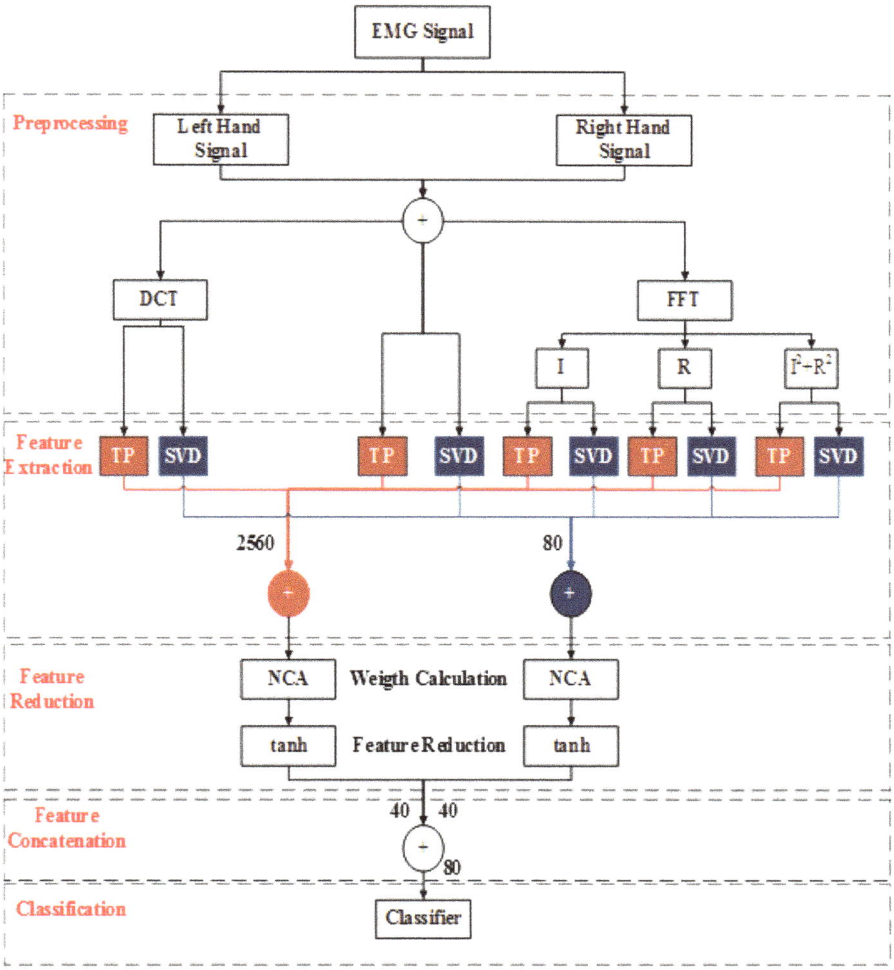

Figure 2.1. The block diagram of the SN.

2.4.1 Pre-processing

The steps of the pre-processing phase are presented below.

Step 1: Concatenate channel-1 and channel-2 sEMG signals.

$$S^C = S^1 \mid S^2 \tag{2.2}$$

where S^C, S^1 and S^2 are first channel, second channel and concatenated signals, respectively. | is concatenation operator.

To prevent memorization and show success of the proposed SN, sEMG signals recorded from channel-1 and channel-2 are concatenated. By using this strategy, 30 samples are obtained for each hand movement. In the literature, many methods have used this strategy.

Step 2: Apply DCT to concatenated signal to obtain transform coefficients.

$$C = \mathrm{DCT}(S^C) \tag{2.3}$$

where C is DCT coefficient of the signal and DCT(.) is function of the discrete cosine transform.

Step 3: Apply FFT to concatenated signal to obtain transform coefficients.

$$[IR] = \mathrm{FFT}(S^C) \tag{2.4}$$

$$S^F = I^2 + R^2 \tag{2.5}$$

where I, R and S^F are imaginary, real and Fourier signals, respectively. FFT(.) generates imaginary and real signals.

After this phase, a total of five signals are constructed, and these are S^C, C, I, R and S^F.

2.4.2 Feature extraction

In this phase, SVD and TP are employed as feature extractors. These extractors are applied to the generated five signals. The steps of the SVD-based feature extraction process are presented below.

Step 1: The input signals are shaped into two-dimensional signals. For instance, the length of the used signals in this study are 6000. We reshaped them into 60 ×100. This step is called a vector-to-matrix transformation.

Step 2: The obtained matrix is divided into 15 × 25 sized non-overlapping blocks.

Step 3: SVD is applied onto each 15 × 25 sized block.

$$[USV] = \mathrm{SVD}(\text{block}) \tag{2.6}$$

where U, S, V are components of the SVD and SVD(.) is singular value decomposition function.

Step 4: Store maximum singular value as a feature.

$$\mathrm{feat}_L^S(i) = \max(S),\ i = \{1, 2, \ldots, 16\},$$

$$L = \{S^C, C, I, R, S^F\} \tag{2.7}$$

where feat_k^S represents ith feature of a signal by SVD. As seen in equation (2.5), the SVD based method extracts 16 features from a signal. This feature extraction method is applied to S^C, C, I, R and S^F signals. Hence, 80 features are extracted in this phase. The final feature of this phase is called feat^S.

The second feature extractor is TP. TP uses nine sized non-overlapping windows and ternary functions to extract features. The main problem of TP is to set threshold value. To adjust an automatic threshold value, standard deviation is used in this chapter. The definition of the automatic threshold calculation strategy is given in equations (2.8)–(2.10).

$$\text{thr} = h \times \text{SD}(\text{signal}),\ h = \{0.1, 0.2, \ldots, 1\} \tag{2.8}$$

$$\text{SD}(\text{signal}) = \frac{1}{n-1}\sqrt{\sum\nolimits_{i=1}^{n}(\text{signal}_i - \overline{\text{signal}})^2} \tag{2.9}$$

$$\overline{\text{signal}} = \frac{\sum_{i=1}^{n}\text{signal}_i}{n} \tag{2.10}$$

where $\overline{\text{signal}}$ is mean of the signal, SD(.) is function of the standard deviation, thr represents threshold value and h is multiplier. The pseudo code of the 1D-TP is shown in Algorithm 2.1

Algorithm 2.1: Pseudo code of the 1D-TP

```
Input: Signal (S) with size L, threshold value (t)
Output: Feature vector of the TP (feat^TP) with length of 512.
Load signal.
for i=1 to L-8 do
    window = S(i:i + 8); // Divide signal into 9 sized non-overlapping windows.
    center = window(5); // Assign center value.
    counter = 1; // Assign counter to calculate lower and upper signals.
    L(i) = 0; U(i) = 0; // Define Lower and Upper values.
    for j=1 to 9 do
        if j != 5 then
            if window(j) − center < −t then
                L(i) = L(i) + 2^(8−counter);
            else if window(j) − center > t then
                H(i) = H(i) + 2^(8−counter);
            end if
            counter = counter + 1;
        end if
    end for j
end for i
Extract histograms of the L and U.
Concatenated the histograms extracted and obtain feat^TP.
```

TP is tested using this standard deviation based threshold point search method. Therefore 10 threshold point and results of them are given in the experimental results. The steps of the TP based feature extraction technique are provided below.

Step 1: Load signals which are S^C, C, I, R and S^F.

$$\mathrm{feat}^{\mathrm{TP}}_{S^C} = \mathrm{TP}(S^C) \tag{2.11}$$

$$\mathrm{feat}^{\mathrm{TP}}_{C} = \mathrm{TP}(C) \tag{2.12}$$

$$\mathrm{feat}^{\mathrm{TP}}_{I} = \mathrm{TP}(I) \tag{2.13}$$

$$\mathrm{feat}^{\mathrm{TP}}_{R} = \mathrm{TP}(R) \tag{2.14}$$

$$\mathrm{feat}^{\mathrm{TP}}_{F} = \mathrm{TP}(S^F) \tag{2.15}$$

Step 2: Apply TP and extract 512 features each signal. TP function is given in Algorithm 2.1.

where $\mathrm{feat}^{\mathrm{TP}}_{S^C}$, $\mathrm{feat}^{\mathrm{TP}}_{C}$, $\mathrm{feat}^{\mathrm{TP}}_{I}$, $\mathrm{feat}^{\mathrm{TP}}_{R}$ and $\mathrm{feat}^{\mathrm{TP}}_{F}$ are TP features of the generated signals in the preprocessing phase. TP(.) is ternary pattern function and it extracts 512 features from each signal.

Step 3: Concatenate features of each signal to obtain final TP features.

$$\mathrm{feat}^{\mathrm{TP}} = \mathrm{feat}^{\mathrm{TP}}_{S^C} | \, \mathrm{feat}^{\mathrm{TP}}_{C} | \, \mathrm{feat}^{\mathrm{TP}}_{I} | \, \mathrm{feat}^{\mathrm{TP}}_{R} | \, \mathrm{feat}^{\mathrm{TP}}_{S^F} \tag{2.16}$$

2560 features are extracted from an sEMG signal by using TP-based feature extractor.

As a result, the two type features are extracted utilizing the developed SN. These are SVD- and TP-based features. 80 and 2560 SVD and TP features are extracted. These features are reduced to 80 features.

2.4.3 Feature reduction

In this phase, we utilized an NCA [47] based novel feature reduction method which generates weights of the features. The generated weights and tangent sigmoid function based method is applied onto features for reduction. Tangent sigmoid function is a widely used activation function in the literature. The mathematical description of it is shown in equation (2.17).

$$\mathrm{tansig}(l) = \frac{e^{l} - e^{-l}}{e^{l} + e^{-l}} \tag{2.17}$$

where l represents input parameter of the tangent sigmoid and tansig(.) is tangent sigmoid function. The pseudo code of the proposed feature reduction technique is given in Algorithm 2.2.

Algorithm 2.2: The pseudo code of the proposed NCA and tangent sigmoid based feature reduction method

Input: Concatenated features ($feat^C$) with length of M, reduction factor is k
Output: Reduced features ($feat^R$) with length of M/k.

```
1: w = NCA(feat^C) // Generates weights (w) using NCA
2: counter = 1; // Define counter. This counter is used as index of the reduced feature.
3: for i=1 to M step by k do
4:    p = 0; d = 0; // Define variable to calculate weighted mean value.
5:    for j=0 to k-1 do
6:        p = p + w(i + j) * feat^C(i + j);
7:        d = d + w(i + j);
8:    end for j
9:    feat^R(counter) = tansig(p/d);
10:   counter = counter + 1;
11: end for i
```

As seen in the Algorithm 2.2, NCA is employed to generate weights of the features. The NCA is generally utilized as feature selection approach. The weights generated are used for feature ranking. NCA is a non-parametric method and it uses distance metrics to generate weights. The generated weights are used to calculate weighted average value of the features then the tangent sigmoid function is applied to the average values calculated. In this study, TP and SVD features are reduced separately.

2.4.4 Feature concatenation

In the feature concatenation phase, the reduced TP and SVD features are concatenated to obtain final features. After the concatenation process, the length of the final feature is obtained as 80.

$$\text{feat}^F = \text{feat}^R_{\text{TP}} | \text{feat}^R_{\text{SVD}} \tag{2.18}$$

where $\text{feat}^R_{\text{SVD}}$, $\text{feat}^R_{\text{TP}}$ and feat^F are reduced SVD features, reduced TP features and final features, respectively.

2.4.5 Classification

In the classification phase several classifiers are employed. These classifiers are SVM [42, 43], LDA [48, 49], KNN [48, 49] and ANN [50]. The used SVM uses medium Gaussian kernel. The employed SVM has a Gaussian kernel function, with a box constraint level one, multi-kernel scale 8.9. Covariance structure of the used LDA is full. In the KNN, *k* is selected as 10 and distance metric is chosen as Euclidean distance. In the used KNN, distance weights are calculated by using squared inverse. To obtain testing results of all of the samples, 10-fold cross validation is employed.

2.5 Results and discussions

2.5.1 Dataset

In this article, a basic hand movements dataset is utilized. This dataset is publicly available and widely used for hand movement recognition experiments and it can be downloaded from the UCI website [51]. This dataset consists of sEMG signals of five subjects consisting of three females and two males who are 20–22 years old. A two-channel Delsys Bagnoli™ Handheld EMG set was located on the arm. To acquire the sEMG data, six basic hand movements were presented by subjects. The used hand movements are cylindrical (CY), hook (HO), lateral (LA), palmar (PA), spherical (SP), and tip (TI). This dataset contains 180 sEMG signals for each hand and person because each movement was repeated 30 times. The frequency of the sEMG data is 500 Hz and the sEMG signals are stored with 6 s. Therefore, each signal has 3000 values [51].

2.5.2 Experimental results

In order to test performance of the developed SN, a widely known sEMG signals dataset is utilized. The simulations of the proposed framework are implemented using MATLAB 2018a. The cases are defined to comprehensively evaluate the proposed SN. These cases are constructed by using Gaussian SVM, LDA, ANN and KNN. To evaluate the performance of the classifier, total classification accuracy which is given below is used [52].

$$\text{Accuracy (\%)} = \frac{\text{TP} + \text{TN}}{\text{TP} + \text{TN} + \text{FP} + \text{FN}} \times 100 \tag{2.19}$$

where TP, TN, FP and FN are true positives, true negatives, false positives and false negatives, respectively. An iterative threshold value calculation strategy for TP is used in each case. This strategy uses a standard deviation-based equation. The cases defined and their results are given below.

Case 1: In this case, the Gaussian kernel SVM is employed as classifier. The results of Case 1 are listed in table 2.1. The best rates achieved were 98.88%, 100.0%, 100.0%, 100.0% and 99.44% for F1, F2, F3, M1 and M2 subjects, respectively. The best threshold value for TP is 0.4 × SD(signal).

Case 2: In this case linear discriminant analysis is utilized as classifier (table 2.2). The best accuracy rates were equal to 95.0%, 98.88%, 100.0%, 99.44% and 100.0% for F1, F2, F3, M1 and M2 subjects, respectively. By using 0.5 × SD(signal) as threshold values, two 100.0% classification rates were achieved.

Case 3: In this case KNN (k = 10 and distance metric is Euclidean) is utilized as classifier. The best accuracy rates achieved were 98.88%, 100.0%, 98.88%, 99.44% and 99.44% for F1, F2, F3, M1 and M2 subjects, respectively. The results of this case are listed in table 2.3.

Table 2.1. The classification accuracy results of case 1.

Subjects	0.1SD	0.2 SD	0.3 SD	0.4 SD	0.5 SD
F1	98.88%	97.22%	98.33%	97.77%	98.88%
F2	100.0%	99.44%	100.0%	100.0%	99.44%
F3	98.88%	99.44%	98.89%	100.0%	100.0%
M1	99.44%	99.44%	100.0%	100.0%	99.44%
M2	98.33%	98.88%	98.33%	98.88%	99.44%

Subjects	0.6 SD	0.7 SD	0.8 SD	0.9 SD	1 SD
F1	97.77%	96.66%	98.33%	96.66%	98.33%
F2	100.0%	100.0%	99.44%	99.44%	99.44%
F3	99.44%	99.44%	98.88%	99.44%	98.88%
M1	98.88%	99.44%	98.88%	98.88%	99.44%
M2	99.44%	99.44%	98.33%	98.33%	98.33%

Table 2.2. The classification accuracy results of case 2.

Subjects	0.1 SD	0.2 SD	0.3 SD	0.4 SD	0.5 SD
F1	91.67%	93.89%	95.00%	91.67%	92.78%
F2	98.33%	97.22%	98.88%	99.44%	98.33%
F3	98.33%	98.88%	97.78%	98.88%	100.0%
M1	98.83%	98.88%	99.44%	98.88%	98.88%
M2	100.0%	99.44%	100.0%	100.0%	100.0%

Subjects	0.6 SD	0.7 SD	0.8 SD	0.9 SD	1 SD
F1	93.33%	90.56%	92.22%	92.78%	93.33%
F2	98.33%	98.33%	98.88%	98.88%	98.88%
F3	99.44%	98.88%	96.67%	97.78%	97.78%
M1	98.33%	98.88%	99.44%	98.88%	99.44%
M2	100.0%	100.0%	100.0%	100.0%	100.0%

Case 4: In this case, ANN is utilized as classifier. The hidden layer size of the ANN is 50 and tangent sigmoid is used as an activation function. ANN achieved best performance according to results because it achieved 100.0% classification accuracy for four subjects which are F1, F2, F3 and M2. As seen from table 2.4, the best classification rates were calculated as 100.0%, 100.0%, 99.44% and 100.0% for F1, F2, F3, M1 and M2 subjects, respectively.

Table 2.3. The classification accuracy results of case 3.

Subjects	0.1 SD	0.2 SD	0.3 SD	0.4 SD	0.5 SD
F1	98.88%	95.00%	97.22%	95.00%	97.22%
F2	100.0%	99.44%	99.44%	100.0%	99.44%
F3	96.11%	97.78%	97.78%	97.78%	98.33%
M1	99.44%	98.33%	99.44%	98.88%	98.88%
M2	97.78%	97.78%	98.33%	98.33%	99.44%

Subjects	0.6 SD	0.7 SD	0.8 SD	0.9 SD	1 SD
F1	96.11%	94.44%	95.56%	95.56%	97.22%
F2	99.44%	100.0%	100.0%	99.44%	100.0%
F3	98.88%	97.22%	97.22%	98.33%	98.33%
M1	98.88%	98.33%	98.33%	97.78%	98.33%
M2	98.33%	97.22%	97.78%	97.78%	97.78%

Table 2.4. The classification accuracy results of case 4.

Subjects	0.1 SD	0.2 SD	0.3 SD	0.4 SD	0.5 SD
F1	97.22%	95.55%	100.0%	96.11%	98.33%
F2	100.0%	100.0%	99.44%	100.0%	100.0%
F3	100.0%	97.22%	98.33%	97.78%	97.22%
M1	96.66%	98.88%	98.88%	99.44%	98.33%
M2	96.66%	99.44%	98.88%	100.0%	98.33%

Subjects	0.6 SD	0.7 SD	0.8 SD	0.9 SD	1 SD
F1	97.78%	96.11%	98.33%	96.11%	95.55%
F2	99.44%	99.44%	100.0%	98.88%	98.88%
F3	98.33%	98.33%	98.33%	97.22%	95.00%
M1	98.88%	97.78%	97.78%	99.44%	98.33%
M2	100.0%	98.88%	98.33%	98.88%	97.78%

In order to understand success of the developed framework in a better way, besides accuracy we employed $F1$-score, sensitivity, specificity and geometric mean parameters as well. The mathematical notations of them are given below [52].

$$F1\text{-score} = \frac{2\text{TP}}{2\text{TP} + \text{FP} + \text{FN}} \tag{2.20}$$

$$\text{Sn} = \frac{\text{TP}}{\text{TP} + \text{FN}} \tag{2.21}$$

$$\text{Sp} = \frac{\text{TN}}{\text{FP} + \text{FN}} \tag{2.22}$$

$$\text{Gm} = \sqrt{\text{Sn} \times \text{Sp}} \tag{2.23}$$

where *F*1, Sn, Sp and Gm are *F*-score, sensitivity, specificity and geometric mean, respectively. The best results are listed in table 2.5.

As seen from table 2.5, the proposed SN achieved high *F*1-score, sensitivity, specificity and geometric mean. The used dataset is also a homogenous dataset. Therefore, we obtained these results which are listed in table 2.5. Also, the area under curve (AUC) was calculated as 100%.

As seen in table 2.5, the proposed SN extracts distinctive features, because the used conventional classifiers can achieve high success rates in a short time.

The successful machine learning methods generally have many layers and they should manage parameters efficiently. Hence, the computational complexities of these methods are very high. The proposed method has low computation cost because it is calculated as $O(pn) \cong O(n)$ where p defines a constant number and p is also number of used methods. Also, the average execution time of the SN is given in table 2.6 step by step.

This table proves that the developed model is very fast and lightweight. The success of the proposed method clearly indicates that the developed SN can achieve high accuracy rates using a larger sEMG dataset. Also, the computational complexity of the developed model is calculated to evaluate the proposed method. The computational complexity of the proposed SN is shown in table 2.7 step by step [53].

Table 2.5. *F*-score, sensitivity, specificity and geometric mean values of the developed model for each subject.

Subjects	F1-score	Sn	Sp	Gm
F1	100.0%	100.0%	100.0%	100.0%
F2	100.0%	100.0%	100.0%	100.0%
F3	100.0%	100.0%	100.0%	100.0%
M1	100.0%	100.0%	100.0%	100.0%
M2	100.0%	100.0%	100.0%	100.0%
Average	100.0%	100.0%	100.0%	100.0%

Table 2.6. The average execution time of the developed SN for an sEMG signal.

Step	Time (seconds)
Load signal	2.11×10^{-4}
Pre-processing and feature extraction	0.0383
The proposed NCA and tansig based feature reduction	0.0089
Training using 10-fold cross validation	0.1614

In table 2.7, L, S and T are length of the signal, length of the SVD features and length of the TP features. According to table 2.7, the computational complexity of the proposed SN is mainly based on length of the signal. Thus, the computational complexity is calculated as $O(n)$.

2.5.3 Discussion

In this article, the proposed method uses DCT, FFT, SVD, TP and NCA-based feature reduction methods. These are effective methods and by using the proposed SN, their positive effects for the signal processing are directly used. The proposed SN extracts distinctive features and they can be basically classified. To obtain performances of the SN, three classifiers are used. The best classifier among them is the ANN which achieved 100.0%, 100.0%, 99.44% and 100.0% for F1, F2, F3, M1 and M2 subjects, respectively. The best classification accuracies of the developed model are also the best accuracies of the state-of-the-art methods. The results are also listed in table 2.8.

According to table 2.8, the proposed SN achieved the best results for all subjects.

Table 2.7. The computational complexity of the proposed SN.

Steps of the proposed SN	Computational cost
1: Concatenate sEMG signals of the right and left hands	$O(L)$
2: Apply DCT to signal	$O(L)$
3: Apply FFT to signal and generates three transformation signals	$O(3L)$
4: Apply TP to DCT, FFT signals and original signal	$O(5L)$
5: Apply SVD to DCT, FFT signals and original signal	$O(5L)$
6: Concatenate TP features	$O(5T)$
7: Concatenate SVD features	$O(5S)$
8: Reduce TP features	$O(5T)$
9: Reduce SVD features	$O(5S)$
10: Concatenate reduced features	$O(S + T)$
Total cost	$T(L, S, T) = O(15L + 11T + 11S)$

Table 2.8. The comparison of the proposed SN with state-of-the-art.

Subjects	Iqbal *et al* [54]	Sapsanis *et al* [55]	Akben *et al* [56]	Ruangpaisarn and Jaiy [57]	Nishad *et al* [7]	The proposed SN
F1	82.78	87.25	93.04	96.67	98.33	100.0
F2	87.67	88.05	86.66	98.88	97.78	100.0
F3	83.11	85.53	97.0	96.67	99.44	100.0
M1	90.0	90.42	99.23	98.88	98.88	100.0
M2	90.0	94.80	97.66	100.0	98.33	100.0
Average	86.71	89.21	94.72	98.22	98.55	100.0

2.6 Conclusions and suggestions

A novel feature extraction framework called SN is presented in this chapter. The main aim of the SN is to combine efficient methods in order to classify signals with a high accuracy rate. The proposed SN uses DCT, FFT, TP, SVD, and a novel NCA-based feature reduction method to achieve high success rates. Several classifiers are also used to create different cases with several parameters. The results obtained were compared to the other state-of-the-art methods and the developed model achieved an average accuracy of 100.0%. This result is approximately 1.45% higher than the previous studies. The computational complexity of the developed model is equal to $O(n)$. Moreover, the developed method is a cognitive method because it does not use any optimization technique. The effective methods are used together to achieve high accuracy rates. According to the experimental results, a cognitive, lightweight, and high accurate feature extraction framework is presented. The proposed SN resulted in high performance using conventional classifiers. Although the used dataset in the experiments is small, the proposed method can be tested on big datasets. ANN achieved better performance and it proved that the proposed SN could achieve a high success rate using a large dataset. Hence, a deep feature extraction method is presented for the recognition of basic hand movements using sEMG signals. The proposed SN is the first framework for basic hand movement recognition as far as we know. Novel physiotherapy devices and smart mechanical hands and gloves can be developed using the proposed SN for amputees. The proposed SN is also an extendable method. The main aim of the SN is to combine effective methods such as FFT, DCT, SVD, TP, NCA to achieve better classification performance. The proposed SN framework can be applied to other signals such as ECG, EEG, and speech, etc.

References

[1] Begg R, Lai D T and Palaniswami M 2007 *Computational Intelligence in Biomedical Engineering* (Boca Raton, FL: CRC Press)

[2] Lee S, Kim M-O, Kang T, Park J and Choi Y 2018 Knit band sensor for myoelectric control of surface EMG-based prosthetic hand *IEEE Sens. J.* **18** 8578–86

[3] Stango A, Negro F and Farina D 2014 Spatial correlation of high density EMG signals provides features robust to electrode number and shift in pattern recognition for myocontrol *IEEE Trans. Neur. Syst. Rehabil. Eng.* **23** 189–98

[4] Ma J, Thakor N V and Matsuno F 2014 Hand and wrist movement control of myoelectric prosthesis based on synergy *IEEE Trans. Human-Mach. Syst* **45** 74–83

[5] Subasi A, Alharbi L, Madani R and Qaisar S M 2018 Surface EMG based classification of basic hand movements using rotation forest *Advances in Science and Engineering Technology Int. Conf. (ASET)* (Piscataway, NJ: IEEE) 2018 pp. 1–5

[6] Noce E, Bellingegni A D, Ciancio A L, Sacchetti R, Davalli A and Guglielmelli E *et al* 2019 EMG and ENG-envelope pattern recognition for prosthetic hand control *J. Neurosci. Methods* **311** 38–46

[7] Nishad A, Upadhyay A, Pachori R B and Acharya U R 2019 Automated classification of hand movements using tunable-Q wavelet transform based filter-bank with surface electromyogram signals *Future Gener. Comput. Syst.* **93** 96–110

[8] Yabuki Y, Tanahashi K, Hoshikawa S, Nakamura T, Kato R and Jiang Y *et al* 2016 Development of new cosmetic gloves for myoelectric prosthetic hand by using thermoplastic styrene elastomer *Int. Conf. on Intelligent Autonomous Systems* (Berlin: Springer) pp 269–82
[9] Shi W-T, Lyu Z-J, Tang S-T, Chia T-L and Yang C-Y 2018 A bionic hand controlled by hand gesture recognition based on surface EMG signals: a preliminary study *Biocybern. Biomed. Eng.* **38** 126–35
[10] Enoka R M 2019 Physiological validation of the decomposition of surface EMG signals *J. Electromyog. Kinesiol.* **46** 70–83
[11] Ryu J and Kim D-H 2017 Real-time gait subphase detection using an EMG signal graph matching (ESGM) algorithm based on EMG signals *Expert Syst. Appl.* **85** 357–65
[12] Junior J D C and de Seixas J M 2019 A template subtraction method for reducing electrocardiographic artifacts in EMG signals of low intensity *Biomed. Signal Process. Control* **47** 380–6
[13] Jochumsen M, Waris A and Kamavuako E N 2018 The effect of arm position on classification of hand gestures with intramuscular emg *Biomed. Signal Process. Control* **43** 1–8
[14] Chowdhury A, Raza H, Meena Y K, Dutta A and Prasad G 2019 An EEG–EMG correlation-based brain-computer interface for hand orthosis supported neuro-rehabilitation *J. Neurosci. Methods* **312** 1–11
[15] Tavakoli M, Benussi C and Lourenco J L 2017 Single channel surface EMG control of advanced prosthetic hands: a simple, low cost and efficient approach *Expert Syst. Appl.* **79** 322–32
[16] Tavakoli M, Benussi C, Lopes P A, Osorio L B and de Almeida A T 2018 Robust hand gesture recognition with a double channel surface EMG wearable armband and SVM classifier *Biomed. Signal Process. Control* **46** 121–30
[17] Sumathi S and Paneerselvam S 2010 *Computational Intelligence Paradigms: Theory and Applications Using MATLAB* (Boca Raton, FL: CRC Press)
[18] Bagga P and Hans R 2015 Applications of mobile agents in healthcare domain: a literature survey *Int. J. Grid Distrib. Comput.* **8** 55–72
[19] Grimson J, Stephens G, Jung B, Grimson W, Berry D and Pardon S 2001 Sharing health-care records over the internet *IEEE Internet Comput.* **5** 49–58
[20] Pölsterl S, Conjeti S, Navab N and Katouzian A 2016 Survival analysis for high-dimensional, heterogeneous medical data: exploring feature extraction as an alternative to feature selection *Artif. Intell. Med.* **72** 1–11
[21] Caballé N C, Castillo-Sequera J L, Gómez-Pulido J A, Gómez-Pulido J M and Polo-Luque M L 2020 Machine learning applied to diagnosis of human diseases: a systematic review *Appl. Sci.* **10** 5135
[22] Kononenko I 2001 Machine learning for medical diagnosis: history, state of the art and perspective *Artif. Intell. Med.* **23** 89–109
[23] Gokgoz E and Subasi A 2015 Comparison of decision tree algorithms for EMG signal classification using DWT *Biomed. Signal Process. Control* **18** 138–44
[24] Subasi A 2013 Classification of EMG signals using PSO optimized SVM for diagnosis of neuromuscular disorders *Comput. Biol. Med.* **43** 576–86
[25] Subasi A 2015 A decision support system for diagnosis of neuromuscular disorders using DWT and evolutionary support vector machines *Signal Image Video Process.* **9** 399–408
[26] Subasi A 2012 Medical decision support system for diagnosis of neuromuscular disorders using DWT and fuzzy support vector machines *Comput. Biol. Med.* **42** 806–15

[27] Coelho A L and Lima C A 2014 Assessing fractal dimension methods as feature extractors for EMG signal classification *Eng. Appl. Artif. Intell.* **36** 81–98

[28] Al-Faiz M Z and Miry A H 2012 Artificial human arm driven by EMG signal *MATLAB* **1** 365

[29] Tsai A-C, Hsieh T-H, Luh J-J and Lin T-T 2014 A comparison of upper-limb motion pattern recognition using EMG signals during dynamic and isometric muscle contractions *Biomed. Signal Process. Control* **11** 17–26

[30] Xing K, Yang P, Huang J, Wang Y and Zhu Q 2014 A real-time EMG pattern recognition method for virtual myoelectric hand control *Neurocomputing* **136** 345–55

[31] Phinyomark A, Quaine F, Charbonnier S, Serviere C, Tarpin-Bernard F and Laurillau Y 2013 EMG feature evaluation for improving myoelectric pattern recognition robustness *Expert Syst. Appl.* **40** 4832–40

[32] Kim K S, Choi H H, moon C S and Mun C W 2011 Comparison of k-nearest neighbor, quadratic discriminant and linear discriminant analysis in classification of electromyogram signals based on the wrist-motion directions *Curr. Appl. Phys.* **11** 740–5

[33] Subasi A 2019 Electromyogram-controlled assistive devices *Bioelectronics and Medical Devices* (Amsterdam: Elsevier) pp 285–311

[34] Kurzynski M, Krysmann M, Trajdos P and Wolczowski A 2016 Multiclassifier system with hybrid learning applied to the control of bioprosthetic hand *Comput. Biol. Med.* **69** 286–97

[35] Wojtczak P, Amaral T G, Dias O P, Wolczowski A and Kurzynski M 2009 Hand movement recognition based on biosignal analysis *Eng. Appl. Artif. Intell.* **22** 608–15

[36] Rechy-Ramirez E J and Hu H 2015 Bio-signal based control in assistive robots: a survey *Digit. Commun. Netw.* **1** 85–101

[37] Khayam S A 2003 *The Discrete Cosine Transform (DCT): Theory and Application* (East Lansing, MI: Michigan State University) 114

[38] Katoh K, Misawa K, Kuma K-i and Miyata T 2002 MAFFT: a novel method for rapid multiple sequence alignment based on fast Fourier transform *Nucleic Acids Res.* **30** 3059–66

[39] Golub G H and Reinsch C 1971 Singular value decomposition and least squares solutions *Linear Algebra* (Berlin: Springer) pp 134–51

[40] Xu W-H, Zhao X-L and Ng M 2019 A fast algorithm for cosine transform based tensor singular value decomposition. arXiv preprint arXiv:190203070

[41] Ren J, Jiang X and Yuan J 2013 Relaxed local ternary pattern for face recognition *IEEE Int. Conf. on Image Processing* (Piscataway, NJ: IEEE) pp 3680–4

[42] Khunarsal P, Lursinsap C and Raicharoen T 2013 Very short time environmental sound classification based on spectrogram pattern matching *Inf. Sci.* **243** 57–74

[43] Peng Y-T, Lin C-Y, Sun M-T and Tsai K-C 2009 Healthcare audio event classification using hidden Markov models and hierarchical hidden Markov models *IEEE Int. Conf. on Multimedia and Expo* (Piscataway, NJ: IEEE) pp 1218–21

[44] Mika S, Ratsch G, Weston J, Scholkopf B and Mullers K-R 1999 Fisher discriminant analysis with kernels *Neural Networks for Signal Processing IX: Proc. 1999 IEEE Signal Processing Society Workshop (cat no 98th8468)* (Piscataway, NJ: IEEE) pp 41–8

[45] Prasath V, Alfeilat H A A, Lasassmeh O and Hassanat A 2017 Distance and similarity measures effect on the performance of *k*-nearest neighbor classifier – a review. arXiv preprint arXiv:170804321

[46] Wang Z, Liu Y and Griffin P J 2000 A combined ANN and expert system tool for transformer fault diagnosis *IEEE Power Engineering Society Winter Meeting Conf. Proc. (Cat No 00CH37077)* (Piscataway, NJ: IEEE) pp 1261–9

[47] Goldberger J, Hinton G E, Roweis S and Salakhutdinov R R 2004 Neighbourhood components analysis *Adv. Neur. Info. Process. Syst.* **17** 513–20

[48] Vapnik V 1998 The support vector method of function estimation *Nonlinear Modeling* (Berlin: Springer) pp 55–85

[49] Vapnik V 2013 *The Nature of Statistical Learning Theory* (Berlin: Springer Science & Business Media)

[50] Yegnanarayana B 2009 *Artificial Neural Networks* : (New Delhi: PHI Learning Pvt. Ltd)

[51] https://archive.ics.uci.edu/ml/datasets/sEMG+for+Basic+Hand+movements#

[52] Tuncer T, Dogan S, Pławiak P and Acharya U R 2019 Automated arrhythmia detection using novel hexadecimal local pattern and multilevel wavelet transform with ECG signals *Knowl. Based Syst.* **186** 104923

[53] Papadimitriou C H 2003 *Computational Complexity* (New York: Wiley)

[54] Iqbal O, Fattah S A and Zahin S 2017 Hand movement recognition based on singular value decomposition of surface EMG signal *IEEE Region 10 Humanitarian Technology Conf. (R10-HTC)* (Piscataway, NJ: IEEE) pp 837–42

[55] Sapsanis C, Georgoulas G, Tzes A and Lymberopoulos D 2013 Improving EMG based classification of basic hand movements using EMD *2013 35th Annual Int. Conf. IEEE Engineering in Medicine Biology Society (EMBC)* (Piscataway, NJ: IEEE) 5754–7

[56] Akben S B 2017 Low-cost and easy-to-use grasp classification, using a simple 2-channel surface electromyography (sEMG) *Biomed. Res.* **28** 577–82

[57] Ruangpaisarn Y and Jaiyen S 2015 SEMG signal classification using SMO algorithm and singular value decomposition *2015 7th Int. Conf. Information Technology Electrical Engineering (ICITEE)* (Piscataway, NJ: IEEE) *;* pp 46–50

IOP Publishing

High Performance Computing for Intelligent Medical Systems

Varun Bajaj and Irshad Ahmad Ansari

Chapter 3

Analysis of IoT interventions to solve voice pathologies challenges

Wahengbam Kanan Kumar, Mithlesh Prasad Singh, Aheibam Dinamani Singh, Rajesh Kumar and Kishorjit Nongmeikapam

Speech is the simplest mode of expression, and any alteration of the vocal cord disrupts its smooth flow. Speech disorders increase vocal exhaustion, pressure, dysphonia, roughness, glottal attack, sore throat, etc. Disruption of a smooth voice in most situations leads to a wide range of psychiatric disorders resulting from stigmatization from peers and the community. It can have detrimental effects in the search for jobs, as well as on social and academic terms. Speech disability also results from brain damage, hearing loss, stroke, and developmental delay. A variety of aspects of voice pathology research are the subject of the present chapter. Applications for the Internet of Things (IoT) and related research work are analyzed in depth. Detailed background information on electroglottography is highlighted, which includes its development, production of vocal folded tone, glottal closure and instant opening, quantitative analysis in terms of frequency and amplitude. Information on some of the most common datasets among researchers are also highlighted. Finally, two separate parts dealing with several important acoustic feature extraction techniques, along with significant pathological voice analysis and identification techniques, are also discussed in great detail.

3.1 Introduction

The most important way to exchange ideas and feelings between two people is by speaking. It is also the simplest and most concise way to convey one's viewpoint, considering that it contains a variety of non-verbal opinions. Creating a voice from one's body is nevertheless a complicated process. Some major organs and tissues play an important role in the three-stage voice production process. They are—(a) generating air volume pressure, (b) supplying vibration, and (c) resonance. Collectively, the rib cage, diaphragms, lungs, and muscles in the abdominal region

doi:10.1088/978-0-7503-3815-8ch3

create an articulate air volume pressure that generates a ‘pitch’ by continuous oscillation of the vocal folds. It is the characteristics and structures of the vocal tract and the vocal folds that produce sounds that are unique to all. The ‘pitch’ that is derived from the vocal fold lingers in the nasal cavities, and the throat that has a distinct acoustic structure is another source of individuality for any voice. There are three distinct layers in the laryngeal vocal fold, that is, the vocal ligament, the mucosa, and the vocal fold. Since these tissues are tender, they can be continuously affected by air pressure and release the mucosal waveform. The ability of the mucosa to produce pitch rates determines whether the voice is regular or abnormal.

For speech specialists such as phoniatricians, a voice has several characteristics of an individual, such as mental well-being, physical trauma, vocal pathologies in the vocal fold, the person’s gender, emotional state, etc. A deviation from the normal vocal attributes of a person as opposed to those who share the age group and gender can be defined as a problem of laryngitis or other vocal fold disease. Vocal fold disease is caused by gradual alteration in the voice synthesizing organs and tissues in the body. These changes may be due to over-manipulation of the vocal cords, frequent intake of medications, or neurological disorders. Abuse of vocal cord can lead to conditions such as unilateral nerve paralysis, laryngeal cancer, polyp, nodule, and folding for a prolonged period of time. These situations can be defined by the hoarseness of one’s voice. In addition to self-abuse, an unhealthy lifestyle may contribute to an increase in vocal disorders [1, 2]. Singers, mothers of children and educators are people who unknowingly abuse their vocal cords. The reasoning is that they have to say words constantly during the work plan. Such excessive use of the voice fold leads to more rigidity over time. The vagus nerve, which is responsible for the proper functioning of the larynx, is also highly likely to be dysfunctional. This condition is known as unilateral nerve paralysis, which is usually noticed from the speaker’s breathing phonation sound. Other issues are also reported, such as air deprivation, trouble swallowing and mild coughing [3]. Irregularity occurs in the vocal box or larynx due to repetitive abuse due to the nature of the work that can contribute to breathing and harsh vocals. Physical features, including elasticity, shape and volume, associated with vocal folds, are modified when disorders, including gastric reflection or anterior-to-posterior (A–P) squeezing, begin. This leads to an unusual variant of vibration. Swelling of the vocal folds are caused by gastric reflux and laryngitis. While muscle tension damage is caused by constant A–P squeezing.

3.1.1 Pathology assessment

The invasive technique used to diagnose pathologies in human laryngeal arrangement is an age-old and modern procedure that is still popular throughout the world. Examples of the two endoscopic procedures required to insert large instruments into the human body in order to map the internal structure include laryngostroboscopy and operational microlaryngoscopy. Intrinsic anxiety and pain are caused to the patient under surveillance. In the past, scientists have also developed non-invasive approaches to minimize pain to a certain degree. In one such scenario, electroglottography (EGG) is done where a person’s voice is analyzed. Patients have been able to ease the pain to some degree. There is, however, a problem with teaching individuals to use these machines, which, if applied on a mass scale, would result in pointless costs. Economical, non-invasive and automated diagnosis of voice signal pathologies for thorough study of glottal signals is a trend for research enthusiasts. It is the future of speech pathology detection. The glottal signal is produced between the vocal fold and the vocal tract. Considering the success of deep learning [4] in various areas of artificial intelligence (AI), the number of studies in the classification of voice pathology will increase further [5–9]. Deep learning is becoming a better option against common classifiers such as decision trees, support vector machine (SVM), k-nearest neighbors (KNN), decision trees, naive bays, etc. Handcrafted speech or acoustic features have been of primary importance for voice pathology detection for the last few decades and cannot therefore be ignored.

Deep learning models such as the Recurrent Neural Network (RNN) and the Long Short-Term Memory (LSTM) are also used. Prediction scores generated using handcrafted machine learning features and deep learning classifiers can also be combined to further improve accuracy [9]. It can therefore be concluded that computer-based voice analytics of these types should be further researched before they are widely used as screening methods to classify laryngeal pathology.

3.1.2 Internet of things in voice pathology

Healthcare is one of the most common sectors for internet of things (IoT) applications. Some potential uses include chronic disease management, smart fitness-tracking wearables, remote patient monitoring, etc. Nowadays, a boom in smart watches that use sensors to monitor different types of everyday fitness activities and uploading to IoT-based smartphones is widespread. Intelligent medical devices and imaging devices are also main components of IoT. Over the coming years, the integration of more miniaturized low-power sensors with better machine learning (ML) algorithms will significantly enhance the cost-effectiveness of these smart IoT products. This will further revolutionize the experience of the consumer. Authors of [10] argued that suppliers view IoT as a tool for remotely reducing the downtime of smart devices. IoT also provides strategic resource planning to ensure that more patients will make the most of their services. Premature testing, health-related problems, chronic diseases and real-time monitoring are expected to be promoted by emerging wireless technologies [11, 12]. A thorough understanding of current IoT research in health applications is expected to help many stakeholders involved in additional research at this point in time. ML has been used to test clinical parameters and their combinations for prediction purposes, such as extracting health knowledge for outcome studies, comprehensive patient treatment, therapeutic planning and support, and predicting disease progression [13, 14].

ML incorporation in the medical sector provides medical professionals with the opportunity to function effectively, create, and enhance the quality and reliability of medical care [15]. Biomedical signals can also be done with real hardware in order to recognize physiological changes in the human body in a variety of different ways.

Some instances are—drowsiness detection [16–18], emotion recognition and identification [19–21], motor imagery classification [22, 23], schizophrenia detection [24], focal electroencephalography signal identification [25–28], sleep apnea, [29] etc.

Various aspects of speech signals can be used in the healthcare sector to diagnose a variety of disorders. Because of the nature of work and poor social practices, certain people are vulnerable to voice hazards, the pathological voice signal is an important topic here [30–32].

The present literature review chapter also focuses on the implementation of IoT-based hardware, features extraction forms, ML and deep learning mechanisms used in the field of voice pathology sensing. While voice pathology is a significant field, it has not attracted significant attention and, therefore, a lack of research on the diagnosis of voice diseases is urgently needed in this area. Laryngeal cancer is one of the most common head and neck cancers in the world [33]. Today, laryngeal cancer is the most severe disease that not only alters the patient's ability to talk, but also has the potential to cause death [34].

A new and effective method or strategy for early detection of this cancer through the voice of patients is therefore crucial if early cancer treatment has a good chance of recovery. Unfortunately, the majority of researchers and developers are concerned with discerning a voice as either a regular (healthy) voice or a pathological voice, for example [35–37], where there is no clear detection of a voice abnormality. These technologies are also affected by poor predictive accuracy and processing time in ML algorithm pathology monitoring approaches. However, the following chapter offers a detailed study of recent research and methods in the field of voice pathology. The chapter also discusses a multitude of challenges that should be addressed in future studies.

The authors of [38] proposed a new health tracking framework by combining IoT with the internet. The research presented a case study of a voice pathology monitoring system in which voice signals are captured and transmitted to the host controller through various IoTs. Signals are identified by the patient identification number in order to preserve the authenticity of voice signals. With reduced computational time, the proposed voice pathology detection is extremely accurate. Appropriate monitoring of health through IoTs and cloud technologies will expand the pathological monitoring framework. In [39] there is offered a framework for smart health monitoring connected to smart cities and smart devices for fully transparent and cost-effective healthcare. The authors proposed an approach involving two inputs: EGG and speech signal. The input devices are cloud-linked and the signals received are transmitted to the cloud. These signs are categorized as normal or pathological. The final decision to decide the next step is to notify the physicians of the findings obtained from the signals. The Gaussian mixture model is implemented in the Saarbruecken Voice Database (SVD). Analysis has shown that the accuracy of the suggested approach is over 93%. The author of [40] proposes a health monitoring system to address the needs of the elderly with a view to continuing treatment. Two inputs, speech and video, monitor the status of the patient in this proposed system. Installed in smart homes, microphones and video cameras capture and send data to the cloud. Both sensors record the words and videos of the patient. The information is stored in the cloud and the classification of voice signals, whether the patient is nervous, normal or in pain, will depend on the patient's situation.

An algorithm for remote detection of voice fold pathology using voice consistency is introduced in [41]. The method uses a linear classification system to measure pitch disturbance, amplitude disturbance and harmonic noise associations of speech samples. The findings show that 89.1% accuracy can be achieved in a controlled setting. However, when the electronic speaker output is used, it falls to 74.2%. The authors classify voices as normal, neuromuscular, physical, and mixed. The significance of this study is that it combines telephony and server-side speech processing to diagnose pathological voices from a remote location. It incorporates telephony and voice processing on the server side in order to evaluate pathological voices from a distant region.

This chapter aims to address the different voice disorders and ML techniques that are used to create automated systems and to present them in detail. Section 3.1 presents the introduction. Section 3.2 offers a description of the phases of production of EGG. The specifics of different voice pathology databases are discussed in section 3.3. Section 3.3 addresses different handmade features using automated voice disorder classification technology for ML. Section 3.4 addresses the classification methods for deep learning-based voice disorders.

3.2 Electroglottography

This technology is low-cost, non-invasively measuring changes in the relative vocal fold area during the production of laryngeal voices. EGG was introduced 30 years ago [42, 43] in the late 1980s and early 1990s [44–49] and has passed through a golden age of growing scientific interest. A high frequency, low ampere current is transmitted between two electrodes located on either side of the thyroid cartilage. Vocal fold vibration transmits changes to the vocal fold contact analysis (VFCA), allowing the EGG signal to vary by VFCA. The lack of spatial information during the calculation of EGG is a crucial weakness. Vocal fold vibration is a complex three-dimensional phenomenon that is mapped to a time-variable value, that is, VFCA. Differences in vibrational features, such as inferior-superior or front-posterior [50], are difficult to resolve. The concept of a multi-channel EGG estimate was demonstrated by [51]. Three years later, two channels using different modulation frequencies were used to capture both horizontal and vertical signals [52]. The concept of a multi-channel EGG was also explored in [53] by setting up a system to decode 36 multiplexing current paths with two 2×3 electrode grids. The ability of the device to monitor vertical and horizontal larynx positions during singing and swallowing was demonstrated by limited pilot data obtained using the prototype of this design. In a different method, the developers of [54] replaced multiplexing time division with frequency division multiplexing. By proposing an electrical impedance tomography (EIT) procedure, Liu *et al* [55] have broadened the concept of collecting spatial information from a non-invasive physiological voice signal outside the EGG. EIT technology appears to be promising in future voice research and diagnostics, although daunting in mathematical and engineering terms.

Two different methods have been used to establish the physiological meaning of the EGG waveform and its landmarks, using experimental evidence from controlled experiments and using analytical techniques. For example, with photoglottography (PGG) [56], videostroboscopy [57], *in vivo* air circulation in glottis [58], some initial empirical multiple-signal validations have been carried out. A number of outstanding contributions in the 'golden era' provided a sufficient understanding of the landmarks of the EGG waveform and its connection with the vocal fold vibration [45, 47, 49, 59–63]. These investigations used some form of time-synchronous laryngeal imagery, using a fast video imaging technique with frame rates of up to 5000 fps. The authors of [64] who used the first EGG signal derivative have further verified their findings.

The most prominent characteristics of the EGG waveform are hypothesized moments of interaction or decontact of the vocal fold. The 'knee' in the EGG waveform represents another signature [59]. It is a convex dislocation on the side of the waveform [45]. This EGG feature found during the decontact phase of the glottal cycle corresponds to the opening along the top edge of the glottis. [45, 65] discussed the relationship between the presence or absence of an EGG 'knee' and the spectral acoustic waveform characteristics and [66] suggested an intelligent algorithm for detecting 'knee' and other EGG waveform inflexions.

EGG (de) contacting versus glottal opening and closure. EGG is often not used and interpreted in itself as a VFCA measurements process, but instead as a non-invasive approximation quantification that theoretically emulates glottal airflow of high-speed video (HSV) recordings. The explanation would be that the reliability of relationship between the laryngeal air flow varies from time to time since it is dictated by the dynamics of the vocal fold's vibration, and the sound quality generated by the larynges. The localized pressure gradient that occurs through a mostly abrupt ceaseflow of the laryngeal flux, at the glottal closure incidence, constitutes a significant proportion of that tone. The timing of the occurrence of glottal closures—commonly known in the speech processing domain as 'glottal closure instants' (GCIs)—is a significant component towards voice quality, and a corresponding physiological measure would therefore be beneficial. To a minor extent, the same reasoning applies to glottal openings (GOIs) [67–69]. Findings from early work indicate that positive dEGG peaks are well-related to that of the GCI [60, 70], while the authors have reported the GOI, which would have been thought to be more variable might occur at various points throughout the background of the glottis [70]. Therefore, it may be difficult to identify GOIs by using the EGG signal's feature alone. But it may also be inaccurate if GCI is in precise synchronization with the positive dEGG peak. [71] records an error rate of 0.24 ms in the GCIs of ten speakers that has been deduced using inverse-filtered airflow and dEGG positive peaks, respectively. The deviation was 0.68 ms, which would equate to approximately 8.2% of the glottal period in males and approximately 13.6% in females.

3.2.1 Quantitative analysis

A. Fundamental frequency estimation. Since the EGG signal is an indirect physiological proof of the cyclic origin of laryngeal vibrations, it is in reality an ideal candidate for the extraction of fundamental frequencies. Several earlier studies used the EGG in various contexts to establish fundamental frequencies [72]. Proceedings can include-testing dosimetry [73], quantifying timbre in a-cappella quartet performance [74], or researching vocal sensations [75]. The [75] study showed that the fundamental frequency obtained from the acoustic signals has been correlated with the EGG signal as calculated in a database of 8000 voice signals. As a result of this EGG efficiency for fundamental frequency extraction, [76] employed EGG signals to set up a fundamental frequency database derived from running sound. [77] noted that EGG was a better predictor of disturbance parameters compared to acoustic sound. However, it is appropriate to ensure that in EGG signaling devices such as baseline timbres, noise equipment is mitigated. In addition, careful cataloging of algorithms for the extraction of fundamental frequencies may be needed if certain signal properties, such as cycle-by-cycle disturbances and/or subharmonics, are present.

B. Amplitude of the EGG waveform. Different factors such as larynx heights, electrode placement, posture changes, neck size and automatic gain controllers (AGCs) can affect the amplitude of the EGG signal. This leads to the incorrect understanding of the vocal fold contact operation [46, 70, 78, 79]. Research studies often use non-normalized dEGG or EGG parameters for quantitative analysis [80, 81]. The importance of the overall amplitude of the unfiltered EGG signal was discussed in [82] where signal elements below the vibration level of the vocal fold could, in theory, be used to track this function of the vocal fold alteration, that is, systemic changes of the general amplitude may occur in the signal acquired without the AGC. Perhaps because the potential factors actually influence the overall amplitude of the EGG waveform mentioned above, the scientific hypothesis between the vocal fold (pre-)phonation (pre-)phonatoid laryngeal configurations and any possible structural consequences for the EGG amplitude is not currently provided with strong empirical support (e.g., the laryngeal endoscopy). It is therefore important to distinguish between low-frequency alterations under the vibration rate of the vocal fold and in-cycle variations of the VFCA in the 'amplitude' of the EGG signal.

3.3 Voice pathology datasets

The current section discusses some recent and most popularly implemented standardized datasets worldwide.

3.3.1 Voice ICar fEDerico II (VOICED)

[83] suggested a pathological speech dataset called VOice ICar fEDerico II (VOICED). There are 150 pathological and 58 balanced voice recordings with an 85 kHz and a 32-bit resolution. A total of 150 pathological records were given by

98 female and 52 male candidates and 58 safe files were facilitated by 37 females and 21 males. Participants were aged between 18 and 60 years. Three different types of disorders, that is, hyperkinetic dysphonia, hypokinetic dysphonia and laryngitis reflux, were grouped in their datasets under the pathology class. Stiffness of vocal folds, vocal fold nodules, polyps, etc are a form of hyperkinetic dysphonia. Second, the hypokinetic dysphonia community comprises speech disorders such as fold paralysis, laryngitis, and glottis insufficiency. There are signs of pharyngitis, asthma, halitosis and cough at night in the third category. The Voice Database was developed in collaboration with the University Hospital of Naples 'Federico II' by the Institute of High-Performance Computing and Networking of the Italian National Research Council (ICAR-CNR). This repository has uneven samples, namely 150 and 58 for a safe and pathological voice. Each recording has the vowel \a\ voice at a rate of 8000 Hz with a sound and pathological voice. This database is very new and few research studies are currently using it.

3.3.2 Massachusetts eye and ear infirmary

This database has been developed by the MEEI Voice and Speech Lab. It includes more than 1400 voice samples of the continuous vowel /a/ and the first section of the Rainbow Quotation. Kay Elemetrics [84] markets the materials. Two different configurations have been recorded. The sample frequency was 50 kHz for normal samples, compared with 25 kHz or 50 kHz for pathological samples. There are many inconveniences, such as the differing conditions and the sampling rates used to capture natural and abnormal voices. It has been used in a number of research works. This database used a variety of methods to assess voice fitness, including stroboscopy, audio aerodynamics, and medical assessments for the neck and mouth. Numerous voice disorders can be treated by analyzing changes in muscles that can induce and improve the strength of the voice.

3.3.3 Saarbruecken Voice Database

This is an unrestricted and accessible German database with a wide variety of samples. This diversity of samples allows numerous forms of studies to be carried out for various scientific purposes. The database [85] is freely available for download and is maintained by the Saarland University Institute of Phonetics. It includes sustained vowels /a/, /i/, and /u/ with different tonalities: regular, low, high, and low-high-low with a German-language phrase 'Guten Morgen, wie geht es Ihnen?' which implies, 'Good morning, how are you?' These characteristics make it a good database to perform experiments for researchers. Any voices of the SVD database have 16-bit resolutions sampled at 50 kHz.

3.3.4 Arabic voice pathology database

The AVPD dataset of speech recordings was collected by well-experienced phoniatricians at King Abdul Aziz University in Saudi Arabia. Records of speeches were collected over two years from a project funded by the National Science and Technology Plans of Saudi Arabia. Phoniatricians maintained a sampling system such that the flaws in the MEEI database could be mitigated. The database contains continuous vowel records for normal and vocal fold patients. After clinical assessment with laryngeal stroboscopy, a safe and unhealthy vocal fold of individuals was established. In clinical cases, the perceived severity of voice disorders has been assessed at a scale of 1 to 3, with 3 being the worst. On the basis of a panel of three medical experts, each sample was connected to a severity ranking. The database contains three different types of documents. They are three long-lasting vowels with beginning and offset information, single words, including Arabic numerals and some other common terms and a continuous voice. The text has been deliberately selected to cover all Arabic phonemes. The three vowels a, u and i were reported by all speakers, while isolated words and continuous speech were used once to prevent tiring patients. The sampling frequency in the database was 44 kHz and the speech was captured in the computerized speech lab (CSL) software. Several specialist physicians at King Abdul Aziz University Hospital have tested and confirmed the voice disorders recorded in this database [86].

3.4 Acoustic speech features with machine learning for voice pathology classification

There are two subsections in this section. The first one addresses several important speech pathology features extraction procedures. Research works using handcrafted features and ML classifiers are disucssed in the second subsection.

3.4.1 Feature extraction techniques

This is the most critical step in any ML process. This includes the conversion of a voice signal into acoustic features by digital signal processing techniques.

A. **Acoustic analysis.** This is an estimate of the audio metadata in the voice. Acoustic assessment results may be used to determine the severity of a speech disturbance. Any activity related to acoustic voice signal analysis can be as follows. (A) Abnormalities around the basic pitch and the peak amplitude. (B) The frequency range of the noisy signal. (C) Waveform pattern from cycle to cycle. (D) Natural features of the frequency. (E) Properties of signal transformation.

B. **Mel frequency Cepstral Coefficients (MFCC).** Essentially, this is used for the diagnosis of speech deficiency. The key benefits compared to other voice features are that they can fully represent the vocal tract. Once the vocal tract has been precisely established, the phoneme produced by the vocal tract can be precisely determined. The vocal tract is distributed in a short-term continuum envelope, and this envelope is properly represented in the MFCC. The following procedure defines the MFCCs. [87]. (A) Initially, the voice signal (x[n]) is broken up using a short-term Fourier transform (STFT) and a window (w[n]). (B) The magnitude of the signal (say X) is now being weighted by a number of filter frequency responses that are roughly balanced by the frequency and bandwidth of the center of the audio filters called 'mel scale' filters. (C) The next step is to classify the energy in the

STFT that is weighted by the frequency response of each mel scale filter. The energy for each verbal frame is determined at time n and the *i*th mel filter. (D) The discrete cosine is then checked for transformation coefficients or energy-related cepstrum. MFCC is unevenly distributed around various frame indices for pathological voices. Thus, MFCC is commonly used in many works to differentiate between a pathological voice and a regular voice.

C. **Linear Predictive Coding (LPC).** Digital signals have been compressed for efficient storage and transmission using LPC. It is one of the most effective methods of language analysis and has become popular as a formant evaluation tool [88]. The LPC analysis is based on the approximation of the vocal tract as a linear all-pole IIR filter. For a signal segment with a sampling rate of 8 kHz, a voice encoder is used to calculate the optimum excitation, voice pitch time, gain and coefficients. The LPC is based on the mean-square error approach. Using this approach, a linear combination of the earlier samples is used to measure the voice signal. The LPC coefficients vary considerably in some portions of the voice signal. However, the magnitude is not significant for other parts of the voice signal. Pathological speech can be differentiated by a continuum of magnitude from normal voice.
D. **Glottal flow signal.** It can be extracted by inversely filtering a speech signal that eliminates redundant voice artifacts from the mouth and vocal tract and preserves the original message signal released during the glottal flow [89]. The Pitch Synchronous Iterative Adaptive Inverse Filtering algorithm was developed to extract glottal signal attributes as one of the MATLAB toolboxes known as Aparat8. The time domain characteristics that can be obtained from the glottal flux signal are: the closing and opening instants, the opening threshold, the amplitude threshold, the quasi-open threshold, the normalized amplitude threshold, and the speed quotient. Frequency domain parameters are: the difference between the harmonics and its richness factor.
E. **Spectrograms**. The waveform of speech consists of a sequence of events that differ from time to time. This time differential refers to the spectral characteristics that vary considerably over time. This type of fast-time signal cannot be acquired by a single Fourier transform, and instead the [90] STFT is used. The STFT consists of a Fourier transform with a sliding waveform part window. The distribution of the spectral power of a voice varies greatly with time and frequency, so that regular to pathological tones can be distinguished. For a normal voice, the spectral density of power is consistent with time and frequency, but is not consistent with a pathological voice. The spectrogram is also considered to be a strong segregator of pathological voices from ordinary voices.
F. **Formants**. The formant analysis is a powerful voice characteristic studied by researchers. The frequencies that form the vocal tract are the resonance frequencies that change the form factors of the different vocal tracts. Usually, the formant refers to the full spectral resonance contribution. The peaks of the continuum are approximately the same as those produced

by the vocal tract response. In a formant map, there are different peaks on certain frequencies. Peaks are also separated by a certain frequency band and are located in decreasing order of magnitude. Unlike a typical voice, the irregular or pathological voice has many different styles of voice. For example, if a pathological voice is used, any three peaks may be closely placed and of the same magnitude. However, the peaks are located at a constant distance from each other and their amplitude gradually decreases in the ordinary voice [91].

G. **Wavelet transform and analysis.** By integrating continuous wave transforms (CWTs), the problem of resolution faced by the STFT has been mitigated. However, the CWT analysis is carried out in the same way as the STFT with the signal multiplied by a function as the window function used in the STFT. The transformation is calculated in a piecewise manner with different segments of the time-domain signal. However, there are two significant variations between CWT and STFT. The first thing that is not taken into account is the Fourier transformation of the window signals, so the single peak that corresponds to the sinusoid is noticed. Simply put, the negative frequencies are not calculated. Second, when the CWT of all spectral components is measured, the length of the window appears to vary. This is the most critical aspect of the transformation of the wavelet. The transformation of wavelets is a very important and widely used concept in the field of voice pathology. The following is therefore a mathematical illustration of its context principles.

The standard form of a CWT is

$$\mathrm{CWT}_x^{\psi}(\tau, s) = \psi_x^{\psi}(\tau, s) = \frac{1}{\sqrt{|s|}} \int x(t)\psi^*\left(\frac{t-\tau}{s}\right)\mathrm{dt} \tag{3.1}$$

The function is a mother wavelet, which is often referred to as a transformation function. Finally, the signal obtained is due to the induction of two essential parameters, namely translation (τ) and scaling (s) parameters. Wavelet means small waves originating from the main feature known as the mother wavelet. The wavelets are deduced using a finite length window function, whereas the word wave refers to the oscillatory aspect of the function. More simply, the windowed functions or segments of the signal are formed from the mother wavelet [92]. High-frequency and time–frequency attributes correlated with pathological speech are also measured using CWT. Integer time and scale values are used to index the actual valued CWT coefficients [93].

3.4.2 Voice pathology analysis and detection techniques

Machine learning is an essential factor that classifies a speech signal as regular or as part of a particular voice pathology. It uses a range of acoustic and speech features, such as those listed in section 3.4.1, to teach computers how different pathologies look. Over the last decade, various ML and deep learning classifiers have been used for these one-dimensional (1D) features. However, there are also newer algorithms that use time–frequency-based images with advanced dilated fully convolutional architecture to improve the reliability of accurate pathology identification. A number of these aspects have been discussed by researchers in the following section.

A. Short and long duration feature descriptors. A wide variety of long and short feature descriptors have been used for diagnosing voice pathology. Some notable research works that have used long-term features are [86, 94–98]. Some of the features extracted from these long-lasting signals include: amplitude and pitch disturbance quotient, glottal-to-noise excitation ratio, amplitude and frequency disturbance analysis, harmonics-to-noise ratio (HNR), normalized noise energy, etc. Although these feature descriptors have been widely used, they are outperformed by emerging short feature descriptors that do not require a fundamental frequency assessment. It is also extremely difficult to deduce the fundamental frequency of pathological signals due to their non-uniformity. There are several new and notable short feature descriptors that have begun to replace these long ones. Initially, the speech signal is segmented into several frames using a fixed length hamming window(s). Functional vectors such as the MFCC and the linear predictive cepstral coefficient (LPCC) are then extracted for each frame. These feature vectors have been developed specifically to replicate the voice production process and the auditory potential of the human body. These features are used in ML algorithms such as SVM, kNN, Gaussian Mixture Model (GMM), k-means clustering, etc to signal as either regular or abnormal. However, it is also important to state that the LPCC as a linear model has ample capacity to deal with an irregular, very non-linear expression. The MFCC descriptors are very dexterous when dealing with irregular or pathological voice signals. However, considering these positive factors and limitations, these short explanations are not very dexterous when testing the classifiers with samples belonging to other databases [98, 99]. The problem is therefore a lack of generality when dealing with datasets belonging to various regions of the world. For example, the MEEI dataset was collected from patients living in the United States of America and thus the voice of a normal individual of Asian or Middle East descent might be categorized as abnormal. This is due to a lack of a global fundamental pitch that can usually be considered to belong to an odd group worldwide. This aspect prevents the hardware implementation of voice pathology identifiers on a global scale and, as such, is limited to particular regions only. Cepstral descriptor is a notable group of feature descriptors used for pathological voice analysis. Its two versions are the cepstral peak prominence (CPP) and its derivative the cepstral peak prominence smoothed (CPPS). These descriptors have shown great tenacity to diagnose even the most serious dysphonic voice because they are not susceptible to time variance [100, 101]. In a research report, the authors extracted MFCC features from voice recordings belonging to physiological and laryngeal pathological categories to practice using two approaches. The first method used feature vectors to train the SVM, the Discriminant Analysis (DA) and the Gaussian Mixture Model (GMM) individually. However, training them on a case-by-case basis may not have provided a successful result and instead, as a second method, they introduced a standard classification [102].

An investigation to establish a detector for vocal larynx defects by extracting a combination of different feature descriptors from a pathological voice sample was proposed in [103]. The key problem with pathological voice identification and classification tasks is that ML algorithms are only equipped to distinguish between regular and abnormal voice samples. It is therefore a matter of binary classification. While the key problem that delays actual hardware deployment is the inability to pinpoint the exact disease. On similar lines, [103] investigators have conducted a binary classification using 30 and 20 pathological and normal voice samples, respectively. A mixture of different types of feature descriptors, such as the well-known MFCC, Zero-Crossing Rate (ZCR), ZCR mean, and LPC, was used for segmented voice recordings with lengths of 200, 300, 400 and 500 milliseconds. In their work, a threshold level was manually set for each function variety to establish a division between usual and abnormal voice signals.

Speech problems may not simply be due to vocal fold defects, but may also be due to Parkinson's disease, hypernasal lip and palate dysfunction in children/individuals. In this line, another research study [104] proposed a technique to diagnose these disorders as well as vocal fold disorders. They experimented with numerous feature descriptors to include automatic detection, such as simple frequency accuracy measurement, noisy spectrum measurement, non-linear amplitude and signal interference, cepstral features. It has been found that adding consistency measures to fundamental frequency is acceptable for speech disorders of laryngeal and Parkinson's, whereas cepstral features function well with hyper nasal speech. However, implementation with a noisy spectrum can properly diagnose dysphonic speech. It can therefore be established that the use of a single feature type or a combination of different feature vectors to diagnose multiple disorders with a single classifier will not yield a good result. It is therefore very important to investigate the best suited combination of a feature-classifier pair for all major voice pathologies.

The [105] research used time and frequency domain features with multiple type of ML algorithms to identify voice pathologies. Their experimentation led to the conclusion that spectral characteristics were among the most important feature descriptors. While it was discovered that pitch or fundamental frequency was not very significant. It was also realized that residual signal features extracted from a signal filtered using an inverse LPC filter have the highest effect on accuracy.

B. SVM classifier. This is a supervised learning method that uses the framework of support vector statistics to classify a feature vector as an acceptable class [106]. In other words, it uses a function to map the output category to the input vector. An example can be used to better understand the term 'supervised learning' Suppose a programmer creates and labels four folders in the directory as Class-A, Class-B, Class-C, and Class-D. Then they place the unique voice samples for these categories. Using basic programming, they show the machine that the labels for all the samples within it are the folder names. The computer will now be taught that voice samples or vector features extracted from a particular folder belong to a specific collection. ML algorithms use these data and have shown excellent results for high-dimensional data. It has also been reported in many practical applications [107]. Its underlying principle is to create a hyperplane that uses a maximum margin to separate feature vectors from different sets or classes. A set of support vectors is used to demarcate the boundary of the decision. A non-linear or linear hyperplane can be used. To have a very strong class differentiation, the basic principle is to construct an ideal hyperplane. In the diagnosis of laryngeal paralysis, the authors of [108] discussed the effectiveness of the use of entropy and energy-based features. To extract tenable features from voice signals affected by unilateral voice fold paralysis, wavelet decomposition was initially used for this purpose. A total of 32 and 11 active sub-bands were used to obtain entropy and energy characteristics, respectively. Before training with a linear SVM classifier, the authors used genetic algorithms to optimize the vector features. By using SVM with entropy and energy characteristics, they achieved an accuracy of 100% and 93.62%, respectively. The properties of entropy have been shown to be useful for the diagnosis of laryngeal paralysis. In another pathological voice detection technique described in [109], the researchers used sustained vocal samples from the MEEI dataset using a modulation spectrum technique. Specifically, it is a mixture of modulation frequency and harmonies of voice. In addition to the modulation spectrum method, the reduction of dimensionality was also used before the training of vectors with the SVM classifier. A special feature of this extraction process is the observation of a distortion in the amplitude pattern of a voice sample with pathology, which can provide rich cues for detection and accurate classification. A cumulative accuracy of 94.1% has been observed. However, it is important to study their application with other current data sets in order to assess their potential efficacy. They also looked at the performance of other traditional extraction methods and highlighted critical challenges related to pitch estimation, global signal estimation. Wavelet filter banks have also been used to differentiate natural and abnormal voice samples. More specifically, the wavelet filter banks were used to measure eight energy features using the lattice factorization technique. The feature vector extraction technique was applied to a privately collected dataset and to the MEEI dataset. Investigators are said to have reached a classification rate of 100% on their issue of binary classification. However, it remains to be seen if this remarkable precision can be accomplished for multiple pathology databases. A universal classifier that can diagnose voice pathology for patients living in any corner of the world is still a major challenge for researchers prior to any realistic implementation in hospitals [110].

Another landmark research using entropy for the binary classification of healthy and pathological voices was proposed in [111]. They evaluated the efficiency of PCA, LDA and SVM classifiers with different vector extraction techniques, such as wavelet packet transformation (WPT), STFT, CWT. Statistical evaluation showed that using an active subband of 6 with a WPT technique with LDA and SVM learners was able to achieve an overall accuracy of 100%. It can also be concluded that disturbance, inconsistency, and non-linearity of irregular voice and entropy extraction can provide efficient binary classification. Entropy is indeed a good way to measure the statistical randomness of a pathological voice. A multi-class voice pathology classifier that uses a rich feature vector derived from diverse and common speech features has been presented in [112]. The features used together to create a single vector function are MFCC, HNR, pitch and amplitude disturbance,

Mel-frequency, cepstral energy, LP Cosine Transform (LPCT) coefficients, and autocorrelation. Feature vectors belonging to healthy, vocal nodules and diffuse voice lesion samples have been trained with the SVM classifier to provide over 90% overall accuracy. The results of their implementation have also been related to the recommendations of the three phoniatricians. It has been noted that the use of sustained vocals alone for automatic prediction is much more successful than human phoniatrician predictions. Researchers of [37] used low-level MPEG-7 audio with false discovery rate (FDR) features to select and categorize four-class vectors—vocal fold nodules, keratosis, laryngeal paralysis, and polyp. They used the feature vectors to train the SVM classifier and achieved 99.99% accuracy. Authors of [113] proposed a binary classification of stable and pathological voice recordings using the M-band and SVM classifiers. Their technique yielded a combined accuracy of 100% using four and five bands. Voiceprint was also extracted by compressing and averaging MFCC voice recording frames with three sustained voice tones, that is, /a/,/u/and/o/ [114]. Using these features, they conducted a binary classifying discriminatory analysis using the SVM classifier and achieved an overall accuracy of 100%. The authors also claimed that voice printing is more acceptable for the diagnosis of voice pathology with a sustained vowel /u/. A multi-band wavelet analysis for the multi-class classification of voice pathologies in the MEEI dataset was also suggested in [115]. The proposed technique used the fractal dimension (FD) power dimension with a three-level discrete wavelet transformation (DWT). Out of a total of 173 abnormal recordings seen in the MEEI dataset, only 168 recordings were used because the MDVP parameters for 5 recordings were not available. They used FD features with a total of 22 MDPV parameters to achieve a 2.26% increase in accuracy over their previous research work. Research by [116] has shown that features derived from the pathological vocal tract area exhibit inconsistent disturbances over successive frames for continuous voice recordings. The metrics used to determine inconsistency are kurtosis, variance, mean and skewness. These signal disturbances have been exploited to distinguish a safe voice from an abnormal voice. Their approach was based on a natural mechanism for voice production. During their investigation, two important points were identified: (a) the supraglottic tract plays a more prominent role in the voice production process than the remaining regions of the vocal tract; (b) the variance is a more critical parameter than the mean area of the vocal tract. The thorough investigation of the MEEI and SVD voice pathology databases showed an accuracy of 99.22% and 94.7%, respectively. A further MDVP-based detection of speech pathologies of voice recordings from MEEI, SVD and AVPD databases has been proposed in [2]. Three common abnormalities have been considered, that is, vocal fold polyp, cyst, and laryngeal paralysis. Study also used the FDR method for sorting the extracted features. Their research into the use of MDVP features with the SVM classifier resulted in an accuracy of 88.21%, 99.68% and 72.53% for the above three databases, respectively. In another uncommon research, a non-linear Gaussian kernel SVM unsupervised learner was employed in three separate phases to distinguish voice pathologies via a comparative approach.

Three-stage training vectors were developed using line spectral frequency and MFCC features for both continuous speech and sustained vocals in the MEEI database. The first stage was trained to distinguish healthy voice from physiological laryngeal abnormalities, while the second stage was accompanied by a comparison of healthy and neuromuscular laryngeal abnormalities. The unsupervised classifier has been trained to recognize neuromuscular and physiological abnormalities at the third level. The research work indicated an overall accuracy of 98.7% [102]. Physical symptoms of brain and spinal cord disorders, such as tumor, neuron degeneration, spinal cord injury, brain lesions, and other injuries, have been shown to influence the way a person speaks. Such abnormalities were also observed by [117] authors using speech digital signal processing algorithms. This also indicates that voice pathologies can also occur due to physical changes in regions other than the vocal fold. Thus, a speech signal is a rich source of information that can be used to present a drawn portrait of the mental condition of the person. Researchers at [117] pointed out the advantages of using 13 MFCCs using a 20 ms Hamming window and a 10 ms overlay generating 149 frames for each 1.5 s long speech recording. The SVM classifier has been trained with these vector features to differentiate between normal and different abnormal conditions.

C. Gaussian Mixture Model (GMM). This is another commonly used unsupervised classification method that works on the basis of the probability principle. It is commonly used in both voice pathology and speech classifications [118]. As an unsupervised process, the labels of samples are not known beforehand, but are learned iteratively instead. The GMM is based on the idea of the theoretical GMM concept. Authors of [119] have used a Mel-frequency filter bank to remove features from short regular speeches. The goal was to identify the speaker by training the unique vectors of each person with the GMM model. Implementation of live (undistorted) and telephonic (distorted) speech showed a wide range of accuracy of 96.8% and 80.8%, respectively. This has shown that accuracy is also dependent on sound quality. An improved variant of the GMM algorithm known as the GMM-universal Background Model (UBM) was proposed for voice classification in [120]. UBM is adopted after the extraction of the feature vectors. The maximum *a posterior* algorithm (MAP) drives the UBM algorithm using two stages. The parameters are initially evaluated in the MAP algorithm, and then new knowledge is combined with the old ones. The drawback, however, is that they are affected by a different language. In another work [121], authors have trained 11 different MFCC features with the GMM model to differentiate a regular voice from a pathological one. More precisely, they received 60 s-long voice recordings from 30 speakers, after which they applied 32 ms-dimensional hamming windows to each sample. Inside each window/frame, a filter bank of size 12 is used to explore 11 specific MFCC features within the 0–8 kHz range. Feature vectors belonging to regular or pathological groups are trained with GMMs of varying orders. It was known that the highest order GMM implementation gave the highest accuracy. The research work listed in [117] suggested the use of Discrete Wavelet Transform (DWT) to disintegrate a voice sample into three wavelet sub-bands to test the MFCCs individually for each band. A total of 142 and 147 healthy and pathological recorded voice samples were used for the extraction of MFCC features, which were later trained in the GMM-SVM and GMM-UBM classification models. Each recording has a duration of 1.5 s with a sampling frequency of 44.1 kHz. The model that uses the MFCC features extracted from each of the GMM-UBM training sub-bands gave 96.96% accuracy. It is significantly higher than the 85.18% achieved while training GMM-UBM with MFCC features derived from a normal voice, that is, without any DWT disintegration. The main feature highlighted by their technique is the need to overcome the reliance on phonemes such as /a/, /u/ and /i/. MFCC features have been commonly used to classify speakers, speech pathologies, amnesia, Alzheimer's, and emotional and physical trauma in individuals. It is not robust enough as it does not account for the non-linear acoustic structure released from the body during voice development [122]. Due to this aspect, the authors of [122] used an 11 set of non-linear methods with MFCC to extract feature vectors from healthy and abnormal voice samples in the MEEI database. A hybrid training model that utilizes the generative ability of GMM and the discerning capabilities of the SVM classifiers has been introduced. More precisely, the GMM and SVM classifiers are split into two different classification levels. Their methodology showed a significant accuracy of 98.23%. However, it remains to be seen if their strategy is doing well in the light of multiple classification problems.

The SVM classifier has also been trained with a feature descriptor developed by the joint implementation of the Daubechies DWT and the linear cepstral prediction coefficient (LPCC) [93]. Time–frequency analysis was able to effectively identify pathologies in a voice. The use of MFCC and other function vectors with SVM classifiers and GMM for the design of the Automatic Speech Recognition (ASR) model [123] was another recent and landmark research work. More precisely, the authors have developed a Hidden Markov Model Tool (HTK) to detect and identify voice abnormalities. A total of 297 speakers were used in their investigation, of which 176 samples were taken from individuals suffering from five forms of vocal fold disorders, of which 121 are typical individuals. Apart from the MFCC features, PLP, RASTA-PLP and LPC features have also been extracted, forming a special vector function for each voice sample class. The normal and abnormal categories investigation uncovered two distinct things. The implementation of the MFCC and LPC features supported 94.44% and 77.5% accuracy, respectively, whereas the use of PLP and RASTA-PLP feature descriptors provided an accuracy of 94.44% and 89.62% respectively. On the other hand, the pathological classification task performed mean accuracy equal to 76.16%, 87.14% and 87.65%, respectively, when the LPC, RASTA-PLP and MFCC function descriptors are used. The use of PLP feature descriptors provided an accuracy of 88.63%, which is the highest of its feature descriptors. The investigation showed reasonable accuracy for standard samples, although the use of the different features of the descriptors individually resulted in poor accuracy. Manual segmentation of voice samples is a significant downside to the proposed work.

The GMM model was also used in [124] to diagnose spasmodic dysphonia in voice recordings. A total of 39 coefficients of feature descriptors were used in the work, including shimmer, jitter and MFCCs. The researchers also argued that the use of a second MFCC derivative offers an even better diagnostic quality.

D. Mixed ML classifiers. kNN classifier is a simple and efficient ML technique that can divide a feature vector into different categories by using a distance metric. Application in voice pathology detection has also been reported. Examples of some of the features that have been used with kNN are: HNR, shimmer, turbulent noise index, jitter, and normalized first harmonic energy. The use of these features with kNN on the MEEI data set resulted in accuracy of 96.1% [125]. The authors of [126] have used kNN with HNR and energy spectrum features to diagnose pathologies such as adductor, vocal fold nodules, laryngeal paralysis, polyp, and Edema. They extracted HNR features using four different frequency ranges after which they were combined to form a single feature vector. The resulting single vector was extracted for all voice samples and concatenated to represent the HNR features of the specific class. Another feature vector used by the authors is the normalized energy produced by the use of 21 bandpass filters. The second collection of features is an intentional effort to mimic the neural structure of the human auditory system. The two unique features of the kNN classifier showed very similar performance, that is, 94.28% and 92.38% accuracy for HNR and normalized energy characteristics, respectively. Research has shown that these two features can aid in the identification of laryngeal pathologies. It is also computationally less expensive as it needs only short duration signals. While other simple frequency and acoustic features extraction techniques work better with longer period signals, making them more computationally expensive.

Random forest (RF) or decision tree has also been used for speech features for the binary classification of pathological voice signals. The idea of RF is to combine a lot of binary decisions that are made using different bootstrap samples of the original data with random subsets to get an accurate predictor. The advantages of the RF method are that it is robust when additional trees are added and that the error of generalization is of limited value. For example, [127] researchers have developed a combined feature vector using 28 separate speech feature vectors, that is, 10 MFCC features, kurtosis, fundamental frequency, jitter, energy, shimmer coefficients, power factor, amplitude, timing, minimum and maximum signal values using the voice samples in the SVD data collection. The training of these combined and class-specific feature vectors produced 100% accuracy. However, there is a need to analyze a dataset where several pathologies are present.

K-means clustering is an unsupervised technique that assigns hard cluster numbers to data points by iteratively deciding the best value of cluster centers. The Euclidean distance metric is used to evaluate pixels with identical properties after which they are grouped into clusters. The [128] researchers have introduced a k-means clustering concept on the features extracted from the voice samples in the MEEI data collection. Features are measured using non-negative matrix factoring and adaptive time–frequency distribution. Pathological voice is non-uniform or non-stationary in nature and thus affects its distribution over time. Consequently, the crucial problem seen with such a short-length signal extraction technique is the loss of information that is more likely to occur when signals are chopped off.

The research work therefore emphasizes the use of time–frequency (TF) features to capture the dynamics of the pathological voice signal. Their binary classification using a k-means unsupervised clustering technique with these characteristics resulted in a substantial accuracy of 98.6%.

Vowel /a/ recording is very widespread in voice pathology techniques and is widely found in all well-known databases such as MEEI, SVD, and APVD. Undoubtedly, its implementation has achieved reasonable accuracy. However, investigators of [129, 130] used both the running speech and the sustained vowel /a/ recordings found in the APVD data collection. They achieved more than 99% accuracy. The authors of [131] used a signal pre-processing technique known as Voice Activity Detection (VAD) before extracting MFCC features. The VAD module is a form of filter that distinguishes the silent or voiced sections or the noise spectrum present in the signal. The training of the VAD module initially involves the development of a signal mixed with the noise spectrum, after which the useful and noisy regions of the signal are manually annotated. These annotated noisy and useful regions are collectively categorized as the voiced component of the signal. In this way, the classifier identifies the spectra of noise, the clean signal, and the silent part of the signal spectrum. This is a sophisticated and nuanced method. The implementation of the MFCC features with the VAD module on the 117 and 23 abnormal and safe recordings present in the MEEI database resulted in an accuracy of 96%.

Another binary classification technique by [132] qualified Hidden Markov Model (HMM), GMM, and SVM with six separate feature descriptors, namely—Relative Average Perturbation (RAP), shimmer, jitter, soft phonation index (SPI), HNR and Amplitude Perturbation Quotient (APQ). The pathological voice category consisted of numerous laryngeal diseases such as laryngeal cancer, cyst, palsy, Edema, nodule, polyp, and laryngitis. The implementation result showed that the GMM with these feature vectors had the highest accuracy, even higher than the artificial neural network (ANN)-based implementation with which it is compared.

A smartphone-based hardware prototype for diagnosing individual dysphonia has been seen in a landmark and recently published research work [133]. The disorder has a high association with the unhealthy manipulation of vocal cords on a regular basis due to the nature of the work. The key features of this type of condition are non-uniformity in loudness, degradation of pitch and voice quality. It is composed of around 10% of the other voice pathologies that affect individuals worldwide. The investigation demonstrated the efficiency of several features with different ML techniques, such as logistic model tree, support vector descriptors, berry model, decision tree, and instance-based learning. Features that have been used in this work are—HNR, SPI, shimmer, spectral features, jitter, MFCC, RAP, disruption, energy, temporal features, noise, and wavelet features. The comparison of efficiencies was made using popular metrics such as sensitivity, specificity, apart from the use of precision as widely used for other techniques. The investigation concluded that SVM and a decision tree with features could provide very good results.

Real-time implementation of pathological and regular voice differentiation using MFCC, ZCR and LPCC function descriptors with ANN has been proposed in the recently published work [101]. The investigation was performed using patient-derived speech samples. Their methods have used less computing energy. Possible effects on the binary classification of speech samples due to the use of acoustic features such as shaping frequency, capacity, shimmer, reflective coefficients, jitter and residual signal have been investigated in [134]. The feature descriptors were implemented with the Radial Base Functional Neural Network (RBFNN) and the SVM classifier and generated mean accuracy of 91% and 83%, respectively.

Identifying the level of severity of a pathological voice is another problem. Much of the research work focuses on binary classification, and a limited number of research literature exists for automatic diagnosis of severity. In a unique research study [135], a technique was proposed to automatically diagnose the stage of voice disorders. A neural network-based tool with acoustic features derived from the sustained vowel /a/ records found in the SVD database was used for the work. The level of severity was measured by observing the performance of four speech characteristics against those of normal values. Their approach resulted in an overall sensitivity, precision, and accuracy of 1.6%, 95% and 97.9%, respectively. Accuracy was registered at 90% and 95% for normal and pathological groups, respectively.

Binary classification has also been carried out using the Principal Component Analysis (PCA) and the Linear Discriminant Analysis (LDA) of the feature vectors [136]. More precisely, the study carried out the experiment by taking 50 normal and pathological samples from the MEEI database. The vector extraction techniques used in their research work include branch-and-bound, entity, backward and forward. In total, 33 different varieties of features were extracted, but only 22 were chosen for training. To better assess the efficiency of these feature vectors, the authors trained with six different types of classifiers, they are—kNN, SVM, quadratic discriminant classifier, Parzen classifier, ANN, and the nearest mean classifier. The implementation of the proposed extraction vector function, the LDA reduction and the SVM classifier given an accuracy of 94.26%.

E. Deep Learning based voice pathology classification. With the advent of deep learning in the field of computer vision [4], the use of deep learning methods for evaluating medical imaging and signal processing has increased considerably. These techniques have been used in several voice recognition applications, one of which is pathological voice research. Various deep learning algorithms have been introduced in speech pathology, often binary classification, that is, healthy voice and pathology.

Researchers at [137] suggested a deep learning system for the diagnosis of voice signal pathologies. Their work is very special in the sense that they used a dataset that they obtained for training, while testing was performed on samples extracted from the MEEI database. More specifically, their training samples are made up of regular and six types of pathological voice disorders. These samples were obtained from a tertiary teaching hospital. The six diseases included in their dataset are: vocal fold nodules, spasmodic dysphonia, neoplasm, polyp, laryngeal paralysis, and cysts. Sustained vowel sound recordings with a duration of 3 s have been used as a source for the extraction of MFCC feature vectors. Deep Neural Network, Gaussian

Mixture Model (GMM) and SVM Classifiers have been trained with MFCC features and a five-fold cross-validation technique to perform the classification. Testing of the three trained classifiers was carried out using the MEEI dataset. The DNN classifier provided a very strong classification rate for both the male and female groups, that is, 94.26% and 90.52%, respectively. The same classifier also provided a very high overall classification rate of 99.32% for the MEEI database. It is realized from their research work that the use of several neuronal layers and the optimization of weights will allow the DNN to outperform other ML classifiers.

Another recently published research literature [9] dealt with the problem of defining the exact pathology associated with voice dysfunction rather than a simple binary classification. The innovation of the research work is the use of the computer vision (CV) based deep spatial exploitation capability to carry out the proposed multiclass classification. All previous approaches used a range of acoustic/speech-based features for the training of ML algorithms. The use of these handcrafted features to diagnose pathologies has become rather monotonous and overstretched. The work of [137, 138] has also shown that there is a huge amount of untapped potential for deep learning in the field of pathological voice recognition. To this end, the research work of [9] explores the use of multiple techniques such as signal denoiser, multiple time–frequency scalograms, image-based analysis using a dilated fully convolutional neural network, swarm intelligence [139] for iteratively boosting prediction score. Samples were initially extracted from the VOICED dataset, which was followed by a deep learning signal filtering process. The filtered signal corpus was then used to construct morse, bump, and analytical-morlet wavelet time–frequency scalogram image corpuses. Three separate 3D-CNN networks were trained three times each using image corpuses, after which an iterative optimization technique called 'group decision analogy' was applied to improve accuracy. The classification task, which includes four groups, that is, normal, hyperkinetic dysphonia, hypokinetic dysphonia, and reflux laryngitis, showed an overall accuracy of 97.7%, while reflux laryngitis and hypokinetic dysphonia were 100% accurate. The approach has been very effective, but some of the factors that have not been applied are five-fold cross-validation and a methodology that uses a single classifier to minimize training and testing times. It can also be further expanded to handle other voice disorders.

[138] uses multi-layer neural networks to automatically extract useful features from raw input data, which can also be related to as an end-to-end approach. In the end-to-end mode, a raw voice signal or spectrogram is directly used to train a deep learning model to target output labels [140, 141]. Multi-layer neural network disadvantages, however, include over-fitting and a conceivably extended training time due to many model parameters. To fix the downside, CNN-based models were proposed using transfer learning and input voice signal representations such as Mel-spectrogram and octave-spectrogram, which achieved a state-of-the-art output of 97.5% accuracy [142]. Researchers also studied the combination of CNN with long short-term memory (LSTM) networks [143] and, similarly, the combination of LSTM and MLP [144] for pathological voice detection. However, one of the current challenges of using deep learning is the criteria of the models for the amount of

training data. As a result, the use of more sophisticated deep learning approaches without under-fitting or over-fitting is quite difficult. To address this challenge, we can focus on one of the most important recent breakthroughs in the field of deep learning, which is the generative adversarial networks (GANs) for the classification of multi-class voice pathology. Another paper also used the semi-supervised GAN [145] to produce unlabelled data representation from real data samples. It outperformed the conventional CNN-based approach with the same number of training samples. Another study also carried out a combination of GAN and improved Fuzzy C-Means Cluster for Multi-Class Voice Disorder Detection with imbalanced samples, which increased efficiency by 4%–6% [146].

3.5 Discussion and conclusion

Based on this survey, we can summarize our review as follows.

- The unnecessary delay between the data collection and the processing and analysis capacity is often the reason IoT is not fully and efficiently utilized in the healthcare industry.
- The big challenge that any patient faces is the unavailability of doctors and care in severe situations, and in particular when living in rural areas. Therefore, a new architecture needs to be established through the use of IoT devices.
- There are also cases in which, for example, people with a chronic illness need long-term monitoring. Continual supervision is highly necessary in this respect.
- In order to be able to communicate everywhere the IoT healthcare network has to have the potential to facilitate the flow of patients. This will involve an advanced IoT environment that takes into account networking customization without undermining data protection.
- Most studies concentrated on voice disease and its results only distinguish between a voice that is normal and a voice that has a pathological disorder where a full IoT system for the diagnosis of a particular disease, such as laryngeal cancer, is required. Since laryngeal cancer is a life-threatening condition, early diagnosis of laryngeal cancer requires a new and successful system / model.
- Although ML is being used in medical diagnosis, its design must be sufficiently precise to prevent any mistakes in the classification process. In addition, cybersecurity requirements, as well as legal and privacy challenges must be considered for the development of proven algorithms in order to benefit from the faith of patients and healthcare service providers.
- The delayed implementation of the use of ML technologies in medical diagnostics requires more ready acceptance and assistance by organizations and simplification of existing instruments for patients' and doctors' usage.
- There is an absence of a particular data set for a certain illness, like laryngeal cancer, where various voice disorders are found in the currently existing dataset. Moreover, the allocation of samples is highly uneven, making it

difficult to diagnose voicing pathology. The explanation is that the entire data collection, like SVD includes only a single form of voice pathology.

- The SVM classification is found to be the most commonly used, especially in comparison with any other ML algorithms. This can be because it is easier to reach a broad database of pathological voices for analysis, and it may be because the SVM classification is best for high dimensional data and for small datasets. In comparison, deep learning and neural networks require a broad dataset to train the model to increase classification precision.
- Most of the advances suggested in the literature rely on methods of voice characterisation, which they refer to as a technique of extraction of traits. A deep learning methodology may be used to extract deep features, but it requires broad training examples. Although DNNs have become a powerful ML tool, relatively few works have been performed for deep learning since there are no large datasets available.
- Many articles also observed that pathology diagnosis was exceptionally reliable, and has in some cases risen to 100%. That being said, the findings are unique to the used database and the method established for one database cannot be expected to extend to all databases with the same amount of productivity. The cross-database and cross-geographic recognition of vocal fold pathologies would be an issue which needs to be solved.
- The existence of massive standard databases is important for the implementation of a clinical infrastructure in real time. As far as we know, the number of common benchmark bases is small because the construction of a database involves the assistance of physicians who are specialists in voice disorder diagnosis. An integrated framework for a specific hospital may be built using the local database. Clinicians usually use sound files for diagnosis, but they cannot detect or preserve the sound files on the basis of diseases over the long term. It would be of immense advantage to provide an IoT based archive storage medium that archives audio recordings instantly depending on the illness.
- Popular methodologies like HMM, GMM, etc have their own boundaries and merits. They provide good outcomes if the framework relies on text. The GMM is very useful in the preparation of a mixture. GMM is a probabilistic approach that gets fuzzy observation. In comparison, there are drawbacks. For text-independent voice comparison framework, methods such as HMM are not appropriate. It is only good for capturing small voices. If there are a massive number of distributions and large datasets are required, GMM is computationally expensive. In comparison, deep learning approaches supply the speaker with straightforward modeling. They have a comprehensive de-noise learning module. They need an optimal framework, though, and overfitting is a challenge.
- The review of literature has shown that it is often difficult to pick voice recordings. Researchers rely on both voiced and unvoiced sample elements, since the unvoiced portion of the speech samples also has evidence of pathology identification. It is also noticed that a letter, phrase or delay

may be used as a voice sample. For a complete term, intermediate words and a delay should be taken into account.

- The next challenge for scientists is the extraction of features from the samples. The survey indicates that most of the researchers are more optimistic in using the frequency domain functions, although few researchers focus on time-domain measures for a particular pathology. There are also no unusual acoustic characteristics. It is a long calculation, though, and may be vulnerable to the patient's anatomy. Also, standard practice as can be seen in the survey, is the multiple feature analysis. The survey also revealed that the CNN-based time–frequency scalogram of voice pathology detection is a very new technique. However, 2D CNN image-based techniques such as GAN can further develop the model to expand the dataset. The scope for further reducing deep learning time can also be provided by using modeling to fuse multiple time–frequency scalograms, like Morse, Bump and Amor into a single scalogram.

References

[1] Hammami I, Salhi L and Labidi S 2020 Voice pathologies classification and detection using EMD-DWT analysis based on higher order statistic features *IRBM* **41** 161–71

[2] Al-Nasheri A, Muhammad G, Alsulaiman M and Ali Z 2017 Investigation of voice pathology detection and classification on different frequency regions using correlation functions *J. Voice* **31** 3–15

[3] Steffen N, Vieira V P, Yazaki R K and Pontes P 2011 Modifications of vestibular fold shape from respiration to phonation in unilateral vocal fold paralysis *J. Voice* **25** 111–3

[4] Krizhevsky A, Sutskever I and Hinton G E 2012 Imagenet classification with deep convolutional neural networks *Adv. Neur. Info. Process. Syst.* **25** 1097–105

[5] Nongmeikapam K, Wahengbam K, Meetei O N and Tuithung T 2019 Handwritten Manipuri Meetei-Mayek classification using convolutional neural network *ACM Trans. Asian Low-Resour. Lang. Info. Process. (TALLIP)* **18** 1–23

[6] Nongmeikapam K, Kumar W K, Meetei O N and Tuithung T 2019 Increasing the effectiveness of handwritten Manipuri Meetei-Mayek character recognition using multiple-HOG-feature descriptors *Sādhanā* **44** 104

[7] Kanan Kumar W, Nongmeikapam K and Dinamani Singh A 2020 An urban parametric scene parsing technique through an improved multispectral image fusion *Proc. 5th Int. Conf. Computers Management Skills (ICCM 2019)|* (North Eastern Regional Institute of Science & Technology (NERIST)) *(Nirjuli, Arunachal Pradesh, India)*

[8] Devi L M, Wahengbam K and Singh A D 2021 Dehazing buried tissues in retinal fundus images using a multiple radiance pre-processing with deep learning based multiple feature-fusion *Opt. Laser Technol.* **138** 106908

[9] Wahengbam K, Singh M P, Nongmeikapam K and Singh A D 2021 A group decision optimization analogy based deep learning architecture for multiclass pathology classification in a voice signal *IEEE Sens. J.* **21** 8100–16

[10] Baker S B, Xiang W and Atkinson I 2017 Internet of things for smart healthcare: technologies, challenges, and opportunities *IEEE Access* **5** 26521–44

[11] Vasanth K and Sbert J 2014 Creating solutions for health through technology innovation. Texas Instruments [Online]. Available: http://ti.com/lit/wp/sszy006/sszy006.pdf, accessed Dec. 7 2014

[12] Islam S R, Kwak D, Kabir M H, Hossain M and Kwak K S 2015 The internet of things for health care: a comprehensive survey *IEEE Access* **3** 678–708

[13] Fatima M and Pasha M 2017 Survey of machine learning algorithms for disease diagnostic *J. Intell. Learn. Syst. App.* **9** 1

[14] Erickson B J, Korfiatis P, Akkus Z and Kline T L 2017 Machine learning for medical imaging *Radiographics* **37** 505–15

[15] Magoulas G D and Prentza A 1999 Machine learning in medical applications *Advanced Course on Artificial Intelligence* (Berlin, Heidelberg: Springer) pp 300–7

[16] Khare S K and Bajaj V 2021 Entropy based drowsiness detection using adaptive variational mode decomposition *IEEE Sensors J.* **21** 6421–8

[17] Budak U, Bajaj V, Akbulut Y, Atila O and Sengur A 2019 An effective hybrid model for EEG-based drowsiness detection *IEEE Sens. J.* **19** 7624–31

[18] Taran S and Bajaj V 2018 Drowsiness detection using adaptive Hermite decomposition and extreme learning machine for electroencephalogram signals *IEEE Sens. J.* **18**(21) 8855–62

[19] Khare S K and Bajaj V 2020 Time–frequency representation and convolutional neural network-based emotion recognition *IEEE Trans. Neural Netw. Learn. Syst.* **32** 2901–9

[20] Khare S K, Bajaj V and Sinha G R 2020 Adaptive tunable Q wavelet transform-based emotion identification *IEEE Trans. Instrum. Meas.* **69** 9609–17

[21] Khare S K and Bajaj V 2020 An evolutionary optimized variational mode decomposition for emotion recognition *IEEE Sens. J.* **21** 2035–42

[22] Chaudhary S, Taran S, Bajaj V and Sengur A 2019 Convolutional neural network based approach towards motor imagery tasks EEG signals classification *IEEE Sens. J.* **19** 4494–500

[23] Bajaj V and Pachori R B 2014 Human emotion classification from EEG signals using multiwavelet transform. *2014 Intr. Conf. on Medical Biometrics* (Piscataway, NJ: IEEE) 125–30

[24] Siuly S, Khare S K, Bajaj V, Wang H and Zhang Y 2020 A computerized method for automatic detection of schizophrenia using EEG signals *IEEE Trans. Neural Syst. Rehabil. Eng.* **28** 2390–400

[25] Taran S and Bajaj V 2018 Clustering variational mode decomposition for identification of focal EEG signals *IEEE Sens. Lett.* **2** 1–4

[26] Bajaj V, Taran S, Tanyildizi E and Sengur A 2019 Robust approach based on convolutional neural networks for identification of focal EEG signals *IEEE Sens. Lett.* **3** 1–4

[27] Rai K, Bajaj V and Kumar A 2015 Novel feature for identification of focal EEG signals with K-means and fuzzy C-means algorithms *2015 IEEE Int. Conf. Digital Signal Processing (DSP)* (Piscataway, NJ: IEEE) pp 412–6

[28] Walde S, Rani P, Bajaj V and Sharma D 2016 Time frequency image based features for detection of focal EEG signals *2016 Int. Conf. Signal Processing Communication (ICSC)* (Piscataway, NJ: IEEE) pp 358–62

[29] Yadav S K, Bajaj V and Kumar A 2017 An EMD based approach for discrimination of apnea and normal EEG signals *2017 Int. Conf. Recent Innovations Signal Processing Embedded Systems (RISE)* (Piscataway, NJ: IEEE) pp 191–4

[30] Hariharan M, Paulraj M P and Yaacob S 2010 Time-domain features and probabilistic neural network for the detection of vocal fold pathology *Malaysian J. Comput. Sci.* **23** 60–7

[31] Martinez C E and Rufiner H L 2000 Acoustic analysis of speech for detection of laryngeal pathologies *Proc. 22nd Annual Int. Conf. IEEE Engineering Medicine Biology Society (Cat. No. 00CH37143)* 3 (Piscataway, NJ: IEEE) pp 2369–72

[32] Bone D, Lee C C, Chaspari T, Gibson J and Narayanan S 2017 Signal processing and machine learning for mental health research and clinical applications [perspectives] *IEEE Signal Process Mag.* **34** 195–6

[33] Korean Society of Thyroid-Head and Neck Surgery Guideline Task Force Ahn S-H *et al* 2017 Guidelines for the surgical management of laryngeal cancer: Korean society of thyroid-head and neck surgery *Clin. Exp. Otorhinolaryngol.* **10** 1–43

[34] Anwer A W, Faisal M, Malik A A, Jamshed A, Hussain R and Pirzada M T 2018 Head and neck cancer in a developing country-a hospital-based retrospective study across 10 years from Pakistan *J. Cancer Allied Spec.* **3** S104

[35] Souza T A D, Vieira V J, Souza M A D, Correia S E, Costa S C and Costa W C D A 2018 Feature selection based on binary particle swarm optimisation and neural networks for pathological voice detection *Int. J. Bio-Inspired Comput.* **11** 91–101

[36] Lee T, Liu Y, Huang P W, Chien J T, Lam W K, Yeung Y T, Law T K, Lee K Y, Kong A P H and Law S P 2016 Automatic speech recognition for acoustical analysis and assessment of Cantonese pathological voice and speech *2016 IEEE Intr. Conf. on Acoustics, Speech and Signal Processing (ICASSP)* (Piscataway, NJ: IEEE) pp 6475–9

[37] Muhammad G and Melhem M 2014 Pathological voice detection and binary classification using MPEG-7 audio features *Biomed. Signal Process. Control* **11** 1–9

[38] Muhammad G, Rahman S M M, Alelaiwi A and Alamri A 2017 Smart health solution integrating IoT and cloud: a case study of voice pathology monitoring *IEEE Commun. Mag.* **55** 69–73

[39] Hossain M S, Muhammad G and Alamri A 2019 Smart healthcare monitoring: a voice pathology detection paradigm for smart cities *Multimedia Syst.* **25** 565–75

[40] Hossain M S 2016 Patient status monitoring for smart home healthcare *2016 IEEE Int. Conf. on Multimedia Expo Workshops (ICMEW)* (Piscataway, NJ: IEEE) pp 1–6

[41] Moran R J, Reilly R B, de Chazal P and Lacy P D 2006 Telephony-based voice pathology assessment using automated speech analysis *IEEE Trans. Biomed. Eng.* **53** 468–77

[42] Fable M 1957 Un procedure electrique percutane d'inscription de l'accolement glottique au cours de la phonation; glottographie de haute fr_equence *Prem. Res.* **141** 66

[43] Fabre P 1958 Etude comparee des glottogrammes et des phonogrammes de la voix humaine, *Ann. Oto-rhino Laryngol.* **75** 767–75

[44] Abberton E R, Howard D M and Fourcin A J 1989 Laryngographic assessment of normal voice: a tutorial *Clin. Linguist. Phon.* **3** 281–96

[45] Anastaplo S and Karnell M P 1988 Synchronized videostroboscopic and electroglottographic examination of glottal opening *J. Acoust. Soc. Am.* **83** 1883–90

[46] Colton R H and Conture E G 1990 Problems and pitfalls of electroglottography *J. Voice* **4** 10–24

[47] Gerratt B R, Hanson D G and Berke G S 1988 Laryngeal configuration associated with glottography *Am. J. Otolaryngol.* **9** 173–9

[48] Kitzing P 1990 Clinical applications of electroglottography *J. Voice* **4** 238–49

[49] Slavit D H, Lipton R J and McCaffrey T V 1990 Glottographic analysis of phonation in the excised canine larynx *Ann. Otol., Rhinol. Laryngol.* **99** 396–402

[50] Childers D G, Hicks D M, Moore G P and Alsaka Y A 1986 A model for vocal fold vibratory motion, contact area, and the electroglottogram *J. Acoust. Soc. Am.* **80** 1309–20

[51] Wan M X, Yan J and Cheng J 1988 Two channel electroglottograph-a new impedance measurement system *Proc. Annual Int. Conf. IEEE Engineering in Medicine and Biology Society* 1288–9 (Piscataway, NJ: IEEE)

[52] Mingxi W and Jingzhi C 1991 Theory and application of field perturbation to electrical impedance technique for medicine *J. Electr. (China)* **8** 324–33

[53] Kob M and Frauenrath T 2009 A system for parallel measurement of glottis opening and larynx position *Biomed. Signal Process. Control* **4** 221–8

[54] Hézard T, Hélie T, Doval B, Bernardoni N H and Kob M 2012 Non-invasive vocal-folds monitoring using electrical imaging methods *100 Years of Electrical Imaging Workshop (Paris)* 1–4

[55] Liu D, Kolehmainen V, Siltanen S and Seppanen A 2015 Estimation of conductivity changes in a region of interest with electrical impedance tomography *Inverse Problems Imaging* **9** 211–29

[56] Fant G, Ondrackova J, Lindqvist J and Sonesson B 1966 Electrical glottography *STL-QPSR* **7** 15–21

[57] Fourcin A J 1974 Laryngographic examination of vocal fold vibration *Ventilat. Phonat. Control Syst.* pp 315–33

[58] Rothenberg M 1981 Some relations between glottal air flow and vocal fold contact area *Asha Rep.* **11** 88–96

[59] Baer T, Löfqvist A and McGarr N S 1983 Laryngeal vibrations: a comparison between high-speed filming and glottographic techniques *J. Acoust. Soc. Am.* **73** 1304–8

[60] Berke G S, Moore D M, Hanson D G, Hantke D R, Gerratt B R and Burstein F 1987 Laryngeal modeling: theoretical, *in vitro*, *in vivo Laryngoscope* **97** 871–81

[61] Gilbert H R, Potter C R and Hoodin R 1984 Laryngograph as a measure of vocal fold contact area *J. Speech Lang.Hear. Res.* **27** 178–82

[62] Hanson D G, D'Agostino M C, USAF M, Jiang J and Herzon G 1995 Clinical measurement of mucosal wave velocity using simultaneous photoglottography and laryngostroboscopy *Ann. Otol. Rhinol. Laryngol.* **104** 340–9

[63] Hertegård S and Gauffin J 1995 Glottal area and vibratory patterns studied with simultaneous stroboscopy, flow glottography, and electroglottography. *J. Speech Lang. Hear. Res.*, **88** 85–100

[64] Henrich N, d'Alessandro C, Doval B and Castellengo M 2004 On the use of the derivative of electroglottographic signals for characterization of nonpathological phonation *J. Acoust. Soc. Am.* **115** 1321–32

[65] Awan S N, Krauss A R and Herbst C T 2015 An examination of the relationship between electroglottographic contact quotient, electroglottographic decontacting phase profile, and acoustical spectral moments *J. Voice* **29** 519–29

[66] Codino J, Torres M E, Rubin A and Jackson-Menaldi C 2016 Automated electroglottographic inflection events detection. A pilot study *J. Voice* **30** 768–e1

[67] Alipour F *et al* 2011 Mathematical models and numerical schemes for the simulation of human phonation *Curr. Bioinfo.* **6** 323–43

[68] Barney A, Shadle C H and Davies P O A L 1999 Fluid flow in a dynamic mechanical model of the vocal folds and tract. I. Measurements and theory *J. Acoust. Soc. Am.* **105** 444–55

[69] Drugman T, Thomas M, Gudnason J, Naylor P and Dutoit T 2011 Detection of glottal closure instants from speech signals: a quantitative review *IEEE Trans. Audio Speech Lang. Process.* **20** 994–1006
[70] Childers D G and Krishnamurthy A K 1985 A critical review of electroglottography *Crit. Rev. Biomed. Eng.* **12** 131–61
[71] Guenason J, Mehta D D and Quatieri T F 2014 Closed phase estimation for inverse _ltering the oral airow waveform, *2014 IEEE Int. Conf. on Acoustics, Speech and Signal Processing (ICASSP)* (Piscataway, NJ: IEEE)
[72] Howard D M 1989 Peak-picking fundamental period estimation for hearing prostheses *J. Acoust. Soc. Am.* **86** 902–10
[73] G. Švec J, S. Popolo P and R. Titze I 2003 Measurement of vocal doses in speech: Experimental procedure and signal processing. *Logoped. Phoniatr. Vocol.* **28** 181–92
[74] Howard D M 2007 Intonation drift in a capella soprano, alto, tenor, bass quartet singing with key modulation *J. Voice* **21** 300–15
[75] Vanello N, Guidi A, Gentili C, Werner S, Bertschy G, Valenza G, Lanata A and Scilingo E P 2012 Speech analysis for mood state characterization in bipolar patients *2012 Annual Int. Conf. IEEE Engineering in Medicine and Biology Society* (Piscataway, NJ: IEEE) pp 2104–7
[76] Kania R E, Hartl D M, Hans S, Maeda S, Vaissiere J and Brasnu D F 2006 Fundamental frequency histograms measured by electroglottography during speech: a pilot study for standardization *J. Voice* **20** 1
[77] Hosokawa K, Ogawa M, Hashimoto M and Inohara H 2014 Statistical analysis of the reliability of acoustic and electroglottographic perturbation parameters for the detection of vocal roughness *J. Voice* **28** 263–e9
[78] Baken R J 1992 Electroglottography *J. Voice* **6** 98–110
[79] Orlikoff R F, Golla M E and Deliyski D D 2012 Analysis of longitudinal phase differences in vocal-fold vibration using synchronous high-speed videoendoscopy and electroglottography *J. Voice* **26** 816–e13
[80] Roubeau B, Henrich N and Castellengo M 2009 Laryngeal vibratory mechanisms: the notion of vocal register revisited *J. Voice* **23** 425–38
[81] Kuang J and Keating P 2014 Vocal fold vibratory patterns in tense versus lax phonation contrasts *J. Acoust. Soc. Am.* **136** 2784–97
[82] Rothenberg M and Mahshie J J 1988 Monitoring vocal fold abduction through vocal fold contact area *J. Speech Lang. Hear. Res.* **31** 338–51
[83] Cesari U, D Pietro G, Marciano E, Niri C, Sannino G and Verde L 2018 A new database of healthy and pathological voices *Comput. Electr. Eng.* **68** 310–21
[84] Corp K E 1994 Disordered voice database, version 1.03 (cd-rom) *MEEI, Voice and Speech Lab* (Boston, MA)
[85] WJ B and Saarbrucken P M 2016 Voice database. Institute of Phonetics, University of Saarland. http://stimmdatenbank.coli.unisaarland.de/
[86] Al-Nasheri A, Muhammad G, Alsulaiman M, Ali Z, Mesallam T A, Farahat M, Malki K H and Bencherif M A 2017 An investigation of multidimensional voice program parameters in three different databases for voice pathology detection and classification *J. Voice* **31** 113–e9
[87] Quatieri T F 2006 *Discrete-Time Speech Signal Processing: Principles and Practice* (New Delhi: Pearson Education India) pp 55–110 2001
[88] O'Shaughnessy D 1988 Linear predictive coding *IEEE Potentials* **7** 29–32

[89] Kohler M, Vellasco M M and Cataldo E 2016 Analysis and classification of voice pathologies using glottal signal parameters *J. Voice* **30** 549–56
[90] Oppenheim A V, Buck J R and Schafer R W 2001 *Discrete-Time Signal Processing* (Upper Saddle River, NJ: Prentice Hall)
[91] Rabiner L and Schafer R 2010 *Theory and Applications of Digital Speech Processing* (Upper Saddle River, NJ: Prentice Hall)
[92] Tan L and Jiang J 2018 *Digital Signal Processing: Fundamentals and Applications* (New York: Academic)
[93] Fonseca E S, Guido R C, Scalassara P R, Maciel C D and Pereira J C 2007 Wavelet time–frequency analysis and least squares support vector machines for the identification of voice disorders *Comput. Biol. Med.* **37** 571–8
[94] Kasuya H, Ogawa S, Mashima K and Ebihara S 1986 Normalized noise energy as an acoustic measure to evaluate pathologic voice *J. Acoust. Soc. Am.* **80** 1329–34
[95] Boyanov B, Ivanov T, Hadjitodorov S and Chollet G 1993 Robust hybrid pitch detector *Electron. Lett.* **29** 1924–6
[96] Gavidia-Ceballos L and Hansen J H 1996 Direct speech feature estimation using an iterative EM algorithm for vocal fold pathology detection *IEEE Trans. Biomed. Eng.* **43** 373–83
[97] Hadjitodorov S and Mitev P 2002 A computer system for acoustic analysis of pathological voices and laryngeal diseases screening *Med. Eng. Phys.* **24** 419–29
[98] Godino-Llorente J I, Osma-Ruiz V, Sáenz-Lechón N, Gómez-Vilda P, Blanco-Velasco M and Cruz-Roldán F 2010 The effectiveness of the glottal to noise excitation ratio for the screening of voice disorders *J. Voice* **24** 47–56
[99] Godino-Llorente J I and Gómez-Vilda P 2004 Automatic detection of voice impairments by means of short-term cepstral parameters and neural network based detectors *IEEE Trans. Biomed. Eng.* **51** 380–4
[100] Benmalek E, Elmhamdi J and Jilbab A 2017 Multiclass classification of Parkinson's disease using different classifiers and LLBFS feature selection algorithm *Int. J. Speech Technol.* **20** 179–84
[101] Ali Z, Alsulaiman M, Muhammad G, Elamvazuthi I, Al-Nasheri A, Mesallam T A, Farahat M and Malki K H 2017 Intra- and inter-database study for Arabic, English, and German databases: do conventional speech features detect voice pathology? *J. Voice* **31** 386–e1
[102] Cordeiro H, Fonseca J, Guimarães I and Meneses C 2017 Hierarchical classification and system combination for automatically identifying physiological and neuromuscular laryngeal pathologies *J. Voice* **31** 384–e9
[103] Wahed M A 2014 Computer aided recognition of pathological voice *2014 31st National Radio Science Conf. (NRSC)* 349–54 (Piscataway, NJ: IEEE)
[104] Orozco-Arroyave J R, Belalcazar-Bolanos E A, Arias-Londoño J D, Vargas-Bonilla J F, Skodda S, Rusz J, Daqrouq K, Hönig F and Nöth E 2015 Characterization methods for the detection of multiple voice disorders: neurological, functional, and laryngeal diseases *IEEE J. Biomed. Health Inform.* **19** 1820–8
[105] Kons Z, Satt A, Hoory R, Uloza V, Vaiciukynas E, Gelzinis A and Bacauskiene M 2011 On feature extraction for voice pathology detection from speech signals *Proc. 1st Annual Afeka-AVIOS Speech Processing Conf.* (Tel Aviv Academic College of Engineering, Tel Aviv) *(Israel)*

[106] Reynolds D 2009 *Universal background models, Encyclopedia of Biometrics* (New York: Springer) pp 1349–52
[107] Vapnik V 2013 *The Nature of Statistical Learning Theory* (Berlin: Springer Science & Business Media)
[108] Behroozmand R and Almasganj F 2007 Optimal selection of wavelet-packet-based features using genetic algorithm in pathological assessment of patients' speech signal with unilateral vocal fold paralysis *Comput. Biol. Med.* **37** 474–85
[109] Markaki M and Stylianou Y 2011 Voice pathology detection and discrimination based on modulation spectral features *IEEE Trans. Audio Speech Lang. Process.* **19** 1938–48
[110] Saeedi N E, Almasganj F and Torabinejad F 2011 Support vector wavelet adaptation for pathological voice assessment *Comput. Biol. Med.* **41** 822–8
[111] Arjmandi M K and Pooyan M 2012 An optimum algorithm in pathological voice quality assessment using wavelet-packet-based features, linear discriminant analysis and support vector machine *Biomed. Signal Process. Control* **7** 3–19
[112] Uloza V, Verikas A, Bacauskiene M, Gelzinis A, Pribuisiene R, Kaseta M and Saferis V 2011 Categorizing normal and pathological voices: automated and perceptual categorization *J. Voice* **25** 700–8
[113] Saidi P and Almasganj F 2015 Voice disorder signal classification using m-band wavelets and support vector machine *Circuits Syst. Signal Process.* **34** 2727–38
[114] Benba A, Jilbab A and Hammouch A 2016 Analysis of multiple types of voice recordings in cepstral domain using MFCC for discriminating between patients with Parkinson's disease and healthy people *Int. J. Speech Technol.* **19** 449–56
[115] Ali Z, Alsulaiman M, Elamvazuthi I, Muhammad G, Mesallam T A, Farahat M and Malki K H 2016 Voice pathology detection based on the modified voice contour and SVM *BICA* **15** 10–8
[116] Muhammad G, Altuwaijri G, Alsulaiman M, Ali Z, Mesallam T A, Farahat M, Malki K H and Al-Nasheri A 2016 Automatic voice pathology detection and classification using vocal tract area irregularity *Biocybern. Biomed. Eng.* **36** 309–17
[117] Vikram C M and Umarani K 2013 Phoneme independent pathological voice detection using wavelet based MFCCs, GMM-SVM hybrid classifier *2013 Int. Conf. on Advances in Computing, Communications and Informatics (ICACCI)* (Piscataway, NJ: IEEE) pp 929–34
[118] 2012 S. Gaussian-mixture-example https://commons.wikimedia.org/wiki/File:Gaussianmixture-example.svg
[119] Reynolds D A and Rose R C 1995 Robust text-independent speaker identification using Gaussian mixture speaker models *IEEE Trans. Speech Audio Process.* **3** 72–83
[120] Kaiser J F 1990 On Teager's energy algorithm and its generalization to continuous signals *Proc. 4th IEEE Digital Signal Processing Workshop (Mohonk, New Paltz, NY)*
[121] Pravena D and Dhivya S 2012 Pathological voice recognition for vocal fold disease *Int. J. Comput. App.* **47** 31–7
[122] Arias-Londoño J D, Godino-Llorente J I, Sáenz-Lechón N, Osma-Ruiz V and Castellanos-Domínguez G 2010 Automatic detection of pathological voices using complexity measures, noise parameters, and mel-cepstral coefficients *IEEE Trans. Biomed. Eng.* **58** 370–9
[123] Mohammed A, Mansour A, Ghulam M, Mohammed Z, Mesallam T A, Malki K H, Mohamed F, Mekhtiche M A and Mohamed B 2015 Automatic speech recognition of pathological voice *Indian J. Sci. Technol.* **8** 1–6

[124] Fezari M, Amara F and El-Emary I M 2014 Acoustic analysis for detection of voice disorders using adaptive features and classifiers *Proc. Int. Conf. Circuits, Syst. Control* pp 112–7

[125] Hadjitodorov S and Mitev P 2002 A computer system for acoustic analysis of pathological voices and laryngeal diseases screening *Med. Eng. Phys.* **24** 419–29

[126] Shama K, Krishna A and Cholayya N U 2006 Study of harmonics-to-noise ratio and critical-band energy spectrum of speech as acoustic indicators of laryngeal and voice pathology *EURASIP J. Adv. Signal Process.* **2007** 085286

[127] Hemmerling D, Skalski A and Gajda J 2016 Voice data mining for laryngeal pathology assessment *Comput. Biol. Med.* **69** 270–76

[128] Ghoraani B and Krishnan S 2009 A joint time–frequency and matrix decomposition feature extraction methodology for pathological voice classification *EURASIP J. Adv. Signal Process.* **2019** 928974

[129] Mesallam T A, Farahat M, Malki K H, Alsulaiman M, Ali Z, Al-Nasheri A and Muhammad G 2017 Development of the arabic voice pathology database and its evaluation by using speech features and machine learning algorithms *J. Healthcare Eng.* **2017** 8783751

[130] Muhammad G, Mesallam T A, Malki K H, Farahat M, Mahmood A and Alsulaiman M 2012 Multidirectional regression (MDR)-based features for automatic voice disorder detection *J. Voice* **26** 817–e19

[131] Godino-Llorente J I, Fraile R, Sáenz-Lechón N, Osma-Ruiz V and Gómez-Vilda P 2007 Automatic detection of voice impairments from text-dependent running speech using a discriminative approach *5th Int. Workshop on Models and Analysis of Vocal Emissions for Biomedical Applications*

[132] Wang J and Jo C 2007 Vocal folds disorder detection using pattern recognition methods *29th Annual Int. Conf. IEEE Engineering in Medicine and Biology Society* (Piscataway, NJ: IEEE) pp 3253–6

[133] Verde L, De Pietro G and Sannino G 2018 Voice disorder identification by using machine learning techniques *IEEE Access* **6** 16246–55

[134] Sellam V and Jagadeesan J 2014 Classification of normal and pathological voice using SVM and RBFNN *J. Signal Inform. Process.* **5** 1–7

[135] Sabir B, Rouda F, Khazri Y, Touri B and Moussetad M 2017 Improved algorithm for pathological and normal voices identification *Int. J. Electr. Comput. Eng.* **7** 238

[136] Arjmandi M K, Pooyan M, Mikaili M, Vali M and Moqarehzadeh A 2011 Identification of voice disorders using long-time features and support vector machine with different feature reduction methods *J. Voice* **25** e275–e279

[137] Fang S H, Tsao Y, Hsiao M J, Chen J Y, Lai Y H, Lin F C and Wang C T 2019 Detection of pathological voice using cepstrum vectors: a deep learning approach *J. Voice* **33** 634–41

[138] Mayle A, Mou Z, Bunescu R C, Mirshekarian S, Xu L and Liu C 2019 Diagnosing dysarthria with long short-term memory networks *INTERSPEECH* pp 4514–8

[139] Laishram R, Kumar W K, Gupta A and Prakash K V 2014 A novel MRI brain edge detection using PSOFCM segmentation and Canny algorithm *2014 Int. Conf. Electronic Systems, Signal Processing and Computing Technologies* (Piscataway, NJ: IEEE) pp 398–401

[140] Xu K, Zhu B, Kong Q, Mi H, Ding B, Wang D and Wang H 2019 General audio tagging with ensembling convolutional neural networks and statistical features *J. Acoust. Soc. Am.* **145** EL521–EL7

[141] Fonseca E, Gong R and Serra X 2018 A Simple Fusion of Deep and Shallow Learning for Acoustic Scene Classification. arXiv preprint arXiv:1806.07506

[142] Muhammad G, Alhamid M F, Alsulaiman M and Gupta B 2018 Edge computing with cloud for voice disorder assessment and treatment *IEEE Commun. Mag.* **56** 60–5

[143] Harar P, Alonso-Hernandezy J B, Mekyska J, Galaz Z, Burget R and Smekal Z 2017 Voice pathology detection using deep learning: a preliminary study *2017 Int. Conf. Workshop on Bioinspired Intelligence (IWOBI)* (Piscataway, NJ: IEEE) pp 1–4

[144] Millet J and Zeghidour N 2019, May Learning to detect dysarthria from raw speech *ICASSP 2019–2019 IEEE Int. Conf. Acoustics, Speech and Signal Processing (ICASSP)* (Piscataway, NJ: IEEE) pp 5831–5

[145] Tu Y, Lin Y, Wang J and Kim J U 2018 Semi-supervised learning with generative adversarial networks on digital signal modulation classification *Comput. Mater. Continua* **55** 243–54

[146] Chui K T, Lytras M D and Vasant P 2020 Combined generative adversarial network and fuzzy C-means clustering for multi-class voice disorder detection with an imbalanced dataset *Appl. Sci.* **10** 4571

IOP Publishing

High Performance Computing for Intelligent Medical Systems

Varun Bajaj and Irshad Ahmad Ansari

Chapter 4

Deep learning for cuffless blood pressure monitoring

Jamal Esmaelpoor, Zahra Momayez Sanat and Mohammad Hassan Moradi

There is a great motivation to use easy-access bio-signals to alleviate the difficulties and shortcomings of present invasive and cuff-based blood pressure monitoring techniques. Many studies propose methods mainly using photoplethysmogram and electrocardiogram signals. Most of these methods are based on hand-crafted features. Although they take advantage of our previous knowledge, it is highly desirable to propose models that are less dependent on feature engineering.

To this aim, in this chapter, we develop several architectures based on deep neural networks. Through discussing their advantages and drawbacks, we try to develop more appropriate models to meet the demands of the British Hypertension Society and the Association for the Advancement of Medical Instrumentation standards. The building blocks of our models are convolutional neural networks and long short-term memories. We evaluate our models on 200 subjects.

4.1 Introduction

Cardiovascular problems are responsible for the death of almost 50% of all people who die because of non-communicable diseases. Therefore, since blood pressure (BP) is among the most vital physiological indicators that reflect the cardiovascular situation, its continuous measurement is very crucial. It can be a true indicator of many health issues, such as hypertension, heart attack, asthma, and kidney failure [1].

Several methods are available for BP monitoring. The most prevalent techniques are intra-arterial catheter insertion, auscultation, oscillometry, and volume clamping.

The intra-arterial catheter insertion approach requires the insertion of a catheter in a vessel. The method makes accurate and continuous BP reading possible. It was first practiced by Hales *et al* by inserting tubes into some animal vessels in 1733.

doi:10.1088/978-0-7503-3815-8ch4

However, Cushing performed the first invasive method based on the catheter insertion in a surgery room in 1901. In spite of the high accuracy of the method, due to its invasive nature and the difficulties it creates for patients, its application is limited to hospital environments, under the close supervision of experts, and merely for patients who are in critical conditions [2].

Auscultation is an indirect method to measure BP. In this method, a cuff is closed around the brachial artery on the upper arm, then using a mercury sphygmomanometer the pressure in the cuff becomes measurable. Then a stethoscope is employed to make some sounds in the squeezed artery audible [3].

Oscillometry is another cuff-based method. The measurement is based on the oscillation in the inflatable cuff during the deflation. The oscillation starts even when the BP is above the systolic BP and resumes under the diastolic pressure [4].

Cuff-based methods are straightforward and involve pretty simple procedures. However, if the patient is obliged to do them frequently, they cause discomfort. Moreover, different interpretations of important events in these methods might cause significant variability and low accuracy.

Volume clamping is a non-invasive and continuous BP monitoring technique. It considers the dynamic vascular unloading of the arterial walls of the finger vessels. The method uses a finger cuff and a photoplethysmographic sensor in a feedback control loop to keep the blood flow constant. In this condition, the applied cuff pressure has the same value as the BP [2].

Even though volume clamping methods provide a non-invasive and continuous reading of BP, they are most of the time too expensive and complex to use. Therefore, there is a lot of motivation to use easy-access bio-signals like photoplethysmogram (PPG) and electrocardiogram (ECG) to measure BP continuously, non-invasively, and conveniently. In this chapter, we aim to explore the potential of deep neural networks (DNN) to achieve this goal.

This chapter is organized as follows. In section 4.1, we reviewed the available BP monitoring methods briefly. Section 4.2 provides a physiological model for BP. Section 4.3 discusses the data used in this chapter, and the preprocessing steps applied to them. Section 4.4 presents four different DNN architectures and their results. Section 4.5 discusses the models' performances, and finally, section 4.6 concludes the chapter.

4.2 Physiological models

Photoplethysmography is an optical approach to indicate blood volume fluctuations caused by the pressure pulse in the peripheral circulation arteries. This measurement is carried out by illuminating the skin using a light-emitting diode and detecting the reflected or transmitted light by a photodetector [5]. Electrocardiography, however, is a method to detect electrical excitations of the heart. It is detected by placing some electrodes on the prespecified places of the body [6]. Consequently, both PPG and ECG signals contain crucial information related to the cardiovascular system and its BP.

The time delay for the pressure pulse to travel through vessels is known as pulse transit time (PTT). PTT equals the time delay between the proximal and distal arterial pressure pulses and is inversely correlated with the BP value [7].

In this section, we consider a simple model for pressure wave propagation to define the relationship between PTT and BP. An arterial vessel is depicted as a flexible and cylindrical tube in figure 4.1. If we neglect viscosity, the resistance against blood current will be negligible. Compliance (C) that is defined as the ratio between cross-section area variations and pressure changes is defined as follows:

$$C = \mathrm{dA/dP} = 2\pi r^3/(E \times h) \tag{4.1}$$

where r is the radial, and h is the wall thickness. Elasticity is not unique and depends on P, as described in equation (4.2).

$$E(P) = E_0 \times e^{\alpha P} \tag{4.2}$$

Parameters E_0 and α are positive and subject-specific. If we assume that A is constant, the mass and momentum conservation rule results in the following equations.

$$\frac{d(\mathrm{A}dx)}{dt} + Q(x) - Q(x + dx) = 0 \rightarrow \frac{\partial Q}{\partial x} + C(P) \times \frac{\partial P}{\partial t} = 0 \tag{4.3}$$

$$A \times [P(x) - P(x + dx)] = \rho \times dx\frac{dQ}{\mathrm{dt}} \rightarrow \frac{\partial P}{\partial x} + L \times \frac{\partial Q}{\partial t} = 0 \tag{4.4}$$

Here, x and t are space and time, Q is the volume flow rate, ρ indicates blood density, and constant $L = \rho/A$ equals arterial inertance per unit of length. Moreover, C is inversely related to P. The relationship between C and P in central arteries is:

$$C(P) = \frac{A_m}{\pi P_1\left[1 + \left(\frac{P - P_0}{P_1}\right)^2\right]} \tag{4.5}$$

here, A_m, P_0, and P_1 are subject-specified. Equations (4.3) and (4.4) indicate the following form for the pressure pulse in vessels:

$$P(x, t) = f\left(\frac{x \pm t}{\sqrt{\mathrm{LC}(P)}}\right) \tag{4.6}$$

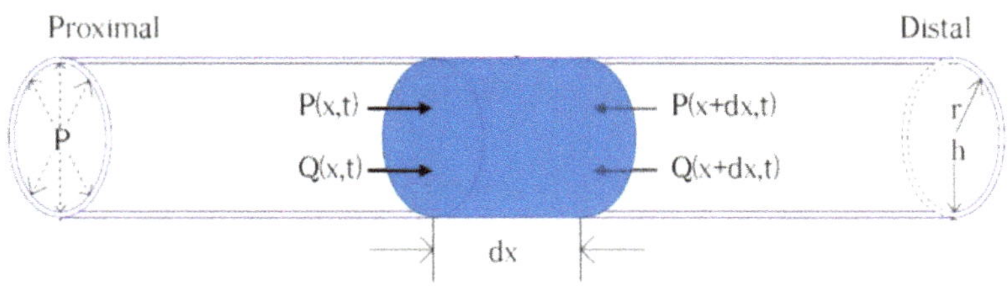

Figure 4.1. Wave propagation in central arteries.

It reveals that the velocity of the pulse in a vessel which is known as *pulse wave velocity* (PWV) equals $[L \times C(P)]^{-1/2}$. Therefore, the time for the wave to pass a length of l (PTT) is:

$$\text{PTT} = l\sqrt{\text{LC}(P)} \tag{4.7}$$

According to equation (4.7), PTT depends on BP inversely. If we assume that C is constant, the PWV becomes:

$$\text{PWV} = \frac{1}{\sqrt{L \times C}} = \sqrt{\frac{\text{AdP}}{\rho \text{dA}}} = \sqrt{\frac{Eh}{2r\rho}} \tag{4.8}$$

This equation is known as the Bramwell–Hill and Moens–Korteweg equation [7].

Besides PWV and PTT, many other studies try to define other hand-crafted features and find out their relationship with BP [8, 9]. In this study, however, we emphasize automatic feature extraction using deep-learning techniques. We believe that similar to many other applications, machine-learning abilities can be utilized for finding appropriate representations of signals for BP estimation. Afterwards, we develop several methods to achieve this goal[1].

4.3 Data source

We use the *Multiparameter Intelligent Monitoring in Intensive Care II* (MIMIC-II) database to implement and evaluate our deep models for BP estimation. It encompasses high-resolution data of a diverse population of patients in the intensive care unit (ICU). The dataset includes clinical documentation, laboratory results, and various physiological waveforms [10].

We consider invasive arterial BP, ECG, and PPG signals of 200 patients (86 women and 114 men) in this research. The mean and standard deviation of the subject ages are 61.6 ± 14.6 years. The sampling frequency of all waveforms is 125 Hz.

Systolic and diastolic BPs[2] in each cardiac cycle are extracted from invasive BP waveforms to use them as target values during the training and validation phases of the models. All selected records contain 51 884 cycles. Figure 4.2 shows the binned-scatter plot and the distribution histogram of the BP. As we expected, the figure indicates the direct correlation between systolic and diastolic BP [11].

4.3.1 Preprocessing procedures

We apply several filters to remove artifacts from signals and improve their quality. Then, PPG signals are segmented to prepare the input data to feed our deep networks. For each input segment, systolic and diastolic BPs are extracted from

[1] In this chapter, we emphasize mostly the PPG waveform for blood pressure monitoring, although, we utilize ECG merely for the segmentation of the PPG records. To find out the role that ECG waveform might play to enhance accuracy, please refer to [9].

[2] The maximum pressure the heart exerts in a cycle is the systolic pressure, and the minimum amount of BP between beats is the diastolic pressure.

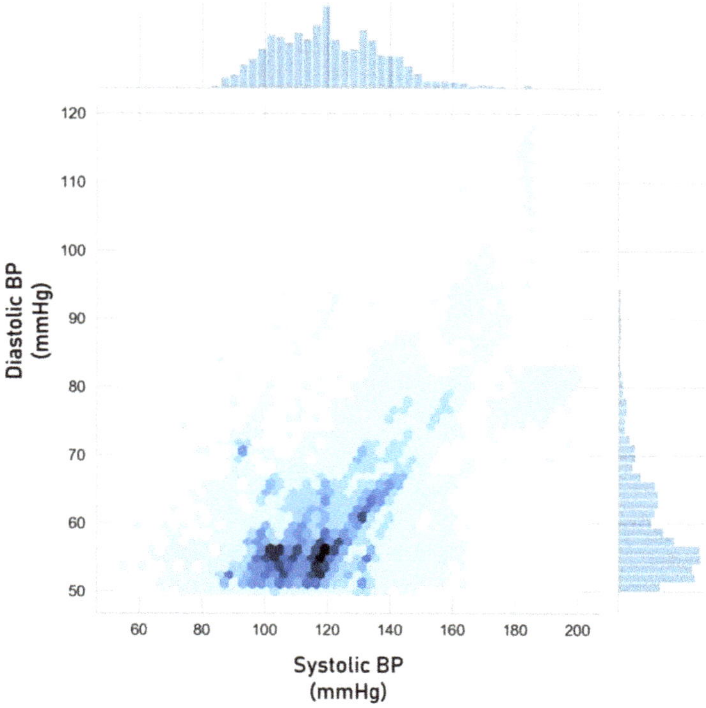

Figure 4.2. Binned-scatter plot and the distribution histogram of systolic and diastolic BP target values.

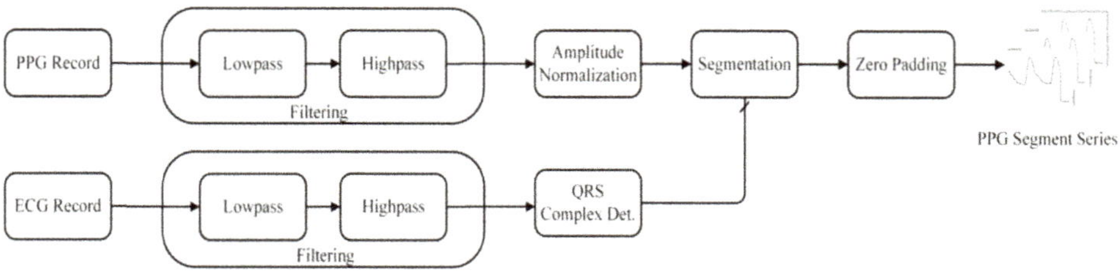

Figure 4.3. Various preprocessing steps to prepare PPG segment series.

corresponding invasive BP waveforms. They would be our target vectors. R-wave occurrences are utilized as the time references during the segmentation procedure. Therefore, each recording turns to an input vector (X) and a target vector (T) as follows:

$$X = \{x_1,\ x_2,\ \dots,\ x_n\} \tag{4.9}$$

$$T = \{t_1,\ t_2,\ \dots,\ t_2\} \tag{4.10}$$

Each element corresponds to a heart cycle. Figure 4.3 depicts various preprocessing steps. Here, we also provide more details.

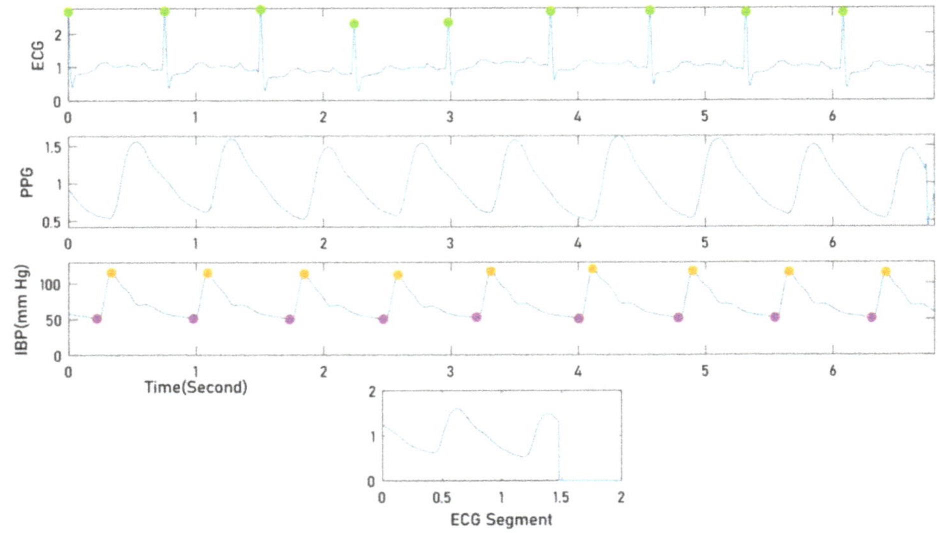

Figure 4.4. A sample for each waveform and the crucial points extracted from each waveform. A PPG segment is also shown at the bottom. Each PPG signal turns to a series of PPG segments.

- We apply two cascaded filters to remove various artifacts like baseline wandering in low frequencies and power-line harmonics and electromyogram noises in high frequencies. The first filter is a low-pass 7-point second-order Savitzky–Golay filter. It smoothes the waveform without disturbing the signal tendency [12]. The second filter is a high-pass Kaiser window FIR filter of order 40 [13]. The overall frequency band of interest is 0.13–40 Hz [5, 14].
- We consider R-peak waves as time-references for the segmentation procedure. We implemented the algorithm presented in [15] to detect the R-peak waves. It is based on the remarkable similarities between the ECG waveform structure and the integrated linear prediction residuals in audio signals.
- If we define the time occurrence of R-peaks as $\{t_1, t_2, \ldots, t_n\}$, the kth segment includes two heart cycles from t_{k-1} to t_{k+1} time-interval. Hence, two successive segments share a PPG cycle.
- Then, the length of each segment (each element of the input vector, X) is adjusted to 250 samples by zero-padding (when its length is smaller than 250), or by discarding some samples (when the length exceeds the length limit). Moreover, the length of each element of the target vector T is two (including invasive systolic and diastolic BP values).

Figure 4.4 shows a sample for each waveform and the crucial points extracted from each waveform. It also depicts a PPG segment at the bottom. Each PPG signal turns to a series of PPG segments after applying these preprocessing steps.

4.4 Deep learning models for blood pressure monitoring

In this section, we propose and implement four different DNNs to estimate BP. In each step, we try to analyze the results and find out the main restrictions of the model. Then we try to provide a solution for the restrictions and enhance the accuracy in the next step. Our models are based on two common and versatile neural networks: long short-term memories (LSTMs) and convolutional neural networks (CNNs).

LSTM networks are a kind of recurrent neural network (RNN). Unlike feedforward neural networks, these types of networks have feedback connections that allow them to process not only current inputs but also previous ones. In other words, they have feedback routes to store current events in their memory states. In theory, classic RNN networks can learn arbitrary long dependencies in the input data. However, the propagating gradient can vanish or explode during the training procedure. LSTM networks solve this problem of vanishing gradient by allowing it to propagate unchanged [16–18].

CNNs are inspired by the connectivity patterns among visual cortex neurons. Each cortical neuron is stimulated by a restricted region of the visual field recognized as the receptive field. The receptive fields, then, partially overlap, and they cover the whole visual field. Moreover, since these networks utilize convolution operations instead of matrix multiplication, they have many fewer parameters and connections. This reality facilitates the training process considerably. They are also more effective in automatically detecting important features in the input data compared with their predecessors [17–19].

In this chapter, two-hundred records were selected from the MIMIC-II database to evaluate our models. After applying preprocessing procedures discussed in section 4.3, each record was divided into three separate parts: the training, validation, and testing sections each claiming 70%, 10%, and 20% of the whole length of the records, respectively. Consequently, the training, validation, and testing sets include 35 965, 10 574, and 5354 cycles, respectively.

4.4.1 LSTM model

Long short-term memories are among the most effective methods for sequence modeling. The clever idea of embedding self-loops to allow the gradient flow for long distances is the key idea of LSTM networks. As the first model, we discuss an approach based on LSTM neural networks here.

- ***Proposed model based on LSTM networks:*** figure 4.5 shows the proposed architecture to estimate systolic and diastolic BPs. It is a two-layer stacked LSTM network. The first LSTM layer encompasses 64 lSTM units, while the second LSTM layer includes 32 units. PPG segment series achieved during segmentation process of PPG signals are fed to the network. Each element in the input series is a vector of dimension 250.

- ***Performance:*** The training and validation data sets were utilized to train the proposed deep LSTM network. Then, the testing set was fed to the network to investigate its performance. Table 4.1 shows the results in terms of the Pearson's correlation coefficient (R), Mean Error (ME), Mean Absolute Error (MAE), Root Mean Square Error (RMSE), and the Standard Deviation of Error (STD).

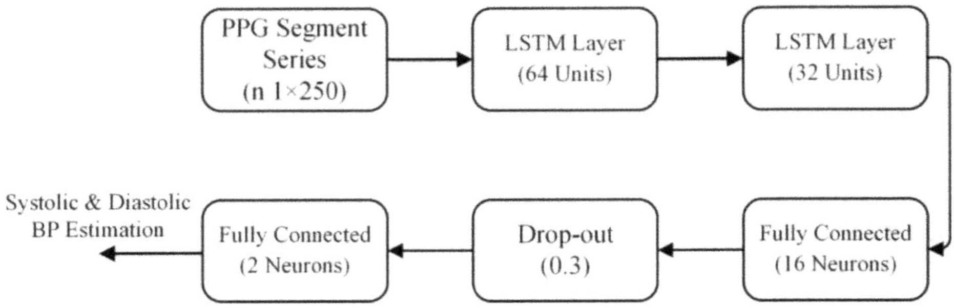

Figure 4.5. The proposed architecture for the first approach based on the LSTM networks to estimate BPs.

Table 4.1. The LSTM based model performance metrics.

Blood pressure	R	ME	MAE	RMSE	STD	Subjects #	AAMI
Systolic BP	0.32	−3.57	15.84	21.92	21.63	200	×
Diastolic BP	0.12	−1.45	8.71	12.26	12.17	200	×

The definition of the Pearson's correlation coefficient is given in equation (4.11). It indicates the relative covariance of the predicted (Y_{est}) and target values (Y_{tar}).

$$R = \frac{\text{cov}(Y_{\text{est}}, Y_{\text{tar}})}{\sigma_{Y_{\text{est}}} \times \sigma_{Y_{\text{tar}}}} \tag{4.11}$$

The table indicates that the algorithm does not meet the Association for the Advancement of Medical Instrumentation (AAMI) standard requirements. This protocol has been used to evaluate various BP monitoring devices. According to this standard, the number of patients must be higher than 85, and the ME and STD should be lower than five mmHg and eight mmHg, respectively [20]. Our results show that the LSTM network is not accurate enough according to the standard.

Another considerable point about the reported results in table 4.1 is the higher value of the Pearson's correlation coefficient for systolic BP compared with diastolic BP despite the reality that the MAE is much higher for systolic BP. To interpret these seemingly contradictory results, we should consider that the correlation coefficient is based on the relative variations instead of absolute values. Therefore, since systolic BP commonly has much higher amplitudes than diastolic BP, the coefficient is bigger for systolic estimations.

Figure 4.6 provides more visual cues about the low performance of the LSTM network. The figure demonstrates the high degree of error in both estimation procedures.

- ***Curse of dimensionality:*** When the input dimension increases, machine-learning problems become exceedingly difficult. It is because the range of input configurations will increase exponentially. This problematic phenomenon is known as the curse of dimensionality [17].

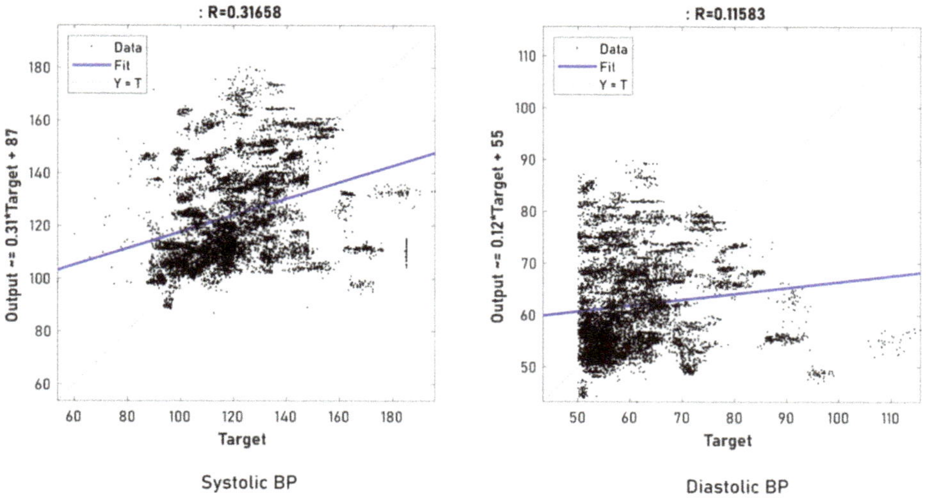

Figure 4.6. The estimation regression plots of systolic and diastolic BPs based on the LSTM model.

Most of the time, the challenge posed by the curse of dimensionality is statistical. When the dimension increases, fewer training samples fall into the exploding number of cells (or defined subspaces) in the input space. Therefore, the number of training samples for various areas in the input space decreases rapidly with increasing dimension. Less training data results in poorer performance inevitably. In such situations, the machine learning algorithm might simply assume that the output corresponding to a new input equals the value for the nearby points, while the further distance between training samples in a high dimensional space reduces the accuracy of such a simplification [17, 21].

As our results in the following sections indicate more clearly, the same problem might have occurred here. Since the input dimension (250) is very high, the LSTM model shows unsatisfactory performance. In the following models, we try to implement strategies to mitigate this problem.

4.4.2 PCA-LSTM model

To find out a solution for the difficulties that the LSTM network had with high-dimension input vectors, we apply Principal Component Analysis (PCA) method. It is an approach to reduce the input dimension.

There are two common ways to illustrate PCA. It can be obtained by the orthogonal projection of the data onto a new space with a lower dimension. The new space is named the principal subspace. The projection is carried out in such a way as to maximize the variance of the projected data.

Another illustration considers PCA as a technique to map our data to a new space with a lower dimension while minimizing the projection cost. Projection cost, here, refers to the mean squared distance between primary data and their projected counterparts [22].

- ***Propose model based on PCA and LSTM networks:*** In this section, we apply PCA to the input data. It organizes the information into principal components. We choose 64 components with the highest amount of information (corresponding to the dimensions with the maximum amounts of variance) to represent our data. Then, we use the new data set to train and evaluate another LSTM network with the same architecture as the previous network.
- ***Performance:*** The new training, validation, and testing sets were used to train and evaluate the LSTM network. Since the input dimension was much lower than the dimension of the original data (64 compared to 250), the network converged much faster during the training phase.

  Table 4.2 and figure 4.7 show the performance of the LSTM network using different metrics. These results confirm a higher estimation precision for the LSTM network based on the new data. Since the training procedure is now easier, we could expect the performance would improve. However, the accuracy is still not high enough to meet the requirements of the AAMI standard.
- ***Information loss:*** Discarding vectors where the data variance is lower will cost us some information loss. This procedure can be considered as a simplistic feature selection approach. Since the process is uncontrolled, it might result in

Table 4.2. The PCA-LSTM based model performance metrics.

Blood pressure	R	ME	MAE	RMSE	STD	Subjects #	AAMI
Systolic BP	0.75	0.35	8.81	12.33	12.33	200	×
Diastolic BP	0.55	0.59	6.02	8.10	8.08	200	×

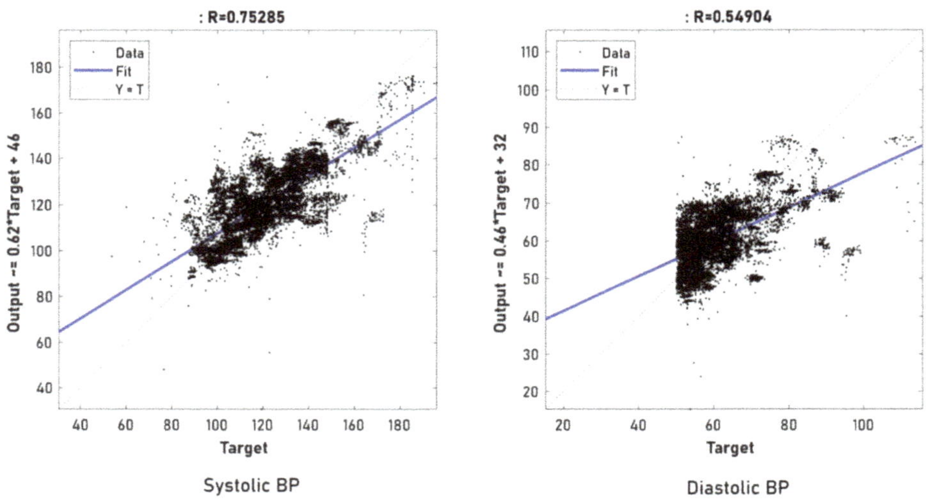

Figure 4.7. The estimation regression plots of systolic and diastolic BPs based on the PCA-LSTM model.

losing very crucial pieces of information. It is because the higher variance of a feature is not a fair indicator of its importance most of the time. For instance, to differentiate people, their nose dimension might be as important as their height, even though the variance of the former feature is much lower [23].

Therefore, we should try to define more appropriate feature selection methods. In the following subsection, we will propose and evaluate an approach based on convolutional neural networks. The network takes responsibility for both feature selection and estimation tasks. Since the network will do both steps simultaneously (the network supervises the performance during the training phase), it can extract features from input data more appropriately.

4.4.3 Convolutional neural network model

Convolutional neural networks are specialized kinds of networks for processing data using specified and grid-like topologies. Examples include time series (like the PPG segments here we use), which can be thought of as one-dimensional data, and images, which can be considered two-dimensional data. CNNs have been enormously successful in various practical applications. They use convolution instead of common matrix multiplications in at least one layer. In traditional fully-connected networks, every output unit interacts with every input unit. This makes them prone to overfitting. CNNs, however, have sparse interactions. It is achieved by making the kernels smaller than the input [17].

In this section, we propose an end-to-end architecture based on CNN networks. We apply segments separately to the network. The network will extract abstractions of the input signal in successive layers. Then, the network uses these extracted representations to carry out the estimation procedure [24].

- ***Proposed model based on CNN networks:*** Figure 4.8 depicts the proposed architecture for the CNN network. The network includes four convolutional

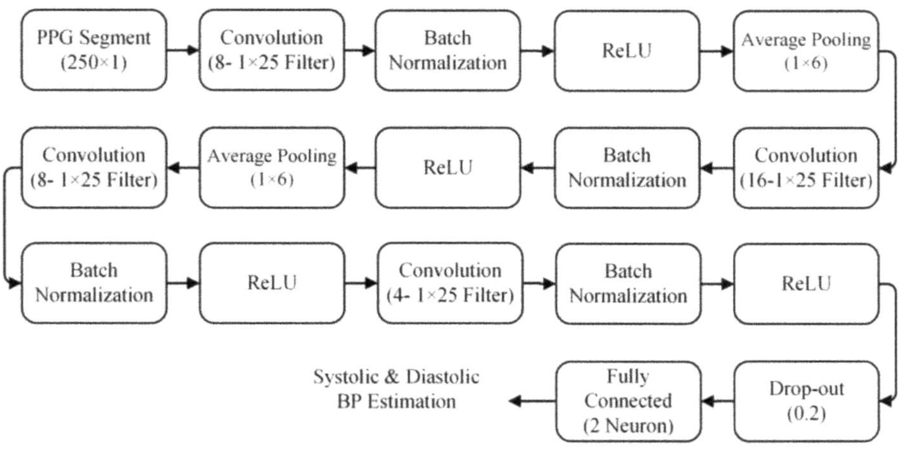

Figure 4.8. The proposed architecture for the CNN network to estimate systolic and diastolic BPs.

layers. More convolutional layers brought no more significant improvement. Batch normalization layers are introduced between CNN layers. They help the training process to speed up and make the network less sensitive to initial conditions. We have employed two average pooling layers for downsampling the data. They carry out the task by dividing the input data into rectangular regions (1 × 6 sections in our work), and then, calculating the average value for each region. A drop-out layer is also added to the network to help it avoid overfitting. The layer sets its input values randomly equal to zero during the training phase. We have chosen the ReLu function as the non-linear function after each convolutional layer to perform threshold operation. Equation (4.12) describes the function.

$$f(x) = \begin{cases} x, & x \geqslant 0; \\ 0 & x < 0. \end{cases} \tag{4.12}$$

- ***Performance:*** The performance of the CNN network is shown in table 4.3. As the results indicate, the performance is improved dramatically. Now, both estimations meet the requirements of the AAMI standard. Figure 4.9 also depicts the regression plot for the estimation results. The high correlation coefficients prove the effectiveness of the new approach based on the abilities of CNN networks for both appropriate feature learning and parameter estimation.

- ***Temporal information loss:*** The CNN network performs the estimation in each time step based on the PPG segment corresponding to that time step. Therefore, it fails to include temporal information carried in the PPG waveform. Undoubtedly, the BP fluctuations do not happen abruptly in each time step. They depend heavily on the previous values of BP too. Despite this fact, the CNN network carries out the estimation merely based on the current information provided to the network. In other words:

$$\text{BP}(t_k) = f(x_k) \tag{4.13}$$

Therefore, if we include temporal variations of the PPG waveform in the estimation procedures, we can expect even further estimation improvement. In the next subsection, we propose a way for embedding this crucial information in the estimation process.

Table 4.3. The CNN model performance metrics.

Blood pressure	R	ME	MAE	RMSE	STD	Subjects #	AAMI
Systolic BP	0.91	−0.01	5.40	7.86	7.86	200	√
Diastolic BP	0.89	−0.01	3.13	4.24	4.24	200	√

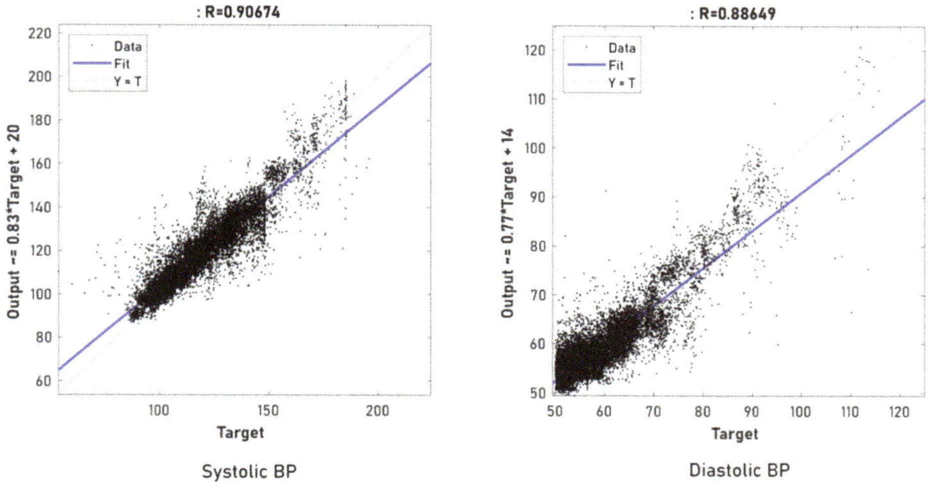

Figure 4.9. The estimation regression plots of systolic and diastolic BPs based on the CNN model.

4.4.4 CNN–LSTM model

In this subsection, we combine the abilities of CNN networks in finding appropriate representations of their inputs with the ability of LSTM networks to memorize temporal information to propose a more optimal architecture for BP estimation.

To achieve these goals, we have designed an end-to-end DNN that includes two stages. The lower stage consists of convolutional layers to extract appropriate morphological indicators from PPG segments. The hidden layers in the upper stage, however, use LSTM units to grasp the time-domain variations of the features extracted by the CNN layers.

- ***Proposed end-to-end CNN–LSTM model:*** figure 4.10 depicts the proposed end-to-end DNN architecture. It includes two hierarchy levels. They are distinguished by larger blue rectangles in the figure. The lower hierarchy level is a CNN network that deploys four convolutional layers, while the upper hierarchy level encompasses a two-layer stacked LSTM network. Both sectors are designed based on the architectures discussed in the previous subsections. The CNN layers are responsible for learning (or extracting) proper machine-learned features from each segment. The LSTM layers, however, will learn the relationship between the segment features of the input series.

Since CNN layers extract features from each PPG segment independently, we need to use a folding layer before applying the input series containing PPG segments. This layer converts a batch of PPG series to a batch of PPG segments. Besides, we should use an unfolding layer to restore the PPG sequence structures after sequence folding to apply them to the LSTM layers.

- ***Performance:*** table 4.4 provides the numerical metrics to evaluate the performance of the end-to-end CNN–LSTM network. If we compare table 4.4

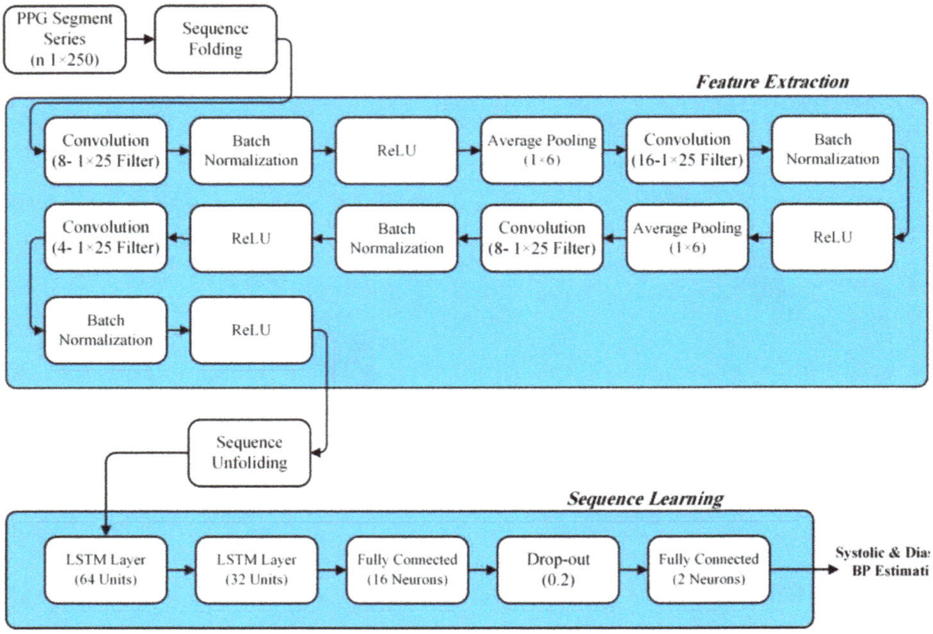

Figure 4.10. The proposed architecture for the end-to-end CNN–LSTM network.

Table 4.4. The CNN–LSTM model performance metrics.

Blood pressure	R	ME	MAE	RMSE	STD	Subjects #	AAMI
Systolic BP	0.92	0.80	4.75	7.30	7.26	200	√
Diastolic BP	0.90	0.53	2.92	3.95	3.92	200	√

with table 4.3, it becomes clear that our decision to add LSTM layers to the CNN networks improves accuracy considerably. It is due to the ability of the new network to find out the time domain dependencies among the PPG segments and use it to calculate BP more precisely. In other words, the estimation process puts into account not only the current information but also all the previous segments:

$$\mathrm{BP}(t_k) = f(x_1, x_2, \ldots, x_k) \tag{4.14}$$

Figure 4.11 depicts the regression plot of the new results. The Pearson's correlation coefficient is the highest for the new model.

4.5 Discussion

In general, proposed approaches for BP monitoring using ECG and PPG signals can be categorized into two groups. The first group includes methods based on physiological models. These methods extract hand-crafted features defined based

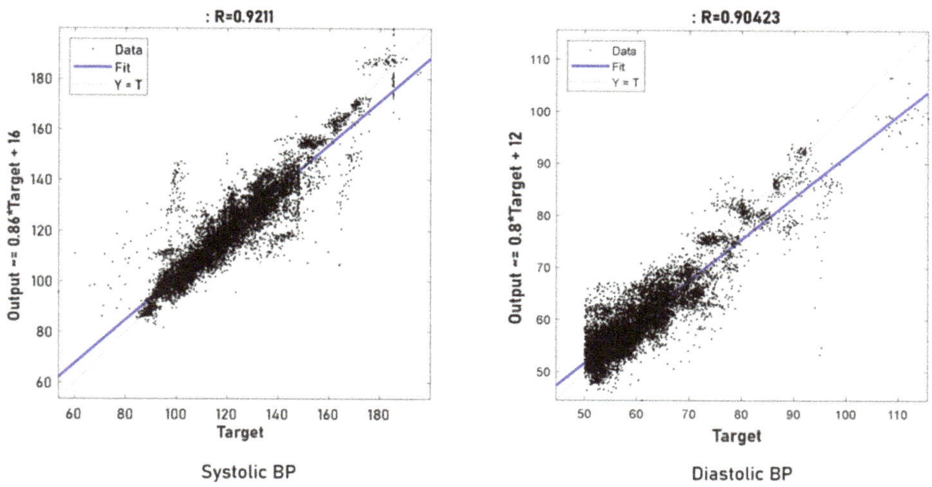

Figure 4.11. The estimation regression plots of systolic and diastolic BPs based on the end-to-end CNN–LSTM model.

on those models for BP monitoring. The other group includes methods that use machine-learning techniques for both feature extraction and estimation[3].

In this chapter, we proposed several models based on state-of-the-art DNN. Step-by-step, we developed our models and made amendments to improve the accuracy. The first model was built upon LSTM layers. However, the high dimension of input vectors caused the performance to deteriorate and made the task exceedingly difficult for the network.

Then, we investigated the effectiveness of the PCA technique to reduce the input dimension and mitigate the curse of dimensionality, althhough, the results indicated that the solution was not effective enough. Since the PCA approach had led to losing crucial information in the PPG waveform, the accuracy was not satisfactory again. It was due to the reality that variance amplitude can't be the right criterion for all situations. Sometimes a feature with low fluctuations can be very decisive.

Therefore, we decided to use a more intelligent approach for feature extraction. Since, convolutional neural networks have made remarkable accomplishments in many applications, such as neural language processing, image and video recognition, and medical image processing, we decided to utilize them to design the third model. This time the results were promising, and they met the AAMI standard requirements.

The architecture based on convolutional neural networks performed the estimation process merely based on the PPG segment corresponding to the time step of interest for BP calculations. Hence, we suggested extending the architecture by adding some LSTM layers in an upper hierarchy to capture time-domain variations too. The approach was effective, and the accuracy improved even further. It was due

[3] For a broader discussion on these approaches, please refer to [9].

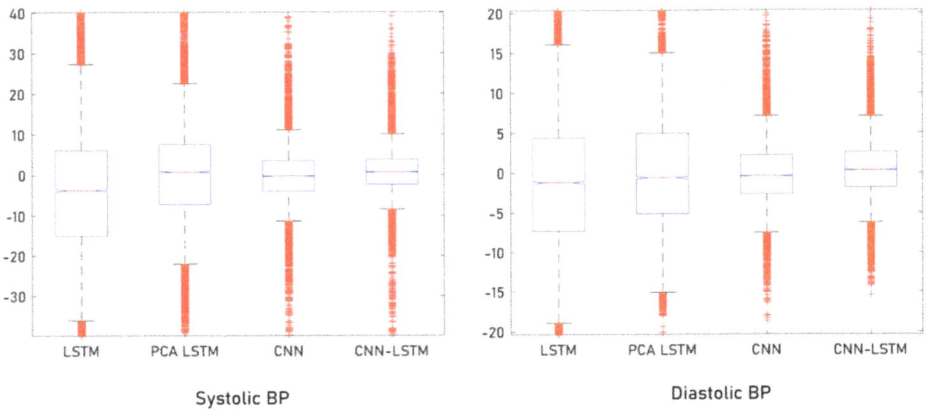

Figure 4.12. Box and Whisker diagram of errors for the proposed models.

to the reality that the LSTM layers could consider temporal information in the calculations.

Figure 4.12 shows the Box and Whisker diagram of errors for the proposed models [25]. Each diagram shows the estimation errors for testing data through their quartiles. Red markers show outliers. It can be seen easily from the figure that the error distribution becomes narrower and more centered around zero as we go through the steps.

Figure 4.13 also depicts the error distribution over systolic and diastolic BP values. The peak values diminish considerably for the methods based on CNN and LSTM networks.

Table 4.5 evaluates the performance of all models based on another new standard. The British Hypertension Standard assigns a grade for a BP monitoring device considering the cumulative percentage of absolute error values under different thresholds [26]. As table 4.5 indicates, the performance improves when more suitable steps are taken to develop the models. Both systolic and diastolic BPs acquire Grade A when we estimate BP based on the CNN–LSTM architecture.

4.5.1 Comparison with other methods

Table 4.6 compares the best results obtained in this chapter based on the end-to-end CNN–LSTM architecture with some other studies. The table encompasses sample models based on both methods based on hand-crafted features (or mentioned as physiological model parameters in some studies) and models based on machine-learned representations of the bio-signals. The table also indicates the number of patients and also the tools used to implement the models.

For a fair comparison of different methods, we should apply the methods on the same data and under similar criteria. However, the table provides some insight into several other models and their relative performance. Considering the number of subjects, the table confirms that our CNN–LSTM architecture provides relatively accurate estimations for both systolic and diastolic BPs.

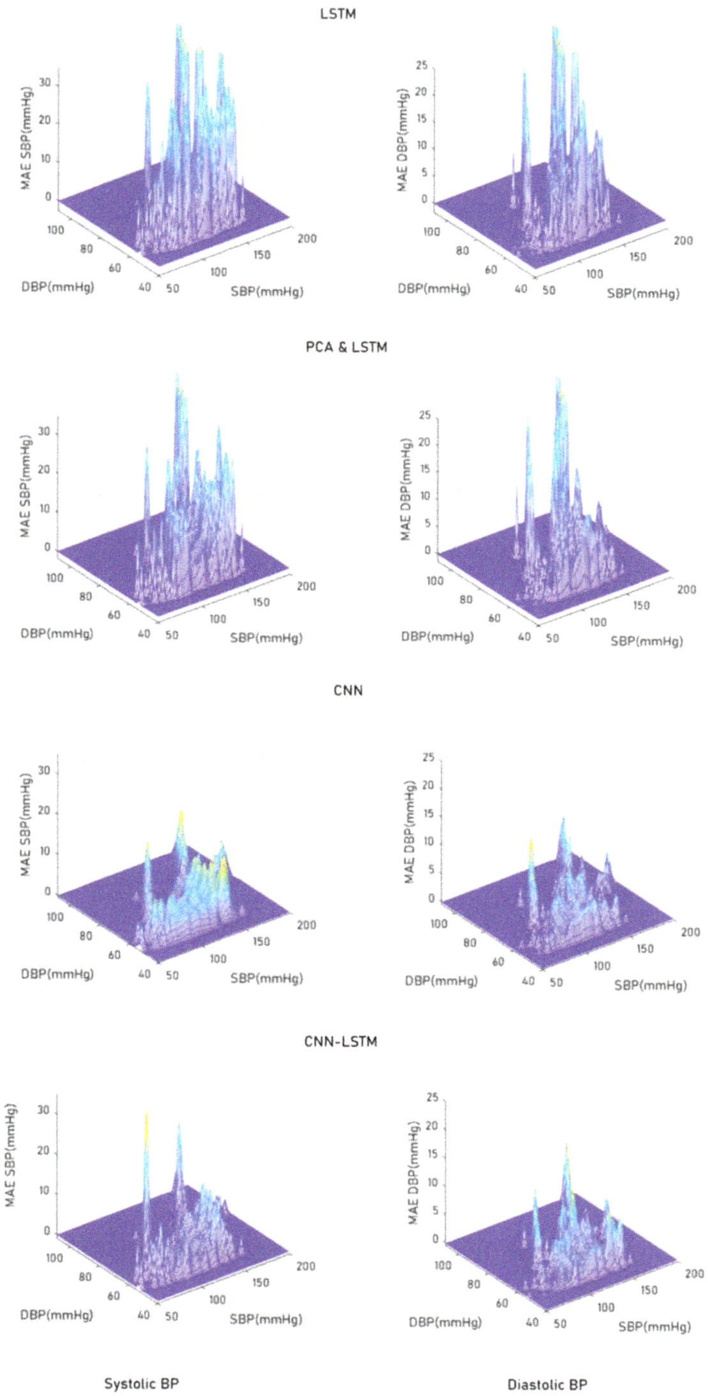

Figure 4.13. Error distribution over systolic and diastolic BP values for all models discussed in this study.

Table 4.5. The performance of all models based on BHS standard.

Estimation model	Blood pressure	Cumulative percentage of error			BHS standard grade
		<5 mmHg	<10 mmHg	<15 mmHg	
LSTM	SBP	26.6%	48.4%	62.2%	***D***
	DBP	43.9%	69.5%	79.8%	***D***
PCA & LSTM	SBP	35.1%	60.5%	72.5%	***D***
	DBP	49.7%	82.3%	93.2%	***C***
CNN	SBP	61.9%	86.5%	93.8%	***B***
	DBP	81.3%	97.3%	99.3%	***A***
CNN–LSTM	SBP	67.9%	90.0%	95.3%	***A***
	DBP	83.5%	97.4%	99.7%	***A***
	Grade A	60%	85%	95%	
	Grabe B	50%	75%	90%	
	Grade C	40%	65%	85%	
	Grade D		Worse Tnan C		

Table 4.6. Comparison with other methods.

Method	Waveform(s)	Subjects	Systolic blood pressure R	RMSE	ME	STD	Diastolic blood pressure R	RMSE	ME	STD
CNN [21]	Two PPGs	14	0.94	—	0.30	4.90	0.93	—	0.10	3.20
ANN-CNN [27]	PPG & ECG	39	0.99	1.56	—	—	0.99	0.85	—	—
FFT-based NNs [28]	PPG	69	—	—	0.06	7.08	—	—	0.01	4.66
Machine Learning [29]	ECG	51	—	10.97	—	—	—	19.34	—	—
CNN–LSTM (Our Results)	**PPG**	**200**	**0.92**	**7.30**	**0.80**	**7.26**	**0.90**	**3.95**	**0.53**	**3.92**

4.6 Conclusion

We proposed several models using DNN for systolic and diastolic BP monitoring. Through discussing the pros and cons of each model, we improved the accuracy in the following steps. We concluded that a proper deep-learning model should consist of at least two vital ingredients: first, an appropriate feature extraction strategy, and second, a suitable method to integrate temporal variations in the estimation algorithms.

Our results propose that convolutional neural networks can be a promising candidate for carrying out feature extraction. Besides, our findings confirm the high efficiency of LSTM networks in learning temporal dependencies among successive PPG segments. Consequently, the proposed end-to-end CNN–LSTM model achieved the best performance among all discussed models. Moreover, its performances for both BP meet the requirements of the AAMI standard, and it acquires Grade A according to the BHS standard.

References

[1] Jamieson D T, Breman J G, Measham A R, Alleyne G, Claeson M, Evans D B, Jha P, Mills A and Musgrove P 2006 *Disease Control Priorities in Developing Countries* (Washington, DC: World Bank)

[2] Kamalzadeh S 2016 PTT-based method for noninvasive beat-to-beat estimation of systolic and diastolic blood pressure *Master Thesis* (Tehran, Iran: Amirkabir University of Technology)

[3] Langewouters G J, Settels J J, Roelandt R and Wesseling K H 1998 Why use Finapres or Portapres rather than intraarterial or intermittent non-invasive techniques of blood pressure measurement? *J. Med. Eng. Technol.* **22** 37–43

[4] Pickering T G *et al* 2005 Recommendations for blood pressure measurement in humans: an AHA scientific statement from the council on high blood pressure research professional and public education subcommittee *J. Clin. Hypertens.* **7** 102–9

[5] Allen J 2007 Photoplethysmography and its application in clinical physiological measurement *Physiol. Meas.* **28** R1

[6] Lilly L S 2012 *Pathophysiology of Heart Disease: A Collaborative Project of Medical Students and Faculty* (Baltimore, MD: Lippincott Williams & Wilkins)

[7] Mukkamala R *et al* 2015 Toward ubiquitous blood pressure monitoring via pulse transit time: theory and practice *IEEE Trans. Biomed. Eng.* **62** 1879–901

[8] Esmaelpoor J, Sanat Z M and Moradi M H 2021 Blood pressure monitoring using photoplethysmogram and electrocardiogram signals *Biomedical Signal Processing for Healthcare Applications* (Boca Raton, FL: CRC Press) pp 123–41

[9] Esmaelpoor J, Moradi M H and Kadkhodamohammadi A 2021 Cuffless blood pressure estimation methods: physiological model parameters versus machine-learned features *Physiol. Meas.* **42** 035006

[10] Saeed M *et al* 2011 Multiparameter intelligent monitoring in intensive care II (MIMIC-II): a public-access intensive care unit database *Crit. Care Med.* **39** 952

[11] Gavish B, Ben-Dov I Z and Bursztyn M 2008 Linear relationship between systolic and diastolic blood pressure monitored over 24 h: assessment and correlates *J. Hypertens.* **26** 199–209

[12] Hargittai S 2005 Savitzky–Golay least-squares polynomial filters in ECG signal processing *Comput. Cardiol.* **2005** 763–6

[13] Chavan M S, Agarwala R A and Uplane M D 2006 Use of Kaiser window for ECG processing, *Proc. 5th WSEAS Int. Conf. Signal Processing, Robotics and Automation (Madrid, Spain)*

[14] Berkaya S K, Uysal A K, Gunal E S, Ergin S, Gunal S and Gulmezoglu M B 2018 A survey on ECG analysis *Biomed. Signal Process. Control* **43** 216–35

[15] Ramakrishnan A G, Prathosh A P and Ananthapadmanabha T V 2014 Threshold-independent QRS detection using the dynamic plosion index *IEEE Signal Process Lett.* **21** 554–8

[16] Reddy B K and Delen D 2018 Predicting hospital readmission for lupus patients: an RNN-LSTM-based deep-learning methodology *Comput. Biol. Med.* **101** 199–209
[17] Goodfellow I, Bengio Y and Courville A 2016 *Deep Learning* (Cambridge, MA: MIT Press)
[18] Esmaelpoor J, Moradi M H and Kadkhodamohammadi A 2020 A multistage deep neural network model for blood pressure estimation using photoplethysmogram signals *Comput. Biol. Med.* **120** 103719
[19] Acharya U R, Oh S L, Hagiwara Y, Tan J H and Adeli H 2018 Deep convolutional neural network for the automated detection and diagnosis of seizure using EEG signals, *Comput. Biol. Med.* **100** 270–8
[20] Alpert B S 2007 Validation of the Welch Allyn spot vital signs blood pressure device according to the ANSI/AAMI SP10: 2002. Accuracy and cost-efficiency successfully combined, *Blood Press. Monit* **12** 345–7
[21] Esmaelpoor J, Sanat Z M and Moradi M H 2021 A clinical set-up for noninvasive blood pressure monitoring using two photoplethysmograms and based on convolutional neural networks *Biomed. Eng.* https://doi.org/10.1515/bmt-2020-0197
[22] Bishop C M 2006 *Pattern Recognition and Machine Learning* (Berlin: Springer)
[23] Potapov P 2017 On the loss of information in PCA of spectrum-images *Ultramicroscopy* **182** 191–4
[24] Bengio Y, Courville A and Vincent P 2013 Representation learning: a review and new perspectives *IEEE Trans. Pattern Anal. Mach. Intell.* **35** 1798–828
[25] Thirumalai C, Vignesh M and Balaji R 2017 Data analysis using Box and Whisker plot for lung cancer *2017 Innovations in Power and Advanced Computing Technologies (i-PACT)* (Piscataway, NJ: IEEE) pp 1–6
[26] O'Brien E *et al* 1990 The British Hypertension Society protocol for the evaluation of automated and semi-automated blood pressure measuring devices with special reference to ambulatory systems. *J. Hypertens.* **8** 607–19
[27] Tanveer M S and Hasan M K 2019 Cuffless blood pressure estimation from electrocardiogram and photoplethysmogram using waveform based ANN–LSTM network *Biomed. Signal Process. Control* **51** 382–92
[28] Xing X and Sun M 2016 Optical blood pressure estimation with photoplethysmography and FFT-based neural networks *Biomed. Opt. Express* **7** 3007–20
[29] Simjanoska M, Gjoreski M, Gams M and Madevska Bogdanova A 2018 Non-invasive blood pressure estimation from ECG using machine learning techniques *Sensors* **18** 1160

Chapter 5

Reliability of machine learning methods for diagnosis and prognosis during the COVID-19 pandemic: a comprehensive critical review

Hamid Reza Marateb, Mohammad Reza Mohebbian, Mehdi Shirzadi, Arezoo Mirshamsi, Shadi Zamani, Atena Abrisham chi, Fatame Bafande and Miguel Ángel Mañanas

COVID-19, the severe acute respiratory syndrome coronavirus (SARS-CoV-2), has been a disaster since 2020. Many papers were published by the medical and computer research communities during the pandemic. However, there are concerns about whether papers with problems in statistical analysis, study design and reported performance indices could help fight the pandemic. Reducing the risk of bias requires proper statistical and validation models. A variety of machine learning methods were proposed in the literature for COVID-19 diagnosis and prognosis, among which deep learning methods were mainly focused on the chest CT-scan. Despite these efforts, there are issues not taken into account hindering their clinical applications. This chapter analyzed the critical STARD/TRIPOD issues of more than 45 machine learning methods proposed in the literature during the pandemic. Strategies were recommended to avoid systematic flaws and improve the clinical reliability of such systems.

5.1 Introduction

Severe acute respiratory syndrome coronavirus (SARS-CoV-2), also known as COVID-19, was not only a disaster in 2020 but continues in 2021 with mutations and more severe clinical outcomes across the world [1]. It has been affecting the entire human society from different perspectives [2–4]. Various machine learning methods have been used for COVID-19 diagnosis, prognosis, and long-term side effects [5–9]. However, most of the proposed methods' quality is low and are not recommended for clinical applications [10, 11]. This is surprising, as there are standards such as TRIPOD (Transparent Reporting of a multivariable prediction model for Individual Prognosis Or Diagnosis) [12] published in the literature that could be extended to limited sample

doi:10.1088/978-0-7503-3815-8ch5

size [13]. We previously discussed the importance of such standards for computer-aided-diagnosis [14]. In this chapter, we specifically analyze the published COVID-19 diagnosis and prognosis papers in terms of validation methods, and the critical issues of the TRIPOD guideline in such papers are discussed.

The following items were listed in the tables for the analyzed papers: reference, research question, input features, classifier, type of validation (internal/external), validation framework, the critical items from STARD [15], TRIPOD [12], and medical data mining [14]: ((1) sample size calculation; (2) sampling method; (3) inclusion and exclusion criteria, missing data handling; (4) proper statistical tests for comparing classifiers; (5) reporting mean and SD of performance indices over test fold when using cross-validation; (6) the confidence interval (CI) 95% of performance indices; and (7) using proper performance indices such as Area Under the ROC Curve (AUC) or Matthews correlation coefficient (MCC), or F_1-score in imbalanced datasets [16]).

5.2 Methods

The analyzed papers were listed based on the publication date as follows: section 5.2.1 (January–March) (table 5.1), section 5.2.2 (April–June) (table 5.2), section 5.2.3 (July–September) (table 5.3), 5.2.4 (October 2020–February 2021) (table 5.4).

5.2.1 January–March

Table 5.1. COVID-19 data mining papers published between January and March 2020.

Reference	Research question	Input features	Classifier or method	Type of validation	Validation framework	Critical STARD items
Li *et al* [17]	Detection of Covid-19 among other pneumonia diseases by deep learning	3D Chest CT	RestNet, max pooling operation, fully connected layer and softmax activation function	External	9-fold cross validation	3,5,7,8
Yuan *et al* [18]	Association of radiologic findings with mortality	CT scans	Features are ground, bilateral sides involved, peripheral and central distribution, and lower zone involvement	Internal	Comparing with RT-PCR findings	5,7
Laguarta *et al* [19]	COVID-19 diagnosis using cough recordings	Cough recordings	Convolutional Neural Network (CNN)	External	Hold-out (20%)	8

5.2.2 April–June

Table 5.2. COVID-19 data mining papers published between April and June 2020.

Reference	Research question	Input feature	Classifier	Type of validation	Validation framework	Critical STARD items
Hu *et al* 2020 [20]	Segmentation of CT Images and COVID-19 Classification	CT radiological features such as GGO and airspace consolidation	CNN	Internal and external	5-fold cross-validation	2,5,7
Apostolopoulos *et al* 2020 [21]	Classification on COVID-19 patients and bacterial pneumonia and normal subject from X-ray images	X-ray images	CNNs with transfer learning	Internal	10-fold cross-validation	8
Ardakani *et al* 2020 [22]	COVID-19 diagnosis using CT images	CT images	Pre-trained deep learning	Internal	80% for training and 20% for validating sets	3,5
Apostolopoulos *et al* 2020 [23]	COVID-19 diagnosis using x-ray images deep learning	X-ray images	CNNs with transfer learning MobileNet v2	Internal	10-fold-cross-validation	2,3
Hasan *et al* 2020 [24]	COVID-19 diagnosis using CT Scans using deep learning	Chest CT-scan	CNN feature extraction and LSTM	Internal	Hold-out (30%)	5
Hurt *et al* 2020 [25]	Deep Learning Localization of Covid-19	Chest radiographs images	Deep learning, U-Net	Internal	—	—
Khan *et al* 2020 [26]	Deep learning of X-ray images and COVID-19 diagnosis	Chest x-ray images	(CoroNet) CNN	Internal and external	4-fold cross-validation	2,8

(*Continued*)

Table 5.2. (*Continued*)

Reference	Research question	Input feature	Classifier	Type of validation	Validation framework	Critical STARD items
Khanday *et al* 2020 [27]	COVID-19 diagnosis using clinical text data mining	212 patients and attributes, such as gender, age, temperature, pO2_saturation, leukocyte count, neutrophil count	Various classifiers such as random forest, support vector machine (SVM), and stochastic gradient boosting	Internal	10-fold cross-validation	2
Ko *et al* 2020 [28]	COVID-19 diagnosis using a single Chest CT Image	3993 chest CT images, and other features such as age, gender, community-acquired pneumonia, hospital-acquired pneumonia	FCONet was developed by transfer learning based on CNN models such as VGG16, ResNet-50, Inception-v3, Xception	Internal and external	5-fold cross-validation	2
Ucar and Korkmaz *et al* 2020 [29]	Diagnosis of the COVID-19 with deep Bayes-SqueezeNet from x-ray images	X-ray images	Bayesian optimization structure (Deep Bayes-SqueezeNet based COVIDiagnosis-Net)	Internal	80%, 10%, and 10% for training, validation and testing	2,8
Singh *et al* 2020 [30]	COVID-19 diagnosis using chest CT images	Extracted features of chest CT images with CNN	Fully connected layers, CNN	Internal	20-fold cross-validation (80% for training, 20% for testing)	5,8

5.2.3 July–September

Table 5.3. COVID-19 data mining papers published between July and September 2020.

Reference	Research question	Input feature	Classifier	Type of validation	Validation framework	Critical STARD items
Goodman-Meza *et al* 2020 [31]	Increasing COVID-19 inpatient diagnostic capacity	Laboratory features includingage, gender, hemoglobin, red blood cell count	Various classifiers including Random Forest, XGBoost, and AdaBoost.	Internal	Hold-out 60%, 10%, and 30% for training, validation, and test	3,4,7
Zhao *et al* 2020 [32]	ICU admission and mortality prediction	Clinical data at admission, including vital signs and demographic	Logistic regression, machine learning	Internal	70% fortraining and 30% for testing	37
Banerjee *et al* 2020 [33]	COVID-19 diagnosis using full blood counts	Full blood counts, including hematocrit, hemoglobin, and laboratory tests	Logistic regression random-forest ANN glmnet	External	10-fold cross-validation	8
Burdick *et al* 2020 [34]	Respiratory decompensation prediction	Various features such as systolic blood pressure (SBP), diastolic blood pressure (DBP), creatinine, and bilirubin	XGBoost Classifier	External	—	3,4
Cie *et al* 2020 [35]	Assessment of COVID-19 severity and prognosis	Chest CT examinations Demographic data, Clinical symptoms, Routine blood test; and Arterial blood Gas	Random forest (RF) U-Net model	Internal	10-fold cross-validation	2,3,5,8

(*Continued*)

Table 5.3. (*Continued*)

Reference	Research question	Input feature	Classifier	Type of validation	Validation framework	Critical STARD items
Liang *et al* 2020 [36]	Critically ill COVID-19 patient's early triage of patients using deep learning	Comorbidities, x-ray abnormalities, age, dyspnea, and some lab tests	LASSO Deep Learning, Survival Cox model, Feedforward neural network	Internal External	10-fold cross-validation Hold-out (20%)	4,7
Ma *et al* 2020 [37]	Mortality risk estimation	CT scans results, comorbidity, symptoms, demographic, laboratory tests, vital signs	Machine-learning methods (Random Forest and XGboost) logistic regression	Internal External	Four-fold cross-validation	4,5
Sun *et al* 2020 [38]	Prediction of severe symptoms	Age, GSH, CD3 ratio, total protein Neutrophil percentage, albumin, CD4 ratio HCRP, Serum myoglobin, CL, Calcium, LDH Retinol binding protein, Acid glycoprotein Neutrophil percentage, Procalcitonin,	Support Vector Machine (SVM)	Internal External	Training (15 severe and 178 mild cases, testing on 11 sever and 132 mild cases)	—
Wu *et al* 2020 [39]	Outcome prediction of COVID-19 patients	Prothrombin activity, and lab tests	Maximum relevance logistic regression. LASSO, minimum redundancy (mRMR)	Internal	5-fold cross-validation	3,7

Zhou Li *et al* 2020 [40]	CT-Scan segmentation and COVID-19 diagnosis	Lung CT scans	3D deep learning models, such as 3D CNN and 3D U-Net	Internal External	5-fold cross-validation	—
Subudhi *et al* 2020 [41]	COVID-19 prognosis	Comorbidities, demographic data, vital signs, outpatient medications, and laboratory test	Random forest, support vector machines, k-nearest neighbor gradient boost, logistical regression, naïve Bayes	Internal External	80% training and 20% testing	4
Sotoudeh *et al* 2020 [42]	Using chest CT to classify H1N1 Influenza and COVID-19	Medical data and chest CT images	Convolutional neural network (CNN)	Internal Eternal	60%, 20%, 20% for training, validation and test sets	3
Dunne *et al* 2020 [43]	COVID-19 diagnosis based on coughs using smart home devices	Audio input of coughs	Mel-frequency cepstral coefficients (MFCC)CNN classification	External	16 audio recordings for training and validation	8

5.2.4 October 2020 to February 2021

Table 5.4. COVID-19 data mining papers published between October 2020 and February 2021.

Reference	Research question	Input feature	Classifier	Type of validation	Validation framework	Critical STARD items
Oulefki *et al* 2020 [44]	Infected region segmentation of lung based on CT-scans images	CT image	Medical image segmentation (MIS), graph cut, and watershed	Internal and external	Validation through several institutions and countries	1,2,8
Javor *et al* 2020 [45]	COVID-19 diagnosis using Deep learning of chest CT	Chest CT images	ResNet50 fastai2 Deep learning framework	Internal	80% for training and 20% for validating sets,	2,8
Nath *et al* 2020 [46]	COVID-19 diagnosis using CT and x-ray images	CT and x-ray images	CNN	Internal and external	Hold-out (20%)	2,3,8
Wang *et al* 2020 [47]	COVID diagnosis using CXR images	13 975 CXR images	COVID-Net, a deep convolutional neural network	External	—	8
Gao *et al* 2021 [48]	CT images segmentation and classification for COVID-19 diagnosis	CT Images	Attention-based dual branch combination network	Internal and external	5-fold cross-validation for internal	3,8
Arvind *et al* 2021 [49]	Forecasting intubation of COVID-19 patients	Systolic BP, diastolic BP, time from admission, pulse and respiratory rate, oxygen saturation, temperature, pH, HCO_3, arterial CO_2, arterial O_2, D-dimer platelet and	Random forest	Internal	Hold-out (70% train and 30% test)	3,4,5,6,7,8

		white blood cell (WBC) count, C-reactive protein, creatinine				
Nayak *et al* 2021 [50]	X-ray images classification for COVID-19 detection	Images	Transfer learning based on VGG-16, AlexNet, GoogleNet, MobileNet-V2, ResNet-34, Inception-V3, SqueezeNet, ResNet-50	Internal	Hold-out (70% train and 30% test)	3,8
Chao *et al* 2021 [51]	Covid-19 detection using image-based and non-image features	First, second and high order features from CT images and combined them with non-imaging features, such as gender, age, temperature, SpO_2, lymphocyte count, WBC, and lymphocyte count-to-WBC ratio	Random forest	Internal	5-fold cross validation	3, 4,5,6,7,8
Canayaz 2021 [52]	Covid-19 detection using x-ray images	Transfer learning for feature extraction based on AlexNet, VGG19, GoogleNet, and ResNet	SVM	Internal	5-fold cross-validation	8
Saha *et al* 2021 [53]	Classification COVID-19 patients and normal subject from Chest x-ray Images	Three different CNN for extract image features and the first fully connected layer for extract features for machine learning classifiers	Decision tree, AdaBoost, Random forest, SVM, CNN	Internal	70% training, 20% validation, 10% test set And Fivefold cross-validation	8

(*Continued*)

Table 5.4. (*Continued*)

Reference	Research question	Input feature	Classifier	Type of validation	Validation framework	Critical STARD items
Pahani *et al* 2021 [54]	Classification COVID-19 patients and normal subject from chest x-ray images	CNN	CNN	Internal	80% for the training and 20% for testing	8
Pham 2020 [55]	COVID-19 diagnosis using x-ray image analysis	Chest x-ray images	CNN transfer learning from AlexNet, GoogleNet, SqueezeNet	Internal	80% training and 20% testing And 80% training and 20% testing	6,8
Di *et al* 2021 [56]	Classification COVID-19 and community-acquired pneumonia from CT images	191 total features. Including infected lesion counting numbers, histogram distribution, lesion area and surface, the first-order intensity statistics and texture features, and demographic variables	Hypergraph learning	Internal	10-fold	5,6
Wu *et al* 2021 [57]	COVID-19 diagnosis and discrimination from common pneumonia and normal controls using CT images	Deep active learning	Deep active learning	Internal	Deep Active Learning with 30% of labeled data. 70% for unlabeled data pool, 10%, and 20% for validation and test	8

Karakanis and Leontidis 2021[58]	Classification of COVID-19 and normal cases and classification of COVID-19, normal cases, and bacterial pneumonia from x-ray images	CNN	CNN	Internal	Hold-out (20%)	—

5.2.5 Machine learning methods

There are usually two COVID-19 data mining research questions answered in the literature, including COVID-19 diagnosis and prognosis. Some examples are provided, and the critical issues are then discussed.

Cai *et al* [35] investigated the application of CT scans for the prediction of clinical outcomes and assessment of disease severity. 99 COVID-19 patients undertook physical examination, chest CT, routine blood test, and arterial blood gas tests on admission (figure 5.1). The clinical data, such as the treatment, outcomes, and disease severity, were collected. Random forest (RF) models were used to investigate CT quantification's validity (moderate, severe, and critical). The length of ICU stays, oxygen inhalation, and hospitalization was also assessed. Prediction of ICU partial versus prolonged recovery showed an AUC of 0.960.

The allocation of resources and focusing on the attention on high-risk patients is a struggling task for physicians. Implementing machine learning algorithms could support physicians in predicting high-risk individuals. Subudhi *et al* [41] developed prognostic ML methods based on electronic health records (figure 5.2). The developed model was validated by the hold-out method (20%). The accuracy of the developed model was 90%. The most important features included lymphocyte, high-sensitivity C-reactive protein (hs-CRP), and lactate dehydrogenase (LDH).

Zoabi *et al* [59] used a gradient-boosting machine model built with a decision-tree to predict COVID-19. The training set included 51 831 subjects (9% positive COVID-19), while the test set was 47 401 subjects (9% positive COVID-19) from the subsequent weeks. The dichotomous input features were age ⩾60 years, gender, contact with an infected subject, cough, fever, sore throat, shortness of breath, and headache. The feature importance was provided in figure 5.3. The proposed model's performance on the prospective test set was assessed as follows: AUC = 0.90 [CI 95%: 0.892–0.905], sensitivity = 87.30%, and specificity = 71.98%. It is one example in which various performance indices were reported, and external validation was used. Moreover, the dataset was not balanced. Thus, the performance of the developed system could be extended to the population. This critical issue is discussed later in this chapter.

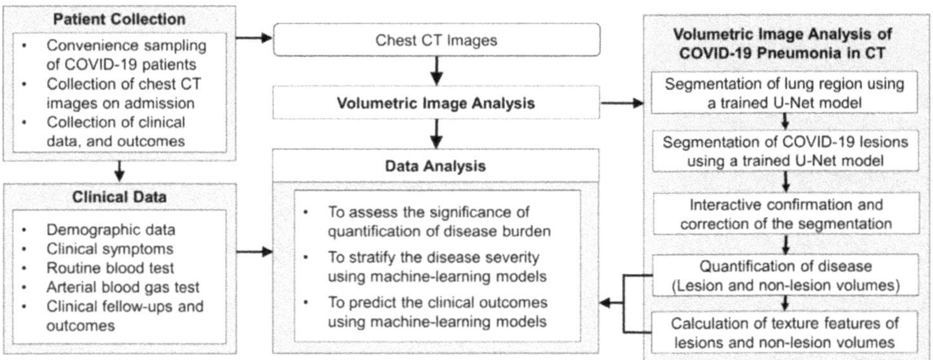

Figure 5.1. The flow chart of the study to assess COVID-19 prognosis and disease severity (reproduced from [35], copyright (2020) with permission from Elsevier).

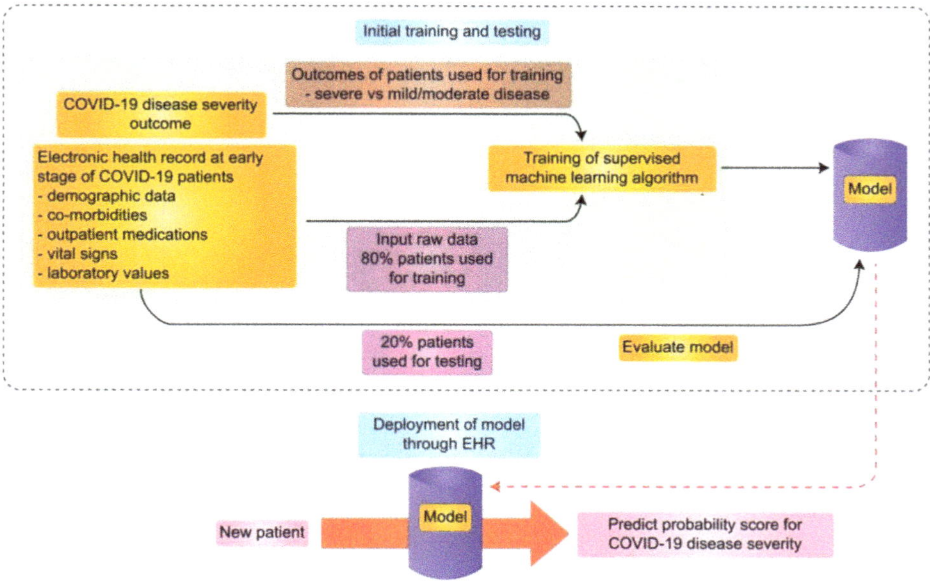

Figure 5.2. Prediction of COVID-19 disease using machine-learning algorithms (reproduced from [41], with the permission of John Wiley & Sons Ltd).

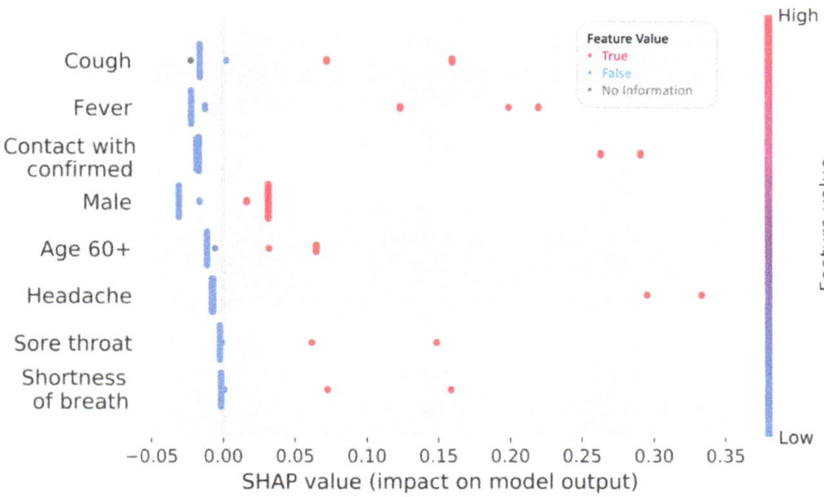

Figure 5.3. SHapley Additive exPlanations (SHAP) beeswarm plot for COVID-19 diagnosis, showing most important features' SHAP values (reproduced with permission from [59] under CC BY 4.0).

Gao *et al* [48] used an attention-based dual branch combination network on CT images for COVID-19 segmentation and classification. In total, 1918 CT scans from 1202 participants (210 395 slices: 498 controls versus 704 patients) were obtained in ten hospitals. The data were split into an internal training set (6130 slices: 75 controls versus 48 patients) from one hospital and an external validation set (204 265 slices:

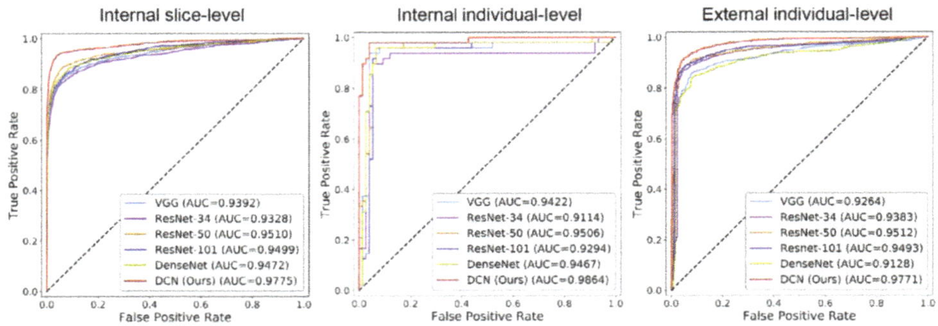

Figure 5.4. Slice-level and individual-level ROC curves on the internal and external datasets (reproduced from [48], copyright (2021) with permission from Elsevier).

423 controls versus 656 patients) from nine other hospitals. For the internal dataset, 5-fold cross-validation was used. It achieved an AUC average of 98% and 97% on individual-level and slice-level, respectively. The external dataset was only for individual-level, and the AUC of 97% was reported (figure 5.4). They used only the internal dataset for the segmentation task, with 5-fold cross-validation, and achieved Dice Similarity Coefficient (DSC) of 99% and 83% for lung and lesion detection. No CI and standard deviation over the test folds were reported.

An algorithm for forecasting intubation of patients diagnosed with COVID-19 was developed by Arvind *et al* [49]. They collected data from 4087 patients from 5 hospitals, wherein 11% of patients were intubated. They used the following features for training a time-series prediction based on Random Forest classifier: Systolic BP, diastolic BP, time from admission, temperature, pulse, respiratory rate, HCO_3, pH, arterial CO_2, oxygen saturation, WBC count, arterial O_2, platelet count, C-reactive protein, creatinine, and D-dimer. Using a hold-out (70% train and 30% test) validation, they achieved an AUC of 0.84 for predicting intubation presence in 72 h. They followed the TRIPOD standard and applied statistical analysis to the results. However, the CI was not reported for the performance indices.

Nayak *et al* [50] used transfer learning for COVID-19 x-ray image classification. Different models such as Inception-V3, MobileNet-V2, AlexNet, GoogleNet, VGG-16, ResNet-50, SqueezeNet, and ResNet-34 were evaluated on the publicly available dataset, and an AUC of 98% was reported for ResNet-34 as the best model using hold-out (70% train and 30% test) validation strategy (figure 5.5). They also did not report the CI or run the proposed method with shuffling data.

Chao *et al* [51] extracted the first, second, and higher-order features from CT images and combined them with non-imaging features, such as age, gender, temperature, white blood cell counts (WBC), SpO_2, lymphocyte count, and lymphocyte count-to-WBC ratio, for predicting COVID-19 (figure 5.6). The evaluation was performed using 5-fold cross-validation, and an AUC of 88% was achieved using random forest. Random forest outperformed the SVM and deep neural networks. The CI was also provided for the performance indices (figure 5.7).

Canayaz [52] examined whether performing preprocessing on CT images could improve the deep learning methods' performance. 364 CT images from two different

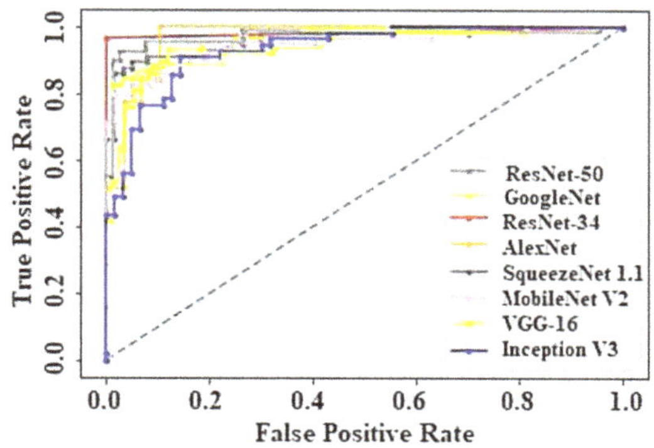

Figure 5.5. ROC curves of eight different CNN models used in this study (reproduced from [50], copyright (2021) with permission from Elsevier).

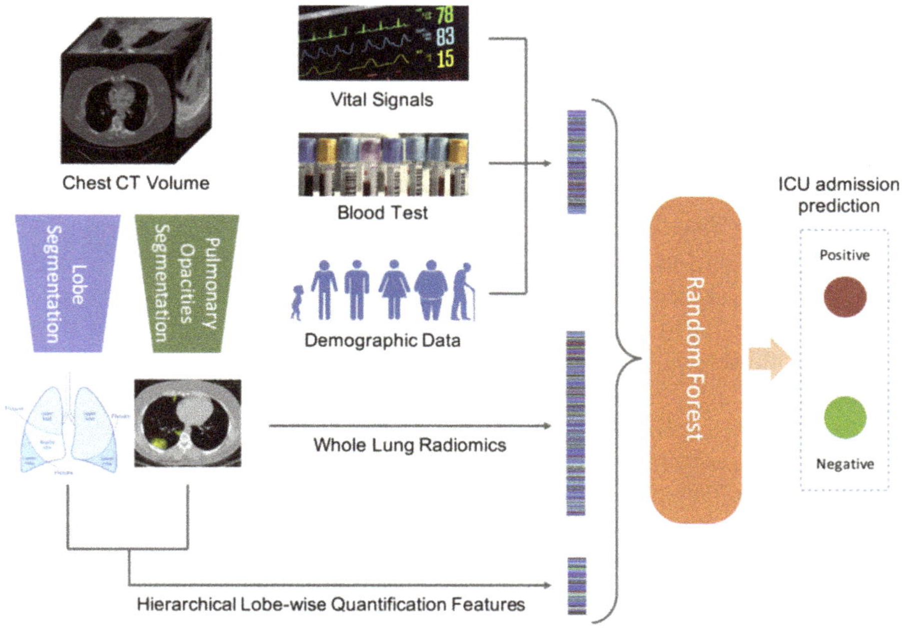

Figure 5.6. Framework of the proposed methods, including the utilized inputs and expected output (Reproduced from [51], copyright (2021) with permission from Elsevier).

sources were used for classifying pneumonia and COVID-19 images. With the help of transfer learning methods, such as ResNet, GoogleNet, VGG19, and AlexNet, features were extracted from images. Finally, the binary particle swarm optimization was utilized for feature extraction, and SVM was used as a classifier that achieved an AUC of 0.99 in a 5-fold cross-validation framework.

Saha *et al* [53] developed EMCNet for the classification of patients with COVID-19 and normal cases. They used 4600 total x-ray images (2300 COVID-19 patients and 2300 normal) collected from different online sources and resized all of them to

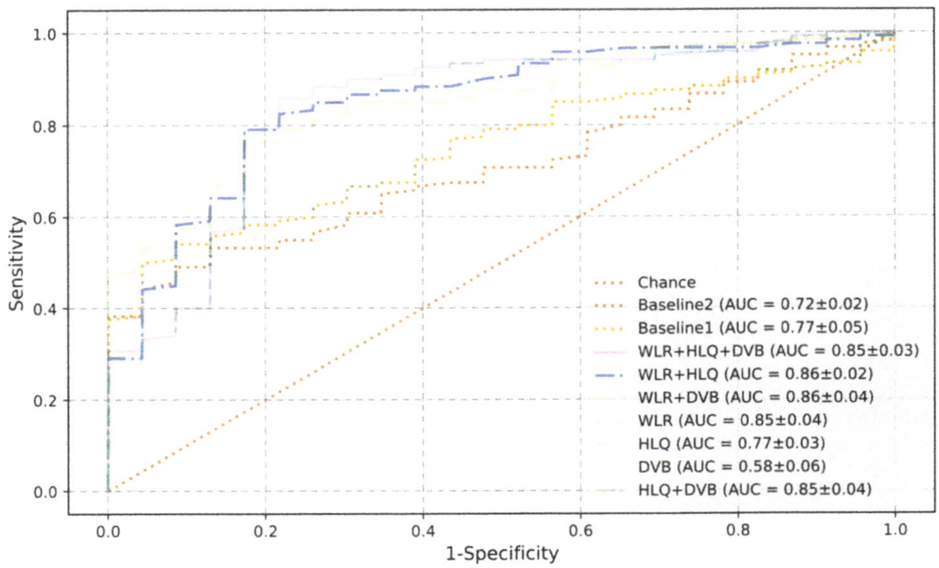

Figure 5.7. ROC curves on Site B dataset (reproduced from [51], copyright (2021) with permission from Elsevier).

$224 \times 224 \times 3$, and then normalized the dataset. The entire dataset was split into 70% training, 20% validation, and 10% for the test set. The EMCNet is a combination of Alexnet, VGG 16, Inception, and ResNet 50 to extract features from images. They used CNN, Decision Tree, SVM, AdaBoost, and random forest for classifying between two classes. They also used ensembling of all of these classifiers with five-fold cross-validation and hard voting. Their ensemble method achieved 100% precision, 97.82% recall, 98.91% accuracy, 98.89% F_1-score, and 0.9894 AUC. They did not follow any specific protocol, and CI was not reported.

Panahi *et al* [54] created Fast COVID-19 Detector (FCOD) for classifying x-ray images of COVID from non-COVID subjects. They used an open-source dataset from Github (https://github.com/ieee8023/covid-chestxray-dataset) and then selected 940 x-ray images of COVID-19 and 940 x-ray images of non-COVID-19. They separated the dataset into two parts: 80% for training and 20% for test. Data augmentation was used, and the size of the training set was then increased to 3760 images. FCOD consisted of several depthwise separatable convolutional layers. Following each layer, a max-pooling layer and a batch normalization layer were used, and a dropout layer was used at the end. They achieved 93% sensitivity, 97% specificity, 97% precision, 96% accuracy, and 96% F_1-score. They did not follow any specific protocol, and CI was not reported.

Pham [55] used transfer learning for the classification of chest x-ray COVID-19 positive from normal subjects (2 classes) and chest x-ray COVID-19 positive from normal subjects and pneumonia (3 classes) (figure 5.8). Three publicly available datasets and then their six sub-datasets were used in this study. The pre-trained AlexNet, GoogleNet, and SqueezeNet were used for classification, and the following

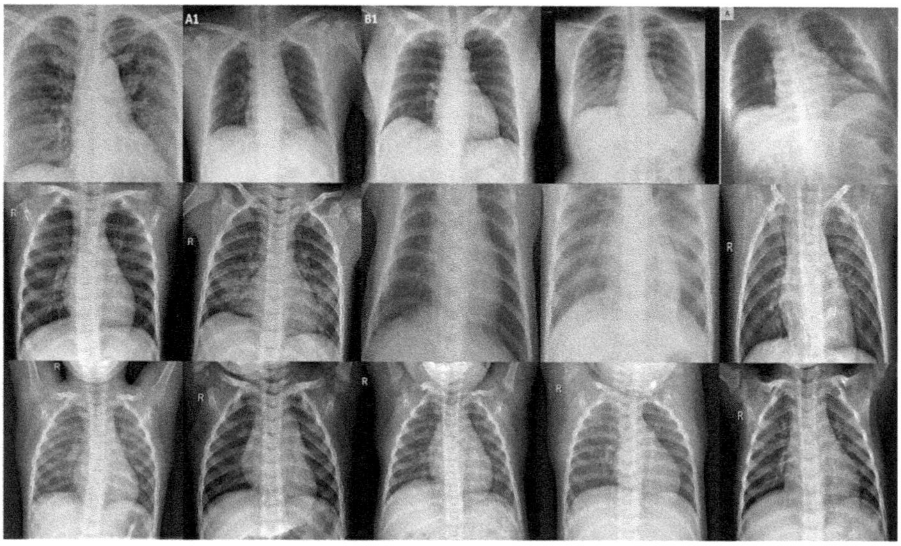

Figure 5.8. Chest x-rays from COVID-19 Radiography Database: COVID-19 (Row 1), viral pneumonia (Row 2), and normal (Row 3) (reproduced from [55] by permission from Springer Nature, copyright 2021).

metrics were reported: sensitivity, specificity, accuracy, F_1-score, precision, and AUC. The hold-out (50%) was used. No specific STARD standard was followed.

Di *et al* [56] classified chest CTs of COVID-19 from community-acquired pneumonia (CAP) with uncertainty-vertex hypergraph construction. They performed segmentation on each image for extracting the lesion area with deep learning-based networks like VB-Net and extracted features for each patient based on histogram distribution, mean and variance in the lesion area, number of the infected lesion, and also demographic variables such as sex and age. Overall, 191 features were calculated for each patient. The dataset had 3330 CT images, among which 2148 belonged to COVID-19 patients, and the remaining 1182 were from CAP patients. They used 10-fold cross-validation. They achieved 89% accuracy, 93% sensitivity, 84% specificity, 90% PPV (precision), and 88% NPV.

Wu *et al* [57] proposed a new algorithm for classifying chest CT images from normal subjects and CAP patients. They used a deep active learning method in which 30% labeled data were used. They used a subset of the CC-CCII dataset that included 962 patients (304 COVID-19, 316 pneumonia, 342 normal). Different augmentation, including affine transformation and color jittering, was used. They used 70% of the data to form an unlabeled dataset and 10% for validation, and 20% for test. First, they extracted the lung section of each image, and then they fed their network with unlabeled data. When the network could not predict the image label, it asked for the label from human experts. Their network included multiple levels of a 3D and 2D convolutional layer, pooling, and dropout. Finally, they compared their method with the state-of-the-art. They achieved 86% accuracy and 96% AUC. They did not report other metrics and did not report any CI, and also, they did not follow any specific standard.

Karakanis *et al* [58] proposed two new models: classifying chest x-ray COVID-19 from healthy control and classifying chest x-ray COVID-19 from pneumonia and healthy control subjects. They followed the protocol proposed by Maguolo and Nanni [60] and explained all their method aspects. Their implementation was published on GitHub. They used public datasets. Synthetic COVID-19 images (#130) were also generated with conditional GAN. The analyzed dataset was 275 COVID-19, 275 pneumonia, and 270 normal subjects. 80% was used for training, while 20% was used for test/validation. They reported 98.7% accuracy, 98.3% specificity, 100% sensitivity for the binary classification and 98.3% accuracy, 98.1% specificity, and 99.3% sensitivity for multi (3 classes) classification. No CI was reported for the performance indices.

5.2.6 Critical issues

Not following the critical STARD, TRIPOD, or medical data mining checklist prevents the COVID-19 diagnosis and prognosis methods' clinical application. Moreover, there are at least two other critical issues to consider.

Balancing the dataset has been used in the literature to improve the performance of the classifiers. The imbalanced datasets are very hard to deal with. For example, Ardakani *et al* [22] reported a comprehensive list of the performance indices and the hold-out validation framework (80% training, 20% test) for COVID-19 diagnosis based on the CT-image deep learning. 86 non-COVID-19 and 34 COVID-19 and patients participated in the study, and finally, 510 non-COVID-19 and 510 COVID-19 CT image patches were analyzed. In addition to the hold-out validation framework that is susceptible to testing hypotheses suggested by the data, the dataset was balanced. The disease's prevalence was not similar to the population, resulting in decreased precision, a.k.a., Positive Predictive Value (PPV), in practice. This issue can be described using the Bayes' Formula:

$$\mathrm{PPV}=\frac{\mathrm{Se}\times p}{\mathrm{Se}\times p+(1-\mathrm{Sp})\times(1-P)} \tag{5.1}$$

where Se and Sp are the sensitivity and specificity of the designed system and P is the prevalence of the disease in the population. In the study of Ardakani *et al* [22], the best method was ResNet-101 with the Se and Sp of 100% and 99.02%, which are very high. If the COVID-19 prevalence is considered 10%, PPV will be 92%. The parameter PPV is the probability that a subject has COVID-19, knowing the diagnosis method's result is positive. Such high Se and Sp values are not usually seen in the literature. Usually, Se and Sp of 80% and 95% are considered appropriate. In a similar prevalence condition, PPV will be only 64%. As a result, when the dataset is balanced, the system's performance must be very high in terms of Se and Sp. Otherwise, the system does not work as expected in practice. Such a balancing procedure was also used in other studies, such as [53].

The other issue is the quality of the peer-review procedure. Due to many submissions to the journals in the pandemic, the peer-review quality reduced,

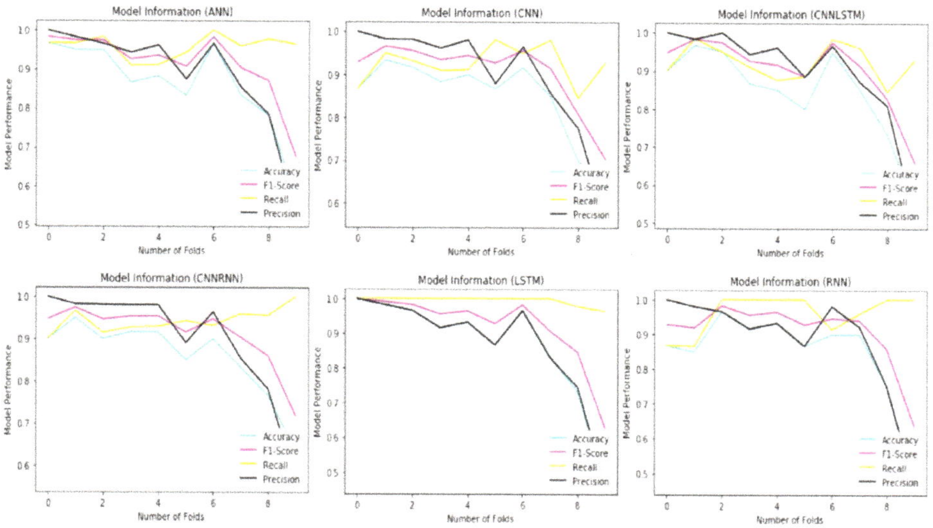

Figure 5.9. The results of deep learning models with 10-fold cross-validation (reproduced from [62], copyright 2020, with permission from Elsevier).

resulting in the retraction of approximately 45 papers when the published papers were re-analyzed by the editors [61]. Although most of the papers were medical papers, it is expected that such a retraction is extended to other multidisciplinary studies such as COVID-19 medical data mining. We provided an example for the explanation. Different deep learning algorithms were compared by Alakus and Turkoglu [62] for COVID-19 diagnosis. 80 COVID and 520 non-COVID patients were examined, and the laboratory data were recorded. Using 10-fold cross-validation, the average AUC, F1-score, accuracy, precision, and sensitivity were reported as 0.625, 91.89%, 86.66%, 86.75%, 99.42% (figure 5.9).

First, CI 95% was not reported for any performance index. It is critical for indices such as AUC (0.625 in this study). If the CI 95% includes 0.5, the user does not benefit from the diagnosis methods more than a random generator in practice. Moreover, it is necessary to report MEAN and SD of the performance indices over test folds to identify each fold's reliability. The SD values were not provided.

Moreover, the specificity of the proposed method was not provided by the authors. However, using the parameters AUC and sensitivity, the specificity of the method is approximately 26%. It is directly related to the type I error and must be reported in the paper. There is also a contradiction in one of the paper figures (figure 5.10), where the AUC of the LSTM was mentioned as 0.83. However, the ROC tells a different story. Such a number was used in other calculations, resulting in some inconsistencies in the paper. Moreover, it is not clear how the accuracy of the method is high (86.66%), knowing that most of the subjects were healthy and the specificity of the system was very low (26%). Such issues must have been identified and corrected during the peer-review procedure.

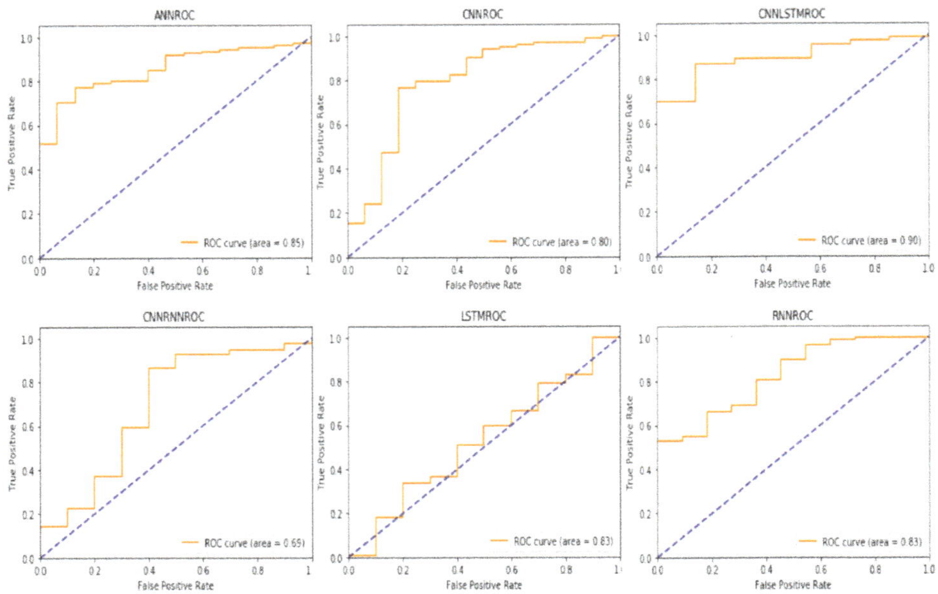

Figure 5.10. AUC values of the entire deep learning models with train-test split approach (reproduced from [62], copyright 2020, with permission from Elsevier).

5.3 Conclusion and future scope

Undoubtedly, the ML methods are valuable tools for medical data mining. However, there are some critical issues to consider to improve their visibility and clinical applications. Tables 5.1–5.4 summarized the critical STARD/TRIPOD issues that were not considered in the published papers. One reason could be that the original STARD or TRIPOD guidelines were not developed for ML and AI methods. This is why their extensions, such as TRIPOD-ML [63] and STARD-AI [64], are underway. Nevertheless, it is possible to use the critical STARD/TRIPOD checklist to improve ML methods' clinical application.

During the pandemics, many papers were published in the literature focusing on all aspects of COVID-19 diagnosis, prognosis, and long COVID. Many journals provided special issues, although some were not related to the journals' aim and scope. Inadequate peer-review procedures and the journals' rush to maintain or improve their impact factor while some clinical journals were the front runners created a situation where publishing was the main issue. Valuable research requires time, and there was no time in the race. This time, the term 'publish or perish' was completely clear. It might be a good idea to have the peer review after the publication of COVID-19 papers, where researchers could comment or discuss the published papers. Publons provided an open community review (https://publons.com/publon/covid-19/?sort_by=date). However, not all of the published COVID-19 papers were included.

Here, we provide a list of critical issues to consider for ML methods for COVID-19 diagnosis and prognosis to improve their clinical application:

- The flow diagram of the study in which the inclusion and exclusion criteria are shown must be provided.
- The sample size calculation and the sampling method must be mentioned.
- Type III error must be avoided. Using only the hold-out validation method could create this problem. Alternative solutions such as repeated hold-out or re-sampling methods are good alternatives.
- When there are repeated measurements from each patient, subject cross-validation must also be provided.
- The mean and SD of the performance indices must be reported over each test fold. A cross-validated confusion matrix could be provided, enabling the statistical comparison between different methods (i.e., the proposed method versus the state-of-the-art).
- The analyzed sample must resemble the population in terms of disease prevalence. Otherwise, the method's performance over balanced datasets must be analyzed and elaborated when using in the population.
- Proper performance indices must be provided when the dataset is imbalanced. Accuracy is a biased estimator in this case.
- A variety of performance indices must be reported. An example is providing the agreement rate between the diagnosis system's output with that of the PCR results, as there are criticisms on using PCR results as the gold standard.
- The CI 95% of the performance indices must be reported, showing the reliability of the estimation.
- Biostatistical knowledge of the biomedical engineers and those working on ML methods in medicine must be improved. An example is the importance of selecting the correct survival models and ML methods when the in-hospital prognosis is performed.

References

[1] Wise J 2021 Covid-19: The E484K mutation and the risks it poses *Brit. Med. J.* **372** n359

[2] Weiner D L, Balasubramaniam V, Shah S I and Javier J RPediatric Policy Council 2020 COVID-19 impact on research, lessons learned from COVID-19 research, implications for pediatric research *Pediatr. Res.* **88** 148–50

[3] Gonzalez T, de la Rubia M A, Hincz K P, Comas-Lopez M, Subirats L, Fort S and Sacha G M 2020 Influence of COVID-19 confinement on students' performance in higher education *PLoS One* **15** e0239490

[4] Carfì A, Bernabei R and Landi Fand Gemelli Against COVID-19 Post-Acute Care Study Group 2020 Persistent symptoms in patients after acute COVID-19 *JAMA* **324** 603–5

[5] Li W T *et al* 2020 Using machine learning of clinical data to diagnose COVID-19: a systematic review and meta-analysis *BMC Med. Inform. Dec. Mak.* **20** 247

[6] Muhammad L J, Algehyne E A, Usman S S, Ahmad A, Chakraborty C and Mohammed I A 2021 Supervised machine learning models for prediction of COVID-19 infection using epidemiology dataset *SN Comput. Sci.* **2** 11

[7] Muhammad L J, Islam M M, Usman S S and Ayon S I 2020 Predictive data mining models for novel Coronavirus (COVID-19) infected patients' recovery *SN Comput. Sci.* **1** 206

[8] Zhang T 2020 Data mining can play a critical role in COVID-19 linked mental health studies *Asian J. Psychiatr* **54** 102399

[9] Wynants L *et al* 2020 Prediction models for diagnosis and prognosis of covid-19 infection: systematic review and critical appraisal *Brit. Med. J.* **369** m1328

[10] Sperrin M, Grant S W and Peek N 2020 Prediction models for diagnosis and prognosis in Covid-19 *Brit. Med. J.* **369** m1464

[11] Glasziou P P, Sanders S and Hoffmann T 2020 Waste in COVID-19 research *Brit. Med. J.* **369** m1847

[12] Collins G S, Reitsma J B, Altman D G and moons K G M 2015 Transparent Reporting of a multivariable prediction model for Individual Prognosis or Diagnosis (TRIPOD): the TRIPOD statement *Ann. Intern. Med.* **162** 55–63

[13] Riley R D, Ensor J, Snell K I E, Harrell F E Jr, Martin G P, Reitsma J B, moons K G M, Collins G and van Smeden M 2020 Calculating the sample size required for developing a clinical prediction model *Brit. Med. J.* **368** m441

[14] Mansourian M, Marateb H R, Mansourian M, Mohebbian M R, Binder H and Mañanas M Á 2020 Rigorous performance assessment of computer-aided medical diagnosis and prognosis systems: a biostatistical perspective on data mining *Modelling and Analysis of Active Biopotential Signals in Healthcare, Volume 2* (Bristol: IOP Publishing) pp 17-1–17-24

[15] Bossuyt P M *et al*and STARD Group 2015 STARD 2015: an updated list of essential items for reporting diagnostic accuracy studies *Brit. Med. J.* **351** h5527

[16] Chicco D and Jurman G 2020 The advantages of the Matthews correlation coefficient (MCC) over F1 score and accuracy in binary classification evaluation *BMC Genom.* **21** 6

[17] Li L *et al* 2020 Using artificial intelligence to detect COVID-19 and community-acquired pneumonia based on pulmonary CT: evaluation of the diagnostic accuracy *Radiology* **296** E65–71

[18] Yuan M, Yin W, Tao Z, Tan W and Hu Y 2020 Association of radiologic findings with mortality of patients infected with 2019 novel coronavirus in Wuhan, China *PLoS One* **15** e0230548

[19] Laguarta J, Hueto F and Subirana B 2020 COVID-19 artificial intelligence diagnosis using only cough recordings *IEEE Open J. Eng. Med. Biol.* **1** 275–81

[20] Hu S *et al* 2020 Weakly supervised deep learning for COVID-19 infection detection and classification from CT images *IEEE Access* **8** 118869–83

[21] Apostolopoulos I D and Mpesiana T A 2020 Covid-19: automatic detection from X-ray images utilizing transfer learning with convolutional neural networks *Phys. Eng. Sci. Med.* **43** 635–40

[22] Ardakani A A, Kanafi A R, Acharya U R, Khadem N and Mohammadi A 2020 Application of deep learning technique to manage COVID-19 in routine clinical practice using CT images: results of 10 convolutional neural networks *Comput. Biol. Med.* **121** 103795

[23] Apostolopoulos I D, Aznaouridis S I and Tzani M A 2020 Extracting possibly representative COVID-19 biomarkers from X-ray images with deep learning approach and image data related to pulmonary diseases *J. Med. Biol. Eng* **40** 1–8

[24] Hasan A M, Al-Jawad M M, Jalab H A, Shaiba H, Ibrahim R W and Al-Shamasneh A R 2020 Classification of covid-19 Coronavirus, pneumonia and healthy lungs in CT scans using Q-deformed entropy and deep learning features *Entropy (Basel)* **22** 517

[25] Hurt B, Kligerman S and Hsiao A 2020 Deep learning localization of pneumonia: 2019 Coronavirus (COVID-19) outbreak *J. Thorac. Imag.* **35** W87–9

[26] Khan A I, Shah J L and Bhat M M 2020 CoroNet: a deep neural network for detection and diagnosis of COVID-19 from chest X-ray images *Comput. Methods Programs Biomed.* **196** 105581
[27] Khanday A M U D, Rabani S T, Khan Q R, Rouf N and Din M M U 2020 Machine learning based approaches for detecting COVID-19 using clinical text data *Int. J. Inf. Technol.* **12** 1–9
[28] Ko H *et al* 2020 COVID-19 pneumonia diagnosis using a simple 2D deep learning framework with a single chest CT image: model development and validation *J. Med. Internet Res.* **22** e19569
[29] Ucar F and Korkmaz D 2020 COVIDiagnosis-Net: Deep Bayes-SqueezeNet based diagnosis of the coronavirus disease 2019 (COVID-19) from X-ray images *Med. Hypotheses* **140** 109761
[30] Singh D, Kumar V, Vaishali and Kaur M 2020 Classification of COVID-19 patients from chest CT images using multi-objective differential evolution-based convolutional neural networks *Eur. J. Clin. Microbiol. Infect. Dis* **39** 1379–89
[31] Goodman-Meza D *et al* 2020 A machine learning algorithm to increase COVID-19 inpatient diagnostic capacity *PLoS One* **15** e0239474
[32] Zhao Z, Chen A, Hou W, Graham J M, Li H, Richman P S, Thode H C, Singer A J and Duong T Q 2020 Prediction model and risk scores of ICU admission and mortality in COVID-19 *PLoS One* **15** e0236618
[33] Banerjee A, Ray S, Vorselaars B, Kitson J, Mamalakis M, Weeks S, Baker M and Mackenzie L S 2020 Use of machine learning and artificial intelligence to predict SARS-CoV-2 infection from full blood counts in a population *Int. Immunopharmacol.* **86** 106705
[34] Burdick H *et al* 2020 Prediction of respiratory decompensation in Covid-19 patients using machine learning: the READY trial *Comput. Biol. Med.* **124** 103949
[35] Cai W, Liu T, Xue X, Luo G, Wang X, Shen Y, Fang Q, Sheng J, Chen F and Liang T 2020 CT quantification and machine-learning models for assessment of disease severity and prognosis of COVID-19 patients *Acad. Radiol.* **27** 1665–78
[36] Liang W *et al* 2020 Early triage of critically ill COVID-19 patients using deep learning *Nat. Commun.* **11** 3543
[37] Ma X *et al* 2020 Development and validation of prognosis model of mortality risk in patients with COVID-19 *Epidemiol. Infect.* **148** e168
[38] Sun L *et al* 2020 Combination of four clinical indicators predicts the severe/critical symptom of patients infected COVID-19 *J. Clin. Virol.* **128** 104431
[39] Wu G, Zhou S, Wang Y, Lv W, Wang S, Wang T and Li X 2020 A prediction model of outcome of SARS-CoV-2 pneumonia based on laboratory findings *Sci. Rep.* **10** 14042
[40] Zhou L *et al* 2020 A rapid, accurate and machine-agnostic segmentation and quantification method for CT-based COVID-19 diagnosis *IEEE Trans. Med. Imag.* **39** 2638–52
[41] Subudhi S, Verma A and Patel A B 2020 Prognostic machine learning models for COVID-19 to facilitate decision making *Int. J. Clin. Pract* **74** e13685
[42] Sotoudeh H, Tasorian B, Tabatabaei S M, Sotoudeh E and Moini A 2020 The feasibility of transfer learning for differentiation H1N1 Influenza from COVID-19 on chest CT *Res. Square* https://doi.org/10.21203/rs.3.rs-40907/v1
[43] Dunne R, Morris T and Harper S 2020 High accuracy classification of COVID-19 coughs using Mel-frequency cepstral coefficients and a convolutional neural network with a use case for smart home devices *Res. Square* https://doi.org/10.21203/rs.3.rs-63796/v1

[44] Oulefki A, Agaian S, Trongtirakul T and Kassah Laouar A 2021 Automatic COVID-19 lung infected region segmentation and measurement using CT-scans images *Pattern Recognit.* **114** 107747
[45] Javor D, Kaplan H, Kaplan A, Puchner S B, Krestan C and Baltzer P 2020 Deep learning analysis provides accurate COVID-19 diagnosis on chest computed tomography *Eur. J. Radiol.* **133** 109402
[46] Nath M K, Kanhe A and Mishra M 2020 A novel deep learning approach for classification of COVID-19 images *2020 IEEE 5th Int. Conf. on Computing Communication and Automation (ICCCA)* (Piscataway, NJ: IEEE)
[47] Wang L, Lin Z Q and Wong A 2020 COVID-Net: a tailored deep convolutional neural network design for detection of COVID-19 cases from chest X-ray images *Sci. Rep.* **10** 19549
[48] Gao K *et al* 2021 Dual-branch combination network (DCN): towards accurate diagnosis and lesion segmentation of COVID-19 using CT images *Med. Image Anal.* **67** 101836
[49] Arvind V, Kim J S, Cho B H, Geng E and Cho S K 2020 Development of a machine learning algorithm to predict intubation among hospitalized patients with COVID-19 *J. Crit. Care* **62** 25–30
[50] Nayak S R, Nayak D R, Sinha U, Arora V and Pachori R B 2021 Application of deep learning techniques for detection of COVID-19 cases using chest X-ray images: a comprehensive study *Biomed. Signal Process. Control* **64** 102365
[51] Chao H *et al* 2021 Integrative analysis for COVID-19 patient outcome prediction *Med. Image Anal.* **67** 101844
[52] Canayaz M 2021 MH-COVIDNet: Diagnosis of COVID-19 using deep neural networks and meta-heuristic-based feature selection on X-ray images *Biomed. Signal Process. Control* **64** 102257
[53] Saha P, Sadi M S and Islam M M 2021 EMCNet: automated COVID-19 diagnosis from X-ray images using convolutional neural network and ensemble of machine learning classifiers *Inform. Med. Unlocked* **22** 100505
[54] Panahi A H, Rafiei A and Rezaee A 2021 FCOD: fast COVID-19 detector based on deep learning techniques *Inform. Med. Unlocked* **22** 100506
[55] Pham T D 2021 Classification of COVID-19 chest X-rays with deep learning: new models or fine tuning? *Health Inf. Sci. Syst* **9** 2
[56] Di D *et al* 2021 Hypergraph learning for identification of COVID-19 with CT imaging *Med. Image Anal.* **68** 101910
[57] Wu X, Chen C, Zhong M, Wang J and Shi J 2021 COVID-AL: the diagnosis of COVID-19 with deep active learning *Med. Image Anal.* **68** 101913
[58] Karakanis S and Leontidis G 2020 Lightweight deep learning models for detecting COVID-19 from chest X-ray images *Comput. Biol. Med.* **130** 104181
[59] Zoabi Y, Deri-Rozov S and Shomron N 2021 Machine learning-based prediction of COVID-19 diagnosis based on symptoms *NPJ Digit. Med* **4** 3
[60] Maguolo G and Nanni L 2020 A critic evaluation of methods for COVID-19 automatic detection from X-Ray images *Inform. Fusion* **76** 1–7
[61] Cortegiani A, Catalisano G, Ippolito M, Giarratano A, Absalom A R and Einav S 2021 Retracted papers on SARS-CoV-2 and COVID-19 *Br. J. Anaesth.*
[62] Alakus T B and Turkoglu I 2020 Comparison of deep learning approaches to predict COVID-19 infection *Chaos Solitons Fractals* **140** 110120

[63] Collins G S and moons K G M 2019 Reporting of artificial intelligence prediction models *Lancet* **393** 1577–9

[64] Sounderajah V *et al* 2020 Developing specific reporting guidelines for diagnostic accuracy studies assessing AI interventions: the STARD-AI Steering Group *Nat. Med.* **26** 807–8

Chapter 6

Forecasting confirmed cases of Corona patients in India using regression and Gaussian analysis

Dhyan Chandra Yadav and Saurabh Pal

Corona virus is a major threat for human life leading to a very deadly life-threatening disease. The infection of this disease is so fast that in a very short span of time it took the whole world under its infection. In this chapter, we analyze the growing dataset of COVID-19 from 30 Jan 2020 to 9 July 2020 and estimate confirmed Covid positive cases and patient deaths.

The cases of this disease originated from Wuhan of China and the exact reason for the origin of this disease has not been explained to date. Experts are constantly experimenting to control this disease in the medical field, but to date no effective medicine to cure the disease immediately has been available. Four different functional models have been utilized for Covid data analysis of Indian Covid patients accessed from Kaggle. In this chapter, we have used linear, logarithmic, polynomial and Gaussian functional models for a COVID-19 dataset.

According to these models, we forecast the number of patients and death for Corona disease for the subsequent 120 days from the actual position of Covid cases at the end of Oct 2020 in India. After the analysis we find the polynomial function model is a very impressive model for forecasting. In this study, we find Covid infection grew in the next 120 days in India.

With the help of the prediction obtained from this research, the Indian Government can take preventive measures for controlling Corona disease such as lockdown and implementing social distancing. Another benefit is to develop medical facilities for providing for such a huge number of patients.

6.1 Introduction

Corona viruses are a complex chain of viruses that generate illness in the human body such as respiratory diseases. The respiratory diseases are mainly two of types:

- Middle East Respiratory Syndrome (MERS-CoV);
- Severe Acute Respiratory Syndrome (SARS-CoV).

A novel corona virus (nCoV) or COVID-19 is a new chain of virus previously unidentified in humans.

'Middle East Respiratory Syndrome' was determined to have been transmitted from dromedary camels to humans and Severe Acute Respiratory Syndrome from civet cats to humans. These two syndromes were determined by various experiments but the novel viruses are not easily identified.

In general, clinically Corona viruses present some symptoms in the infected person but some will not display symptoms. Some symptoms may include:

- respiratory symptoms;
- feeling high fever;
- feeling hard or dry cough;
- trouble with breathing;
- obesity;
- liver damage;
- complexity in chest function.

The World Health Organization (WHO) provide advice or suggestions to people that are at a higher risk of getting severe COVID-19 disease. This includes people who are suffering in old age with serious chronic illnesses such as:

- diabetes;
- cardiovascular disease;
- chronic respiratory disease;
- cancer;
- hypertension;
- chronic liver disease.

The WHO makes suggestions for social care and health protection if any signs and symptoms of COVID-19 illness appear in a healthcare facility.

The WHO suggests preventative measures to protect against the new corona virus such as:

- being up to date on the latest information with COVID-19;
- frequent hand hygiene;
- avoiding touching your body parts;
- use of a medical mask for hands and face;
- keeping social distance from individuals with respiratory symptoms.

They advise people not to avoid but to seek medical care if any illness symptoms appears such as: fever, cough and difficulty breathing. The Ministry of Health and Family Welfare reported in total 767 296 confirmed cases, 495 413 recoveries and 21 129 deaths in India [*mohfw.gov.in*, June 2020]. Although the number of deaths in India is less than China and America, the number of cases of corona-affected people is the highest in Asia [*Hindustan Times, May* 2020]. The government has taken various kinds of decisions to prevent the spread of corona virus infection in India. Symptoms occur only 2 to 14 days after the person is exposed to the virus. These include fever, cough, frequent breathlessness, feeling of excessive difficulty in breathing, feeling of cold, cold as well as insidiousness, muscle pain and tightness, frequent headache, increased sore throat and reduced taste and smell [1]. Covid infection is a dangerous disease for human life. The COVID-19 infection is caused by severe acute respiratory syndrome coronavirus2. The first Covid infected person in India was detected on 30 January 2020. On 22 March, voluntary public curfew for 24 h was followed by the country's residents, and on 24 March the lockdown order was established by the government to last for 21 days. The lockdown order was continued from 14 April to 3 May, then from 3 to 17 May the government allowed some relaxation for people, thus from 1 June the government started the process of lock and unlock in three phases [2, 3]. The WHO and the United Nations have described this as a commendable step to remove infection spread in the country. On 21, 22 and 23 June, India was ranked 56th by the Deep Knowledge Group, out of 200 countries. On 12 January 2020, the corona virus had been caused by respiratory disease in people living in China, which had been reported to the WHO on 31 December 2019 [4, 5]. On 30 January, the first person suffering from Covid infection was confirmed in Kerala, which increased to three new cases by 3 February. On 4 March, 22 new cases were found to be Covid positive, in which 14 new cases were reported by one tourist group in the month of March returning from abroad. A large number of Covid infections spread due to Sikh celebrations in areas like Punjab [6–8]. Similarly, on 31 March, the incident of Tabligi Jamaat religious congregation in Delhi became a big incident. After this incident, 4291 cases of Covid infection were reported [9, 10]. On May, 1225 new cases were reported in Punjab in returning pilgrims from Maharashtra, as a result of which the provision of the Epidemic Diseases Act 1897 came into force in more than a dozen states and union territories. As a result, educational and commercial establishments were temporarily closed and all tourist visas were revoked and canceled [11].We have represented the state details in India for Covid infection and observed the infection position in each state.

From figure 6.1 it is clear that Maharashtra, the West, Gujarat, Tamil, Bihar, Madhya, Delhi, Uttar Pradesh and some other states have highly infected patients while Uttarakhand, Himanchal, Ladakh with some other states have fewer infected patients.

From figure 6.2, it is clear that Maharashtra, Kernataka, Kerala and Uttar Pradesh and some other states have confirmed Indian national patients compared to Uttarakhand, Himanchal, Ladakh etc, states.

From figure 6.3, it is clear that the states Rajasthan and Hariyana have highly infected foreign national patients while Uttarakhand, Himanchal, Ladakh with some other states have fewer foreign national patients.

We have observed persons cured of Covid infection in each state and find Maharashtra, Gujrat, Rajsthan, Tamil, Madhya, Delhi and Uttar Pradesh have high numbers of cured persons compared to other states. In figure 6.4, we have predicted deaths by Covid infection in each state and find highest deaths in Maharashtra, Gujrat, Rajsthan, Madhya, Delhi and Uttar Pradesh.

In this dataset confirmed cases, final death and new cases are described as: new cases = total cases – (total cases of previous days), we have aggregated all the states of India and find major differences between head level analysis and tail level

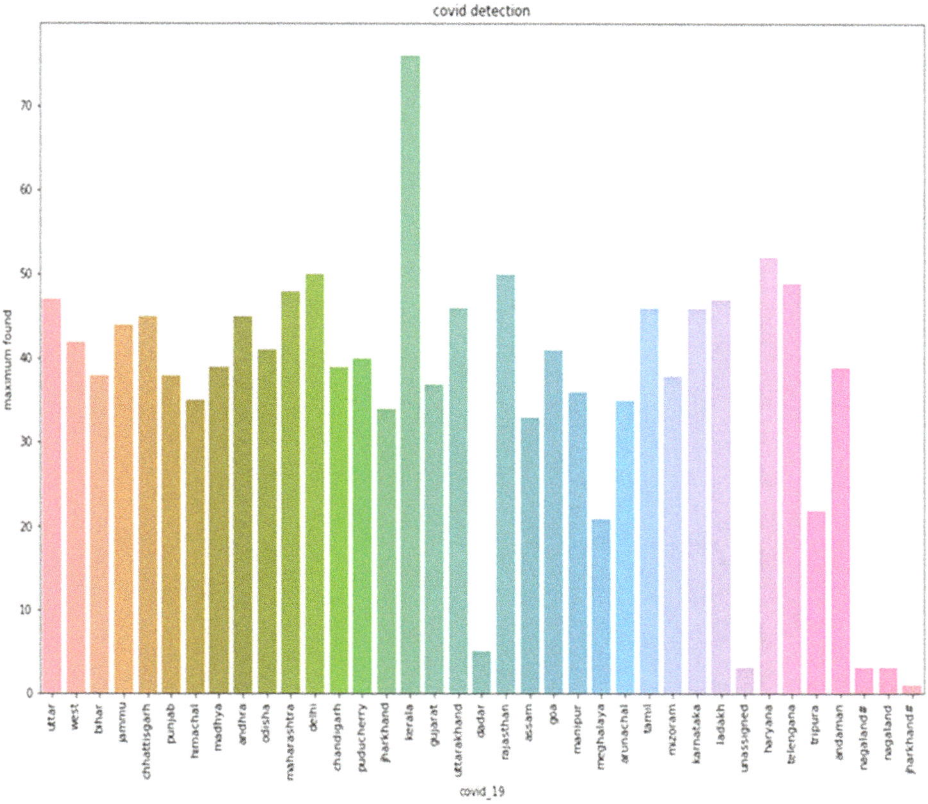

Figure 6.1. Representation of Covid infected patients with state details in India.

prediction. From table 6.1, it is clear that initially we find final deaths and new cases as: 0 and 0–1 increase, respectively.

With the results, it is clear that table 6.2 finds high deaths and new cases due to grow for each day. We have predicted head level from 2020–01–30 to 2020–02–03 and tail level from 2020–07–05 to 2020–07–09.

6.2 Regression analysis in machine learning

Regression machine learning techniques generate a relationship between target and predictor variables. The role of this technique is to generate a time series model find future outcomes from a variable relationship and fit a curve/line to the variables. It provides a significant relationship and strength of impact between variables.

The regression model is a subpart of machine learning. The regression model estimated how strong was the relationship between dependable and one or more independable variables. Machine learning provides a relationship between variables by different functional models. A linear function model generates continuous outcome variables ($f(x)$) for given values of x. These variables make a linear relationship between outcome and given variables [29]. The exponential function

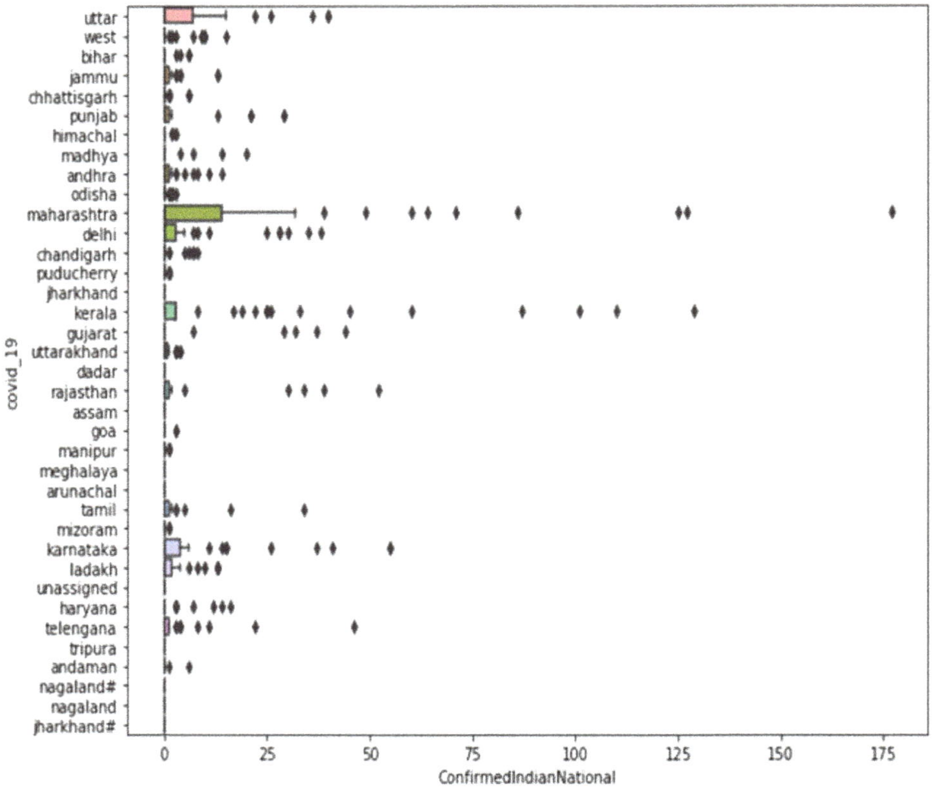

Figure 6.2. Representation of Covid confirmed Indian national patients in India.

measures the growth of population of Covid infected persons. In this chapter we have learned the relationship between the variables of Covid infection. The main purpose of regression function analysis is that the fit of the given regression model means that it should be better than the fit of the mean model. Machine learning can help in decision making to control this disease. Regression functional analysis of COVID-19 disease finds the spread of disease in the next 120 days.

In this section, we propose five regression based models known as linear regression, logarithmic regression, polynomial regression and Gaussian regression methods. The descriptions of these models are given in the equations below:

$$f(x) = a + b \times x \tag{6.1}$$

where a is called the intercept on Y-axis and b is called slope of the line. These two parameters provide help in functional analysis.

$$f(x) = a \log(x) + b \tag{6.2}$$

$$f(x) = ax^3 + bx^2 + cx + d \tag{6.3}$$

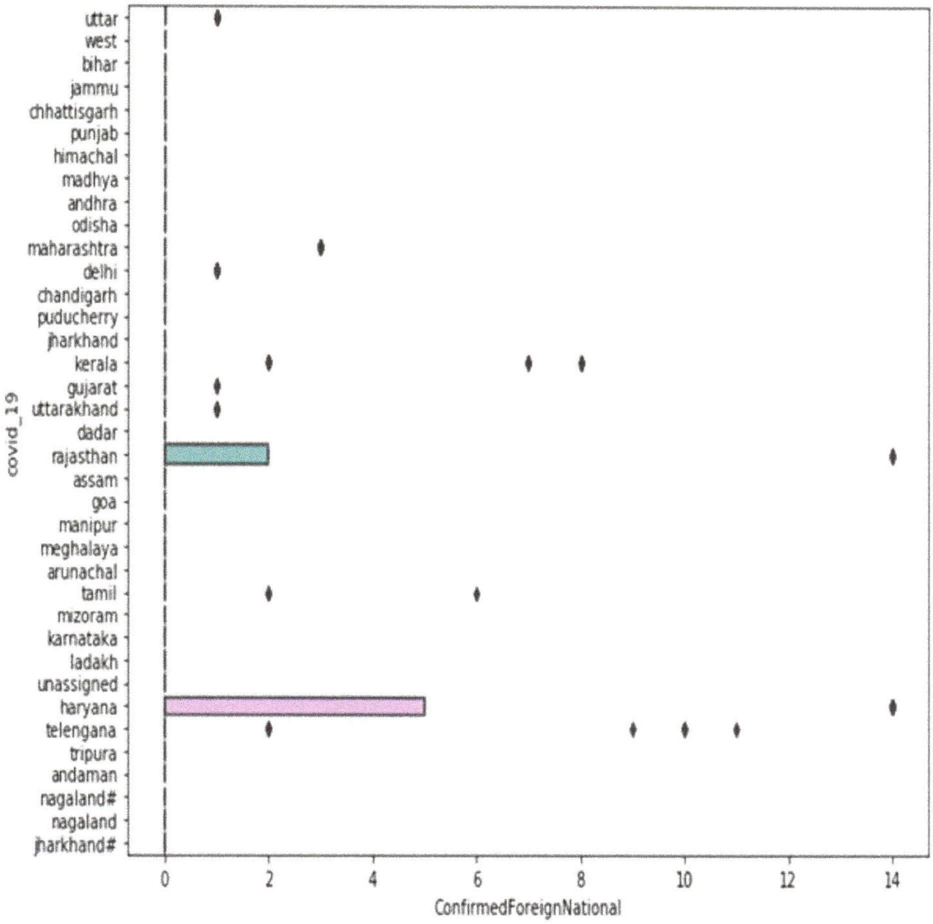

Figure 6.3. Representation of Covid confirmed foreign national patients in India.

The Gaussian regression model calculates the probability distribution of parameters or overall admissible functions that fit the data.

$$f(x) = a + e^{\wedge}\left(-0.5 \times \left(\frac{(x - \mu)}{\sigma^{**}2}\right)\right) \tag{6.4}$$

In statistics, the coefficients of determination are denoted $R2$, the main objective of $R2$ analysis of future outcomes on the basis of relevance feature or testing of the variance by standard ranges from 0 to 1. $R2$ shows how well data points used fit the curve or line. If we use more unnecessary or useless variables then it will decrease. By adjusting $R2$ data points will be added to increase efficiency.

$$(\mathrm{Adj})R2 = 1 - \left[\frac{(1 - R2)(n - 1)}{n - k - 1}\right] \tag{6.5}$$

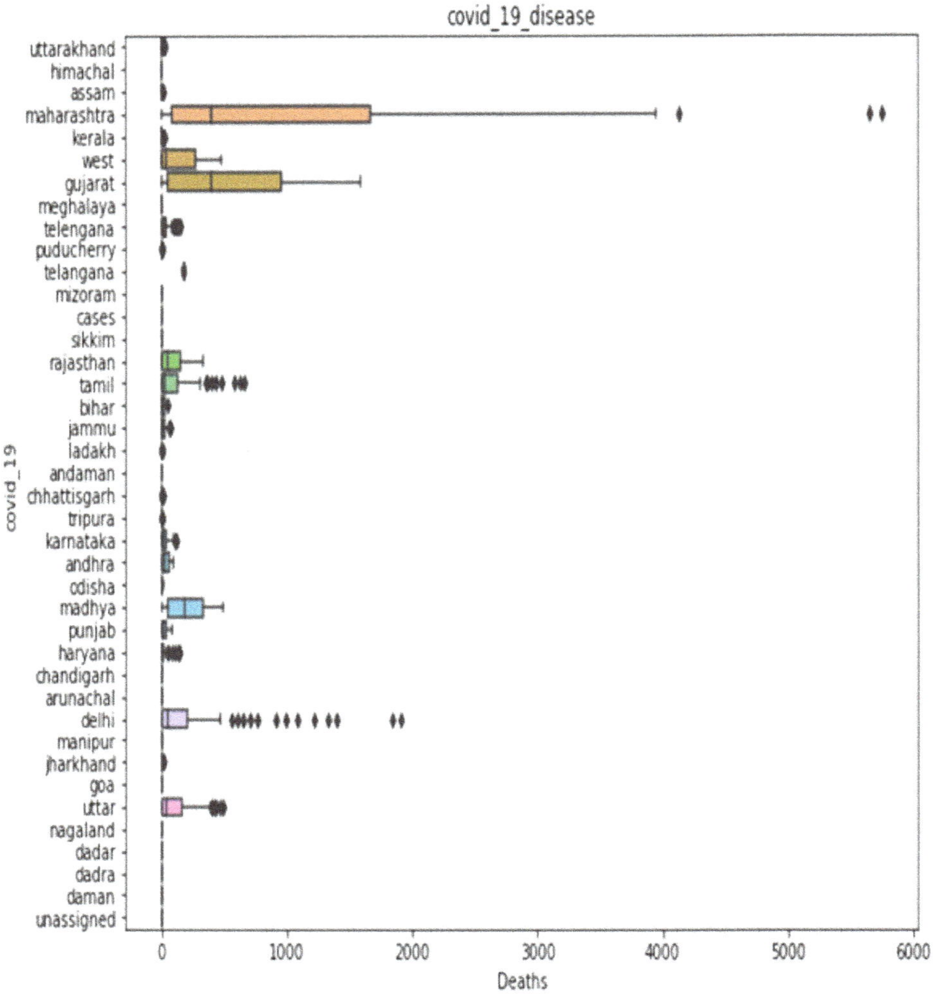

Figure 6.4. Representation of deaths cases by Covid infected patients with state details in India.

where,

- n is the data instances with attributes.
- K is the number of independent regressors.

$$R2 = 1 - \left(\frac{\text{SS regression}}{\text{SS total}}\right) \tag{6.6}$$

where,

- SS regression = sum of squared regression error
- SS total = sum of total error

Equations (6.1)–(6.6) have been taken for better estimates in COVID-19 disease [12–14]. In figure 6.5 the box represents cured patient details by higher and lower level.

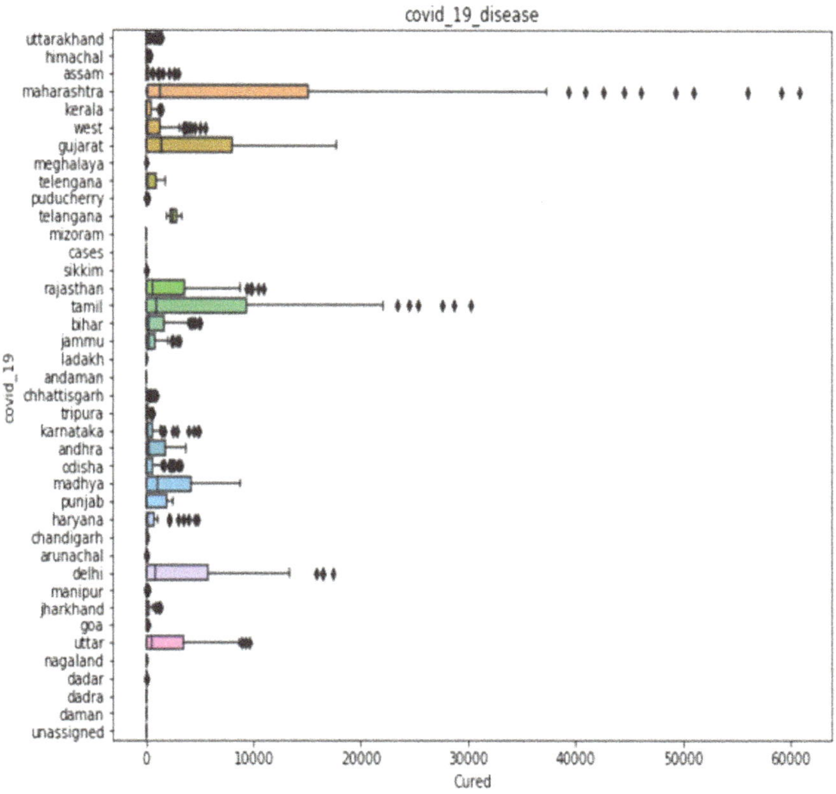

Figure 6.5. Representation of cured patients with state details in India by higher and lower level box plot.

Table 6.1. Representation of computational table for head model of Covid infection.

Date	Confirmed	Final death	new
2020–01–30	1	0	0.0
2020–01–31	1	0	0.0
2020–02–01	2	0	1.0
2020–02–02	3	0	1.0
2020–02–03	3	0	0.0

Table 6.2. Representation of computational table for tail model of Covid infection.

Sl. No.	Date	Confirmed	Final death
158	2020–07–05	673 165	19 268
159	2020–07–06	697 413	19 693
160	2020–07–07	719 665	20 160
161	2020–07–08	742 417	20 642
162	2020–07–09	767 296	21 129

6.3 Related work

The number of confirmed COVID-19 cases by machine learning algorithms was discussed in one study. They used a K-Means machine learning algorithm based on disease prevalence, air population metrics, and healthy system courage to analyse country data. The authors created a model for 155 countries using three PCA parameters and six clusters to show the relevance of group countries [15]. In another research the authors analyzed COVID-19 incidence of Google trends by data mining and deep learning. They used linear regression and long–short-term model to detect the incidence of COVID-19 actual cases. The authors calculated the values of RMSE 7.562 (SD 6.492) and the RMSE of the LSTM 27.187 (SD 28.705) [16]. Other researchers computed the growth and trend of COVID-19 by machine learning and cloud computing. They predicted COVID-19 disease by mathematical model, machine learning and cloud computing on the basis of baseline. The authors proposed the Robust Weibull model and predicted better than baseline [17]. Machine learning algorithms were used to analyse the COVID-19 epidemic in India. The author calculated root mean square error using six regression analysis-based machine learning algorithms models. For forecasting over long time intervals, the author discovered that a 6° polynomial model calculated a significantly lower root mean square error (RMSE) (the standard deviation of the residuals (prediction errors)) [18]. Another research team predicted a comparative analysis of machine learning with soft computing (multilayered perception, adaptive neural network, fuzzy system and ANFIS) for COVID-19. The authors used SIR (susceptible, infectious, recovered) and SEIR (susceptible, exposed, infectious, recovered) models that help for COVID-19 discovery for outlook and found SEIR performed better [19]. The research team analyzed the COVID-19 outbreak in India and used SEIR with a regression model. The authors calculated the values of RMSE for the SEIR model and they found the SEIR model widely predicted the COVID-19 data compared to the regression model. Pandey *et al* measured the values of RMSE 1.52 for SEIR and 1.75 for the regression model [20]. The researchers measured healthy policy in each country by time and intensity in COVID-19. They used deep reinforcement learning and finally they found higher intensity lockdown and travel restrictions public health interventions during COVID-19 [21]. Rustam *et al* discussed forecasting by machine learning to decision making on future courses of action. They used linear regression, Lasso, support vector machine and exponential smoothing in COVID-19 forecasting. Finally, they found exponential smoothing performs best results compare to other algorithms [22]. Wang *et al* discussed COVID-19 infection with symptoms and the effect of infection on the human body. They found the effects of infection are greater in men than women, and no deaths were reported between the ages of 0 and 9 [23]. Other authors considered several cases of pneumonia with unfamiliar etiology in china. The National Health Commission of China reported details on viral pneumonia [24]. The researchers analyzed the details of the novel corona virus and diagnosis of corona virus infection in China. The National Health Commission visited a sea food market and released details of the infected animals, birds and other food sources. After analyzing the infected person details, the commission provided details of human capacity for the virus and exposed infection symptoms with the spread of infection penetrating human lungs through the nose or mouth [25–28]. Authors discussed the origination and transmission of corona virus source. Some authors have studied research work on SARS-CoV and found they focused on raccoons, dogs and palm civets for corona infection [29]. Guan *et al* observed the clinical characteristics of corona virus in China. They considered laboratory confirmed reports of COVID-19 and the patient's status, their death, ventilation and ICU requirements [30]. Ai *et al* discussed the correlation of chest and reverse transcription polymerase chain reaction (RT-PCR) testing in COVID-19 in China. They analyzed blood samples for RT-PCR because without this reaction the authors did not identify virus or risk of infection in patients [31]. Shi and Hu analyzed the risk factors for mortality of adult in-patients in the case of COVID-19. They considered COVID-19 adult patients from Jiny Intan Hospital and Wuhan Pulmonary Hospital in Wuhan, China. They found deaths and disclosed patient details. They used logistic regression to find current smoker versus non-smoker patients [32]. Huang *et al* discussed clinical features of patients infected with COVID-19. They found 41 discharges, 6 deaths and 3 patients in ICU from 16 Dec 2019 to 22 Jan 2020 [33]. Liu *et al* considered factors in COVID-19 disease in hospitalized patients. They found positive/negative and disease progression from 30 Dec 2019 to 15 Jan 2020. They found 11 COVID patients in progress, 67 patients in improvement with 2 deaths negative. They used multivariate logistic regression and calculated the research factor for smokers (OR = 14.28; 95% Cl; 1.58–00; P = 0.018) [34]. One group of authors discussed MERS with Pipistrellus and Perimyotis bats. They found that bats work as a key host and transmitting medium to spread the virus. Another research team analyzed some corona virus cases and found snakes to be a possible host. They compared the similarity of novel corona virus with SARS-like bat virus and found bats could be key reservoirs [35, 36]. Yadav and Pal discussed clinical characteristics of 138 hospital patients with epidemiological clinical characteristics of 99 cases and early transmission dynamics to spread of the disease imminent. They identified infection, quarantine and treatment procedures. The authors discussed COVID-19 symptoms and viral pneumonia. They found non-specified symptoms and revealed chest CT scan pneumonia and a pathogenic test for virus came back positive [37]. Machine learning classification algorithms and regression algorithms have evaluated classification accuracy and variables relationship for future outcomes on various medical datasets [38–44].

6.4 Methodology

In this stage, we have arranged various sections as follows: section 6.2 discussed the dataset and applied linear, exponential, logistic and Gaussian functional models. Sections 6.5 and 6.6 cover the results and discussion and section 6.7 contains the final conclusion.

6.4.1 Data description

In this chapter, we have organized COVID-19 Indian patients' dataset from Kaggle with data word open access website. The COVID-19 dataset contains 3244 instances with 3 attributes from 30 Jan 2020 to 9 July 2020 and estimates confirmed COVID positive cases and patients' deaths in each state of India.

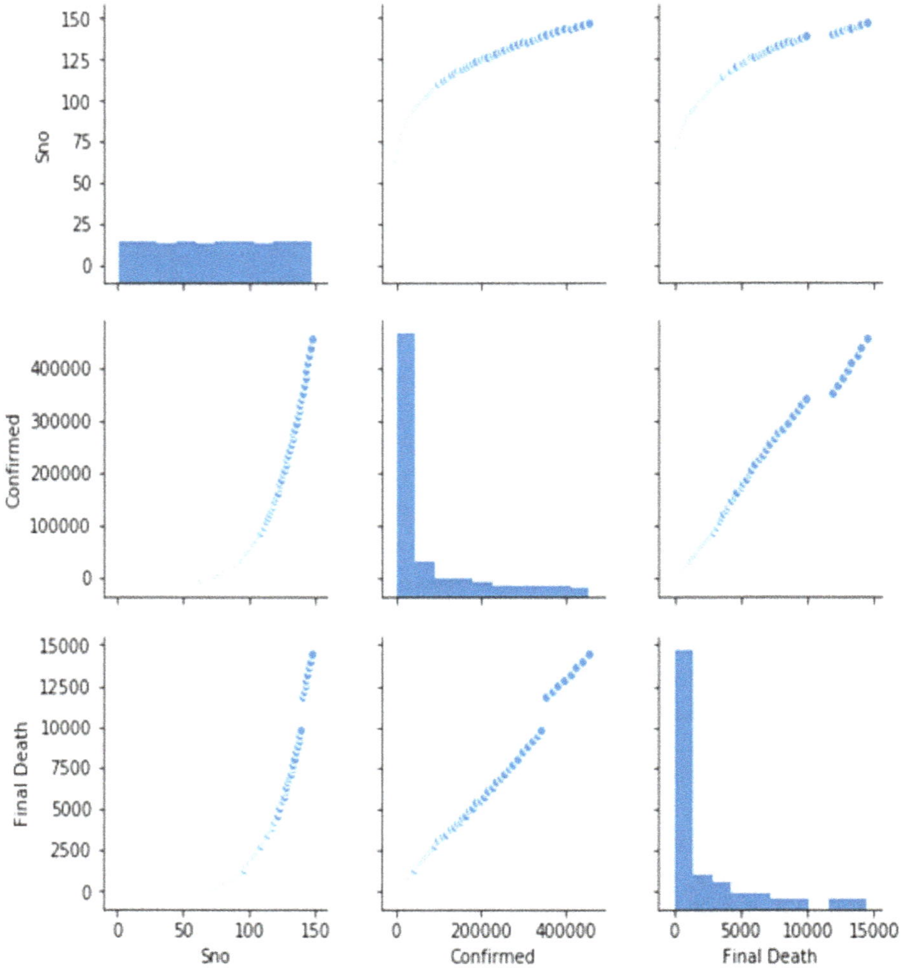

Figure 6.6. Representation of COVID-19 selected attributes distributions between each variable.

In figure 6.6 we represent COVID-19 selected attributes distributions between each variable. The *X*- and *Y*-axis represents attributes names. In order to understand which data they include, check left and bottom axis names in pair plot bar chart.

6.5 Results

Now we have predicted and plotted Covid case series by blue points and three models defined by three different colors red, yellow and black. The red color for linear function of total Covid infection cases, black color for logarithmic function of total Covid infection cases and yellow color for polynomial function (three orders) of total Covid infection cases. These models represent continuous increase of Covid infection cases in each date or growth time in each state and if the growth is stopped

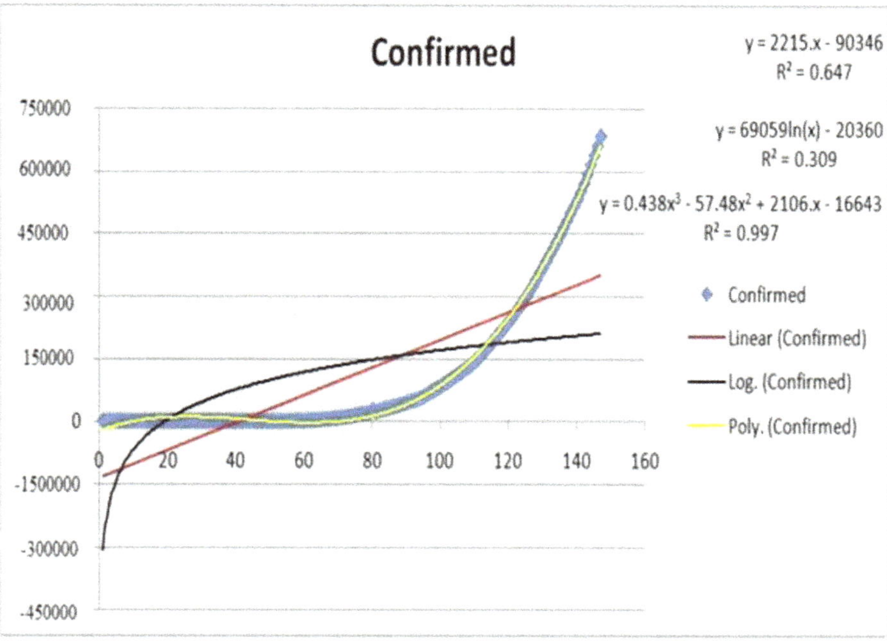

Figure 6.7. Representation of the linear, logarithmic and polynomial regression models for best fitting the growth curve of Covid infection with time.

the curve will be flat. From figure 6.7, we find the polynomial regression model is more suitable among them.

In this study, we used the regression model to estimate confirmed cases of COVID-19. We have used linear, logarithmic and polynomial regression models for best fitting curve. These regression models generate equations for different parameters of COVID-19 dataset and calculate confirmed Covid cases due to no. of days. The proposed functional model is calculated as:

$$y = 2215 \times x - 90346 \quad R^2 = 0.647 \tag{6.7}$$

$$y = 69059 \ln(x) - 20360 \quad R^2 = 0.309 \tag{6.8}$$

$$y = 0.438x^3 - 57.48x^2 + 2106 \times x - 16643 \quad R^2 = 0.997 \tag{6.9}$$

Equations 6.7–6.9 represent linear, logarithmic and polynomial regression models for best fitting curve. Equation (6.7), represents the linear regression model by high parameter values with low $R2$ values ($R2 < 1$) and equation (6.8), represents that the logarithmic regression model is very poor because it has major deviation from the best fit line/curve. In equation (6.9), we find the three-order polynomial regression model measured better results compared with equations (6.7) and (6.8); the three-order polynomial regression model represents high $R2$ value near 1.

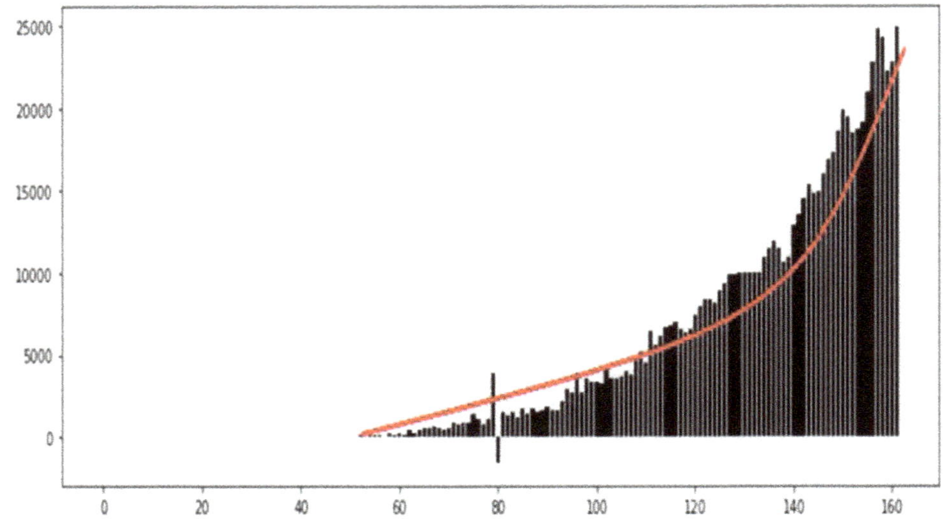

Figure 6.8. Representation of actual data plotted by (black) bar and Gaussian function (red lines).

Now we switch the new cases for random parameter visualization and minimize the fitting errors. The actual data is plotted by black bars and the Gaussian function by red lines. With the results, we find continuous increase in new Covid infection cases with time as shown in figure 6.8.

6.6 Discussion

Now we have used the logistic regression model as a combined model of linear, logarithmic and polynomial regression models for the final forecasting model of Covid infection daily increased cases. The logistic regression model is proposed for future analysis in this experiment. We used two different models for the same dataset, one for major differences between increased times(days) such as: 0–50, 50–100, 100–150, 150–200 etc, and find more than 700 000 infected Covid cases took 160 days, after that the functional model forecasted continuous increase of Covid infection from 700 000 to 1 500 000 with increased time from 162 to 300 days. This shows that number of Covid patients will double within 1 month (figure 6.9).

In another model, we have predicted for minor difference between number of days such as: 0–25, 25–50, 50–75 etc, and found near 700 000 infected Covid cases took between 150 and 200 days, after that the functional model forecasted continuous increase of Covid infection from 700 000 to 1 500 000 with increased time from 160 to 225 days (figure 6.10).

6.7 Conclusion

In this chapter, the COVID-19 dataset contains 3244 instances with 3 attributes from 30 Jan 2020 to 9 July 2020 and estimated confirmed Covid positive cases and patients' deaths in each state of India. We concluded the actual data plotted by black

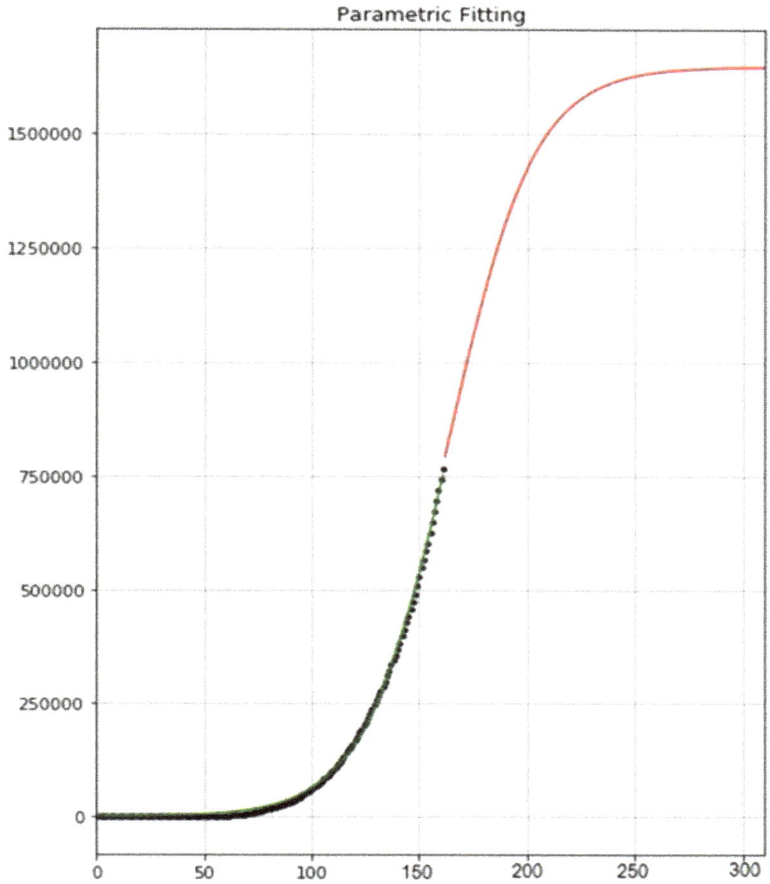

Figure 6.9. Representation of model (green) and forecasting (red) for current and future growth of Covid infection.

bar and Gaussian function by red lines. With the results, we find continuous increase of new Covid infection cases with time. All the measurement was done by linear, logarithmic and polynomial models. We find the polynomial regression model with order three performs better compared to linear and logarithmic regression models. So the polynomial regression model measured forecast for future Covid infection status in India. From the above prediction, we find the polynomial function model is more suitable among them because it has provided more suitable curve fitting compared to the other functional models. We found Covid infection will continuously increase for the next 300 days then it will remain under control, and near 1 600 000 patients will be sick by Covid infection. According to the model the increment rate will be down after 300 days in India. The functional model we have prepared for forecasting over long-term intervals and short-term intervals will help in making decisions for doctors and the government in India. For the future work, we use various regression techniques and measure the variations of different correlated predictors.

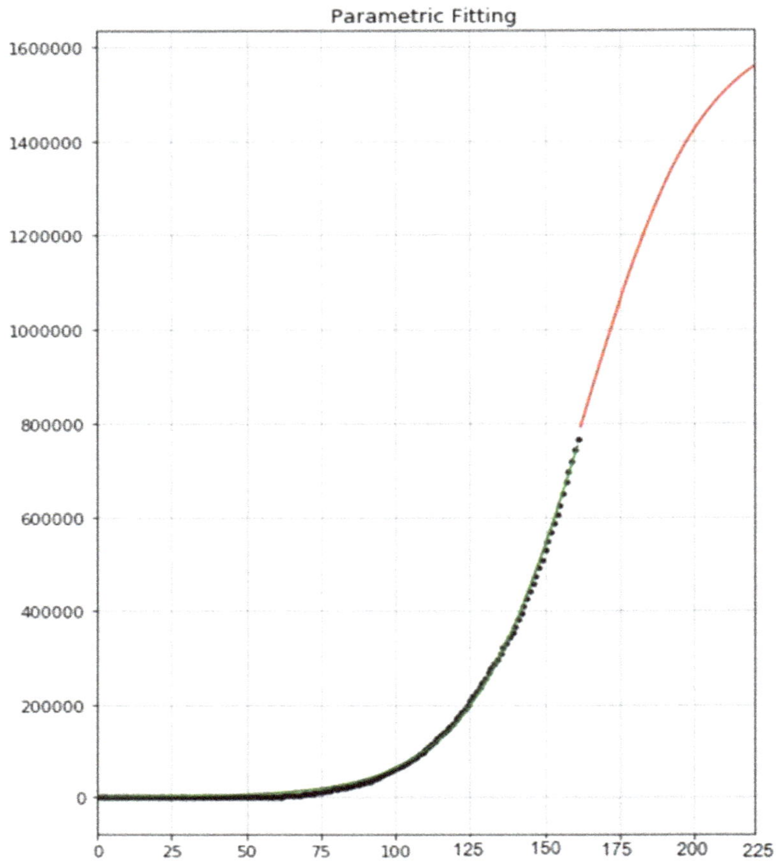

Figure 6.10. Representation of model (green) and forecasting (red) for current and future growth of covid infection.

Acknowledgments

The authors are grateful to Veer Bahadur Singh Purvanchal University, Jaunpur, Uttar Pradesh, for providing financial support to work as Post-Doctoral Research Fellowship.

References

[1] Cui J, Li F and Shi Z L 2019 Origin evolution of pathogenic coronaviruses *Nat. Rev. Microbiol.* **17** 181–92

[2] Regan, Helen, Mitra, Esha, Gupta and Swati 2020 *CNN*

[3] Withnall and Adam 2020

[4] Hindustan Times 2020 Retrieved 2020 May 30

[5] Sharma and Sanchita 2020 Hindustan Times. Retrieved April 3

[6] Reid and David 2020 'CNBC

[7] Patra S 2020 COVID-19: global economic impact of novel Corona virus with special reference to India *Horizon.* **2** 173–84

[8] Das S 2020 Analysis of COVID-19 disease progression in India: under the effect of national lockdown. arXiv preprint arXiv:2004.03147

[9] Krishnan S, Deo S and Manurkar S 2020 50 days of lockdown: measuring India's success in arresting COVID-19 *ORF Special Report* pp 1–12

[10] Chanana N 2020 Corona virus pandemic (2019–2020): preventive actions taken by Indian government *Purakala UGC Care J.* **31** 175–80

[11] Aggarwal V 2020 Effective ways to make corona virus lockdown: Productive and positive *Purakala UGC Care Journal* **31** 1798–807

[12] Sauerbrei W, Meier-Hirmer C, Benner A and Royston P 2006 Multivariable regression model building by using fractional polynomials: description of SAS, STATA and R programs *Comput. Stat. Data Anal.* **50** 3464–85

[13] Kopsaftopoulos F P and Fassois S D 2013 A functional model based statistical time series method for vibration based damage detection, localization, and magnitude estimation *Mech. Syst. Sig. Process.* **39** 143–61

[14] Miles J 2014 R squared, adjusted R squared. Wiley Stats Ref: Statistics Reference Online https://doi.org/10.1002/9781118445112.stat06627

[15] Carrillo-Larco R M and Castillo-Cara M 2020 Using country-level variables to classify countries according to the number of confirmed COVID-19 cases: an unsupervised machine learning approach *Wellcome Open Res.* **5** 56

[16] Ayyoubzadeh S M, Ayyoubzadeh S M, Zahedi H, Ahmadi M and Kalhori S 2020 Predicting COVID-19 incidence through analysis of Google trends data in Iran: data mining and deep learning pilot study *JMIR Public Health Surveillance* **6** e18828

[17] Tuli S, Tuli R and Gill S S 2020 Predicting the growth and trend of COVID-19 pandemic using machine learning and cloud computing *Internet Things* **11** 100222

[18] Yadav R S 2020 Data analysis of COVID-2019 epidemic using machine learning methods: a case study of India *Int. J. Inf. Technol.* **12** 1321–30

[19] Ardabili S F, Mosavi A, Ghamisi P, Ferdinand F, Varkonyi-Koczy A R, Reuter U, Rabczuk T and Atkinson P M 2020 COVID-19 outbreak analysis with machine learning. Available at SSRN 3580188

[20] Pandey G, Chaudhary P, Gupta R and Pal S 2020 SEIR with regression model based COVID-19 outbreak predictions in India. arXiv preprint arXiv:2004.00958

[21] Hyunjung G, Kwak, Ling L and Hui P 2020 Modelling global public health strategies in COVID-19 pandemic using deep reinforcement learning pp 1–14

[22] Rustam F, Reshi A A, Mehmood A, Ullah S, On B, Aslam W and Choi G S 2020 COVID-19 future forecasting using supervised machine learning models *IEEE Access* **8** 101489–99

[23] Wang Y, Hu M, Li Q, Zhang X P, Zhai G and Yao N 2020 Abnormal respiratory patterns classifier may contribute to large-scale screening of people infected with COVID-19 in an accurate and unobtrusive manner. arXiv preprint arXiv:2002.05534

[24] Wang C, Horby P W, Hayden F G and Gao G F 2020 A novel corona virus outbreak of global health concern *Lancet* **395** 470–3

[25] Phan L T, Nguyen T V, Luong Q C, Nguyen T V, Nguyen H T and Le H Q *et al* 2020 Importation and human-to-human transmission of a novel corona virus in Vietnam *N. Engl. J. Med.* **382** 872–4

[26] Parry J 2020 China coronavirus: cases surge as official admits human to human transmission *Br. Med. J.* **368** m236

[27] Li Q, Guan X, Wu P, Wang X, Zhou L and Tong Y 2020 Early transmission dynamics in Wuhan, China, of novel corona virus–infected pneumonia *N. Engl. J. Med.* **382** 1199–207
[28] Kan B, Wang M, Jing H, Xu H, Jiang X and Yan M 2005 Molecular evolution analysis and geographic investigation of severe acute respiratory syndrome corona virus-like virus in palm civets at an animal market and on farms *J. Virol.* **79** 11892–900
[29] Goodfellow I, Bengio Y and Courville A 2016 Machine learning basics *Deep Learn.* **1** 98–164
[30] Guan W J *et al* 2020 Clinical characteristics of corona virus disease 2019 in China *New Engl. J. Med.* **382** 1708–20
[31] Ai T, Yang Z, Hou H, Zhan C, Chen C, Lv W, Tao Q, Sun Z and Xia L 2020 Correlation of chest CT and RT-PCR testing in corona virus disease 2019 (COVID-19) in China: a report of 1014 cases *Radiology* **296** E32–40
[32] Shi Z and Hu Z 2008 A review of studies on animal reservoirs of the SARS corona virus *Virus Res.* **133** 74–87
[33] Huang C *et al* 2020 Clinical features of patients infected with 2019 novel corona virus in Wuhan, China *Lancet* **395** 497–506
[34] Liu W *et al* 2020 Analysis of factors associated with disease outcomes in hospitalized patients with 2019 novel corona virus disease *Chin. Med. J. (Engl.)* **133** 1032–8
[35] Lu R, Zhao X, Li J, Niu P, Yang B and Wu H 2020 Genomic characterization and epidemiology of 2019 novel coronavirus: implications for virus origins and receptor binding *Lancet* **395** 565–74
[36] Wang D *et al* 2020 Clinical characteristics of 138 hospitalized patients with 2019 novel corona virus–infected pneumonia in Wuhan, China *JAMA* **323** 1061–9
[37] Yadav D C and Pal S 2019 Thyroid prediction using ensemble data mining techniques *Int. J. Inf. Technol.* https://doi.org/10.1007/s41870-019-00395-7
[38] Yadav D C and Pal S 2020 Prediction of heart disease using feature selection and random forest ensemble method *Int. J. Pharm. Res.* **12** 56–66
[39] Chaurasia V and Pal S 2020 COVID-19 pandemic: ARIMA and regression model based worldwide death cases predictions. Available at SSRN 3663935
[40] Corona virus lockdown extended till 31 May, says NDMA. Retrieved 2020 May 17
[41] Verma A K, Pal S and Kumar S Prediction of different classes of skin disease using machine learning techniques *Smart Innovations in Communication and Computational Sciences* (Singapore: Springer) pp 91–100
[42] Chaurasia V and Pal S 2020 COVID-19 pandemic: ARIMA and regression model-based worldwide death cases predictions *SN Comput. Sci.* **1** 1–2
[43] Yadav D C and Pal S 2021 Analysis of heart disease using parallel and sequential ensemble methods with feature selection techniques: heart disease prediction *Int. J. Big Data Analyt. Healthcare (IJBDAH)* **6** 40–56
[44] Yadav D C and Pal S 2020 Analysis of heart patients using a tree based ensemble model *Modelling and Analysis of Active Biopotential Signals in Healthcare, Volume 2* ed V Bajaj and G R Sinha (Bristol: IOP Publishing Ltd) pp 10-1–10-23

IOP Publishing

High Performance Computing for Intelligent Medical Systems

Varun Bajaj and Irshad Ahmad Ansari

Chapter 7

A model for advanced patient feedback procedures in diagnostics

Marjo Rissanen, Antti Rissanen and Kalle Saastamoinen

In healthcare, patients' experience is monitored in many ways. However, accuracy of diagnostics is a common concern of healthcare clients. This chapter proposes a model for improved patient feedback in diagnostics. The proposed model is beneficial for organizations because it offers more precise information on patient opinions. Moreover, it helps healthcare consumers formulate and express their opinions quickly and easily about perceived diagnostic phase in their care. This approach combines clients' free-text feedback and structured responses in areas of physician competence and compassion in diagnostics. Breakthroughs in biomedical information processing like advanced data, text mining techniques, and machine learning algorithms are at the forefront of success in controlling information overload and text clustering problems. These aids are beneficial in categorizing free-text feedback and binary answers, as well in analysis and in visualization. The proposed model represents intelligent medical management and such computational intelligence which can benefit patients, doctors, and health organizations. The advantage of the model is its economics for patients but also for quality auditors, and data management sites.

7.1 Introduction

Diagnostic errors result in higher healthcare costs, unnecessary deaths, and mental suffering [1–3]. Diagnostic errors lead easily to increased numbers of doctor visits, longer hospital stays, or to inappropriate treatments [1, 4]. Evaluative information gained from patient feedback plays an essential role in responding to patient concerns and making necessary changes to diagnostic practices. To improve patient safety related to diagnostics, feedback systems focused on diagnostic evaluation should be clear and efficient. Therefore, it would be desirable to distinguish diagnostics connected patient feedback from other general patient feedback into its separate feedback systems to make progress quickly. However, providing specific feedback can be challenging for the patient when it comes to diagnostic practices. Some areas in the diagnostic phase are easier to handle in feedback procedure by clients if the stages and content of the process are presented in simple, easy-to-read formats. Thus to a certain degree structured phases in addition to open text formats are recommendable in diagnostics focused consumer targeted feedback systems. Nowadays also the processing of narrative feedback phases is smoother. Improved artificial intelligence (AI) algorithms and intelligent big data analytics offer more efficient tools to refine open format based material for further analysis.

7.2 Focus on diagnostics

7.2.1 Diagnostic error as a concept

Diagnostic error is defined as 'the failure to establish an accurate and timely explanation of the patient's health problem or communicate that explanation to the patient' [2]. Errors arise 'as a result of actions not taken or as a result of the wrong action taken' [3]. Active errors are made by people, between clinicians, and an object in question [2, 5]. Latent errors result from problems in system or process design and may easily go unnoticed. System-related errors may be associated with communication, care coordination, inefficient processes, or technical failures [2, 5]. In daily practice, diagnostic errors are often unrecognized and under-reported [6, 7]. Health professionals' indifference to report mistakes may be due to fear of penalty or sanction [5, 8]. Individual and systematic factors are some of the most common reasons for the under-reporting of diagnostic errors [7].

7.2.2 Diagnostic errors in healthcare

Medical errors are a critical problem in healthcare. According to statistics, medical errors are assumed to be the leading cause of death in the United States [5]. These errors include e.g., surgical, diagnostic, medication, devices, equipment, system failures, and other problems with healthcare technology. Higher error rates usually occur in stressful environments such as emergency departments, intensive care units, and operating rooms but high error rates are seen also in primary healthcare [9, 10]. Medical errors are often associated with extreme age, high acuity, and new procedures [5, 9, 11]. Communication errors are a common source of medical error [5]. Quality of care is lower among female patients and women report more harm than male patients [9, 12]. Errors related to medication occur in 3–10% of all consultations when drugs are prescribed [9, 13]. Common factors contributing to medication errors include communication, transfer of care, and continuity of care [9].

Diagnostic errors contribute as much 70% of medical errors [14]. Vascular disease, infections, and cancer account for about 75% of diagnostic errors [15]. In a Scandinavian retrospective cohort study [16] in a sample of a total of 4830 cases of preventable harm, 46% were due to diagnostic errors. Cancers represented 37% of all diagnostic errors in primary healthcare. The cases most often missed were colorectal, skin, kidney and bladder, prostate, lung, and breast cancers. Heart disease, fractures, infections, pneumonia, tuberculosis, type 1 diabetes, and pulmonary embolism were the most frequently missed diseases in other disease categories. The most frequently missed diagnoses in Sweden with reported harm were cancers in primary healthcare and fractures in emergency units [16].

7.2.3 Common reasons for diagnostic failures

Skill gaps in bedside examination abilities, poor clinical reasoning skills, and problems in synthesizing information are significant contributors to diagnostic errors [17–19]. Knowledge and skill gaps have been underestimated in this context, while cognitive bias has been overemphasized [17, 20]. In primary healthcare, common reasons for diagnostic errors include failure to order appropriate tests, faulty interpretation, problems in follow-up, failures in referring patients, transfer of care, and insufficient consultation techniques [2, 9].

Education in clinical content knowledge, awareness of bedside history, and correct physical examination skills are examples of factors that can reduce diagnostic errors [7]. In emergency department settings proper diagnostics relates to acuity recognition, information synthesis, and straight communication with patients [21]. More advanced imaging technologies have improved physicians' ability to detect, diagnose, and treat conditions while allowing patients to avoid invasive procedures [22]. However, diagnostic radiology errors, especially shorter viewing times, are clear contributors to adverse outcomes [23–25]. Pathology is an essential step in cancer diagnostics and better integration of quality and safety principles is seen as necessary in error prevention in this area. Diagnostic error prevention in pathology requires, e.g., collaborative teamwork, enhanced training about the diagnostic process, and a safety culture focusing on health information technology and other strategic changes [26]. As is known, proper investigation intensity is critical in healthcare. Many challenges, however, in this area can be met and poor clinical outcomes could be prevented by enhancing diagnostic processes [27, 28].

7.2.4 Preventing diagnostic errors in cooperation with patients

The importance of patient involvement and mutual communication between patients and doctors are emphasized widely in prevention of diagnostic errors. Improved patient access to clinical notes with co-generation and feedback possibilities represent one form of error recovery and shared decision-making [2, 29]. The majority of patients who access their patient records report positive experiences [29]. However, this is only one step toward better patient-centered care. In prevention policies in a Scandinavian study [9], patients emphasized the value of nationwide online medical records, regular comprehensive physical examinations, and clarity in routines for the follow-up. Availability of contact information for doctors and other medical professionals was seen as important in situations of normal test results but remaining symptoms [9]. Healthcare professionals may propose a working diagnosis in cases of uncertainty [2]. When the diagnosis stays unclear, the follow-up care is often inadequate.

7.3 Diagnostics and safety challenges in healthcare

7.3.1 Patient safety and equity challenges

Patient safety is a multidisciplinary goal and a primary task in healthcare. In addition to technological innovations, a hospital culture should emphasize change-positive leadership in clinical practice [30]. Healthcare organizations should promote safety-conscious culture and learn from diagnostic errors [2]. Encouraging transparency about errors can make healthcare safer and foster a culture in which healthcare professionals are supported in identifying and learning from mistakes [2, 31].

In many countries, patient safety is poor, especially among the older patient population, partly due to an inadequate and disorganized healthcare system [32]. In western society, patients who have taken good care of their health may remain relatively healthy until the age of 80. At this age, specific health problems often occur, in which case, there would be a particular need for high-quality care and higher treatment intensity. In spite of that, medical treatment intensity is lower among the older patient population (aged 80 and over) [33]. Old age is easily perceived in healthcare as a so-called 'period of fragility.' However, older adults form highly heterogeneous groups, and their health and functioning may be better than negative stereotypes suggest [34]. This age represents a specific period in life when, in many cases, intensive care may be needed for the first time. The diagnostic process for the older patient population can be challenging due to its multi-problem character [35]. The high prevalence of pain may be considered a normal phenomenon in older age [36, 37]. This complexity can easily result in treating only the symptoms and not the cause of the symptoms.

Also, critically ill elderly patients show favorable clinical outcomes in intensive care. Thus, underlying medical conditions rather than age per se should be considered for determining intensive care [38]. Inaccurate estimates of operative risks however prevent older people from receiving sometimes even standard surgery because they are deemed unfit for demanding treatments [39]. Almost one-half of all critically ill patients with primary central nervous system lymphoma, (PCNSL) admitted to ICU were alive six months after ICU discharge [40]. Frailty-rating scales or simple, standardized tools alone are not acceptable prognostic assets for predicting unfavorable outcomes, for example, in acute care [41–43]. Quality auditing and transparency are needed, especially in elderly care.

One of the key ideas in translational medicine is to improve a patient's health in an ethically acceptable way. Shared decision-making has a solid place in translational design in healthcare; hearing the client's voice is one step toward better equality. Such decision-making means intense collaborative processes between patients and providers [2]. Shared decision-making is about giving weight to the patient's values and opinions, and also when older patients are in question. Thus, tuned feedback systems, suitable for all age groups mean important and vital development areas. The COVID-19 crisis is an area fostering the use of modern information and communication technologies among older adults [34]. Equality in the decision-making process among different age groups refers to the state of ethical values in organizations.

7.3.2 Enhanced patient safety with rational cost control policy

Cost-saving pressures in healthcare may pose a challenge to a doctor's clinical work. Inadequate savings targets in patient care, for instance in the area of diagnostics can disturb clinical practices and be very costly. A common approach to save money is random reduction of laboratory budgets [28]. Diagnostic management teams represent an advanced model for more intensive and meaningful cost-effective processes. In this model professionals with expertise advise colleagues in clinical practice on test selection and interpretation [28, 44].

AI offers more proficient methods for the optimal use of human resources and the planning of logistical processes [45]. Those methods offer new options to find rigorous cost savings opportunities because human resources form in hospitals the most significant cost factor [46]. Thus, personnel costs do not have to be viewed only as fixed costs. This optimization modeling will also be principally taken care of by those resourced for these planning tasks, which is a step forward.

Advanced AI tools and methods have their role to play in sound cost management policy and, therefore, in safety enhancement when enabling doctors to have better focusing primarily on their clinical work. Also, intelligent diagnostic systems like AI-assisted decision support systems can improve diagnostic accuracy and aid in disease management and thus help doctors decrease routine clinical tasks and focus first and foremost on patient care [47, 48]. These systems also do not increase the duration of the doctor consultation or the number of ordered tests [1]. Digital scribes, like AI-powered digital notes enable doctors to fully engage with patients by reducing the time invested by clinicians in the documentation process [49].

7.4 Importance of patient feedback in the diagnostics phase

7.4.1 Need for timely feedback

It is essential that doctors get patient feedback on their diagnostic skills and competence. Overconfidence is more prevalent than low confidence, especially at lower competence levels [50]. Also, extensive experience does not necessarily mean greater diagnostic accuracy [17, 51]. Only a few healthcare organizations have genuinely concentrated on identifying diagnostic errors [2, 52]. Healthcare professionals often do not have the opportunity to hear from health consumers about their diagnostic performance [2, 53, 54]. Time limits may prevent real engagement with customers in the diagnostic process [2, 55]. Clinicians need to be ready to communicate with their customers about the occurrence of diagnostic errors but also may find the feedback on their diagnostic performance uncomfortable [2, 56]. However, in feedback training programs, clinicians found the exercises constructive and helpful [56]. Organization-wide and improved customer complaints coordination may also help individual doctors develop in their self-evaluative processes by enhancing their diagnostic calibration properties [57, 58]. Diagnostic calibration is about self-knowledge and understanding of the limitations of one's knowledge [58].

7.4.2 The role of timely feedback

The purpose of patient feedback systems is to offer high quality health information. Such information can work as an enabler for enhanced organizational and patient outcomes [59]. Patients' opinions about their visits to the doctor offer beneficial information for health professionals and comprehensive awareness of the causes of diagnostic errors with critical, unique insights [6, 60]. Healthcare providers should ensure that systematic feedback on diagnostic performance extends to doctors and care teams involved in care and organizational management [61, 62]. Periodic feedback is necessary for improved diagnostic performance and quality improvement in healthcare but is often absent [17, 53, 63, 64]. Such feedback, however, could be valuable as a regular part of the assessment policy [2].

Diagnostics centered feedback systems should provide evidence-based information on critical areas of clinical practice [2]. Such feedback is welcome from both professionals and healthcare consumers [2]. Healthcare clients' more prominent role in the diagnostics phase means that patients are 'at the center.' Such policy reflects 'rehumanized medicine' [62]. High-quality feedback from diagnostics can mean enhanced organizational and patient outcomes that benefit both patients and doctors by eliminating preventable adverse events and improving the diagnostic process [2, 53, 59, 60, 65].

Patient involvement should thus have a stable position in professional development within the clinical practice. However, this presupposes the existence of such cultural attitudes and values that foster patient-centered care and continuous learning [57, 58]. Even complete re-engineering of services and novel technologies without correct staff engagement do not change policies accurately [30]. Feedback should be part of learning systems that focus on improving diagnostic performance [56]. This helps target individual counseling assistance and aids in identifying doctors who may need educational support or retraining [66].

Patient engagement is a matter of supporting people in benefiting more from the healthcare system [2]. However, this engagement may be challenging for patients and their families [2, 67]. Disease-related stress with lower physical health can prevent people from engaging genuinely in the diagnostic process [2]. Some patients prefer active involvement in all aspects of the decision-making process, while others would instead rely on a doctor's assessment [2]. Feedbacks systems should also allow space for those health consumers who have already experienced a diagnostic error. Such individuals are often ready to share their experiences to enlighten future patients' diagnostic processes [2, 68, 69].

7.5 The challenges of diagnostics-centered clients' feedback

An effective feedback system for the client on the diagnostic process's success controls the quality of care and improved patient safety. Consumer targeted feedback systems are often very comprehensive, focusing on the entire healthcare process. There is a particular need for feedback systems that focus specifically on the patient's view of diagnostics' success and the patient's experience of working collaboratively in this context [46]. Feedback systems that focus on the actual area of diagnostics should be linked closely to the treatment or care process in question. In this way, the doctor in charge could get the patient's view of the diagnosis's correctness and get additional information for evaluative purposes.

It is possible to assess the investigation intensity in the field of diagnostics by patient basis. The number of tests, examinations, and other research and consultation carried out in connection with the diagnostic process reflects the degree of intensity in the diagnostics phase. If the client believes that the degree of investigative intensity of their own case is too low for proper diagnostics, they must have a pathway to address their concerns. The current problem is that feedback on the validity of the diagnosis does not reach the doctor in charge quickly enough. On the other hand, the patient's feedback on the medical performance should be specific enough to allow corrective action to be taken [70].

The feedback of diagnostics should be adequately specified, so that feedback delivery would be easy for the patient and beneficial to clinicians. Therefore, carefully constructed but economical (quick to fill) formats may enhance the process. Free-text comments are useful for service improvement if patient feedback is provided in near-real-time [63, 71]. Due to AI algorithms, the utilization of free-text format is also more efficient. Thus, narrative feedback from the diagnostics phase also has its place as a basis for broader evaluation.

7.6 Enhancing technology acceptance in system development

Healthcare organizations should promote open and transparent environments in which patients can engage in the diagnostic process and share their feedback and concerns with ease [2]. At the same time, feedback systems should be sufficiently detailed, user-friendly, clear, and understandable. Also, there are problems in such areas as survey length, infrequent sampling frequency, and slow feedback. To be useful, patient feedback results should be timely, intelligible, and easy to interpret by all stakeholders. Clarity, ease of use, suitability for frequent use, and multiple features (e.g., feedback with paper, touchscreens, smartphones, tablets, and telephones with automated interactive voice response) are essential characters of a beneficial feedback system [63, 72].

In the technology acceptance model (TAM), the primary determinants for technology acceptance are perceived usefulness and perceived ease of use [73]. The model by Yan *et al* [74], describes aspects connected to the human–computer trust interaction. 'Communication trust' is one incentive for use. It covers areas of 'perceived privacy', 'perceived identity', and 'communication context'. The customer must be able to trust that security issues concerning customer privacy are in order, e.g., in feedback system options [74]. Clients do not even use beneficial healthcare services if they are unsure about their information security [75]. Computer system trust relates to aspects of trustworthiness like 'system and information quality' and aspects of flexible use [74].

Motivation is an action inspiring humans in objective-guided activities and keeping them in motion [76, 77]. Pintrich [78] distinguishes among motivational beliefs for value-, goal-, ability-, and control-connected beliefs. Patients are motivated to give feedback only if they trust their input's validity and the change it enables in their own situation (goal-, control-connected beliefs). The application should represent values that are acceptable to the patient. Although some patients want to leave the responsibility for diagnostics to the doctor, many patients appreciate the opportunity to participate in evaluating their own care, especially in the case of diagnostics (ability-connected beliefs).

7.7 Phases of diagnostics and the requirements for doctors

7.7.1 Requirements for competence and compassion

Patients expect that the doctor has sufficient expertise to provide both right diagnosis and adequate care. Medical 'competence' for a doctor is assumed to include technical capability and willingness to provide needed information. Consumers also expect 'compassion', empathy, and moral support when making healthcare decisions [79]. Effective communication, trust, and an encouraging environment are aspects of mature consultation skills [60]. In surgery and intensive care, physician competence, like technical skills, is often preferred while in the end-of-life vignette, compassion is emphasized. In chronic care, preferences for physician competence and compassion vary. In pediatric cases, a doctor's competence is preferred, but the importance of empathy is also valued [79].

7.7.2 Diagnostic process from the view of doctors

In their self-evaluative actions, many doctors use a variety of often individual-tuned process models. These checklists play a role in improving the diagnostic process [2, 80]. The best process models describe different phases of the diagnostic process. With aid of taxonomic models it is easier to detect what went wrong in diagnostic process. Taxonomic failures can be assessed from several standpoints in the diagnostic process; from access and patient history to the final stages of referrals and follow-up. In each step, embedded sub-categories clarify items for evaluation. In ordering tests, e.g., mistakes may include delays in test ordering or sequencing [61].

Schiff and colleagues [81] divide the diagnostic process into seven stages: (1) access and presentation, (2) history taking/collection, (3) the physical exam, (4) testing, (5) assessment, (6) referral, and (7) follow-up. A patient's clinical history includes documentation of the current health problem, history (medical, family, social), and other needed information like medications [2, 82]. Physical examination skills have a substantial role in diagnostics, but these skills have often been underemphasized in professional education [2, 83]. Diagnostic testing contains areas of laboratory, medicine, anatomic pathology, and medical imaging [2].

7.7.3 Diagnostic process from the view of patients

In principle, patients could evaluate the diagnostic process's success by utilizing traditional steps for the process from their point of view. These steps are self-evident and obvious for health professionals. Partially, these traditional categories can be converted to serve patient feedback by streamlining them to suit the customer perspective. There is also need for such aspects which are relevant especially for customer feedback. Patients typically have some insights into where there were problems in their case. Patients are not necessarily always able to evaluate diagnostic steps with such accuracy as professionals. Still, they typically have ideas about aspects that received less attention or were omitted during the consultancy. Health consumers' concerns also typically focus on poorly organized and administered care like long waiting times, problems in access, and loss of other interaction possibilities with doctors beside formal consultations [84]. Thus, care management issues related to rapid and flexible diagnostics are also worthy of patient feedback.

7.8 A model for instant patient feedback

7.8.1 General principles

When the patient evaluates the level of professionalism, the doctor's competence in diagnostics, it is most manageable for the client to assess this area with a ready-made format. When dealing with attributes of empathy (e.g., listening to patients properly) both open and structured feedback formats may function well. It is essential that the patient's experience and vision are presented in a specified way; the doctor responsible for the diagnostic process can understand the areas for which clients have open questions or remarks. If the patient is encouraged to provide feedback on the diagnostic process's correctness as part of standard practice, giving feedback on the diagnostic process will be more comfortable. Accordingly, the patient feels that he or she is not only providing feedback on the specific aspect of the care process but is also a full participant in assessing the quality of his or her care. With a detailed but reasonably simple questionnaire, patients can give summary feedback on the diagnosis they have received. It is essential that the patient accurately identifies those aspects they believed were deficient in the diagnostic process. The proposed model gives the doctor a better idea of the patient's experience than is typically possible during a limited consultancy session. This information helps the doctor improve their working methods and self-evaluation.

7.8.2 Structure of the model

The proposed model contains three phases (see table 7.1). Phase 1 includes eight structured stand-alone sections focusing on the competence of the doctor. This phase

Table 7.1. Model in three phases.

Phase	Content of the phase	Meaning of the phase/structure
I Fixed format	Competence of the doctor	Eight-item basic or advanced feedback
II Open format	Compassion of the doctor (additional communication)	Free individual feedback text (other information, e.g. pictures)
III User experience	Utility of the feedback system	Development needs of the application

offers two options: immediate feedback items (eight areas of patient feedback—figure 7.1) and an advanced section with multiple options for each of the eight items (figure 7.2).

Patients eager to report more comprehensively about their experience may continue to the advanced section after submitting the first quick-response section (see figure 7.2). Phase 2 contains free space for narrative text (open commentary). Specific aspects related to the doctor's compassion (e.g., empathy, etc), other questions, and remarks and additional material can be delivered in this item. Phase 3 provides an opportunity for patients to present their views on the model's usefulness and design (table 7.1, phase 3). Phase 3 is needed for quality improvement and maturation purposes and is thus useful for any kinds of feedback systems (figure 7.3).

7.8.3 Patient management with the model

The main menu includes essential diagnostic-related sections (see figure 7.1). The patient can check the options that he/she considers to be deficient in ensuring correct diagnostics (marking the item as 'unsatisfactory'). The areas that are not meant to be labeled are assumed to have proceeded as expected from the patient's perspective. After completing the eight areas of assessment (with marking only those sections for

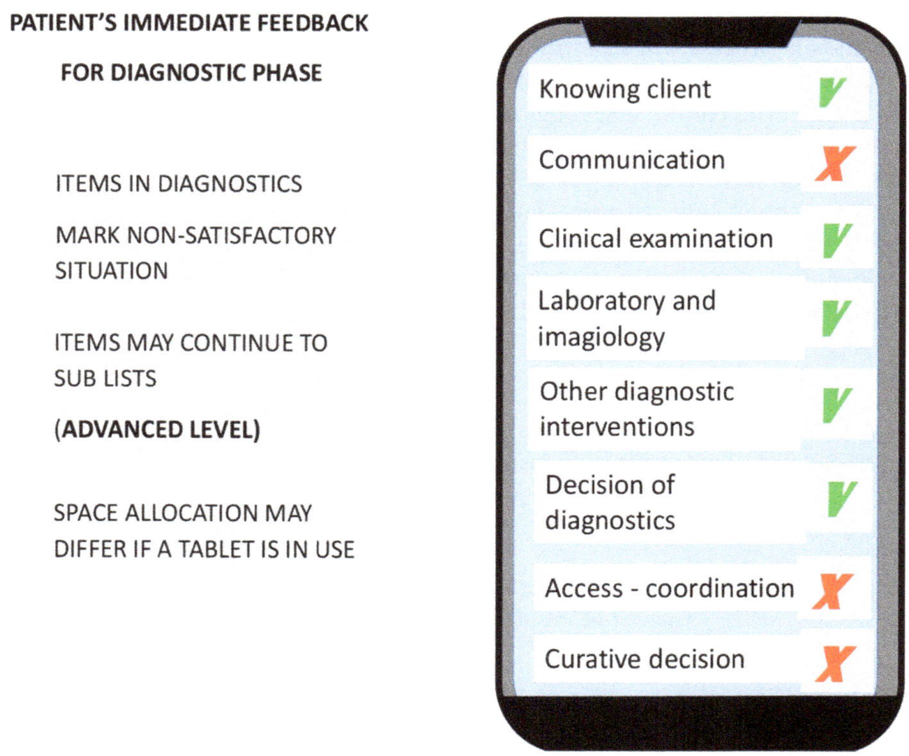

Figure 7.1. Application main menu for quick feedback.

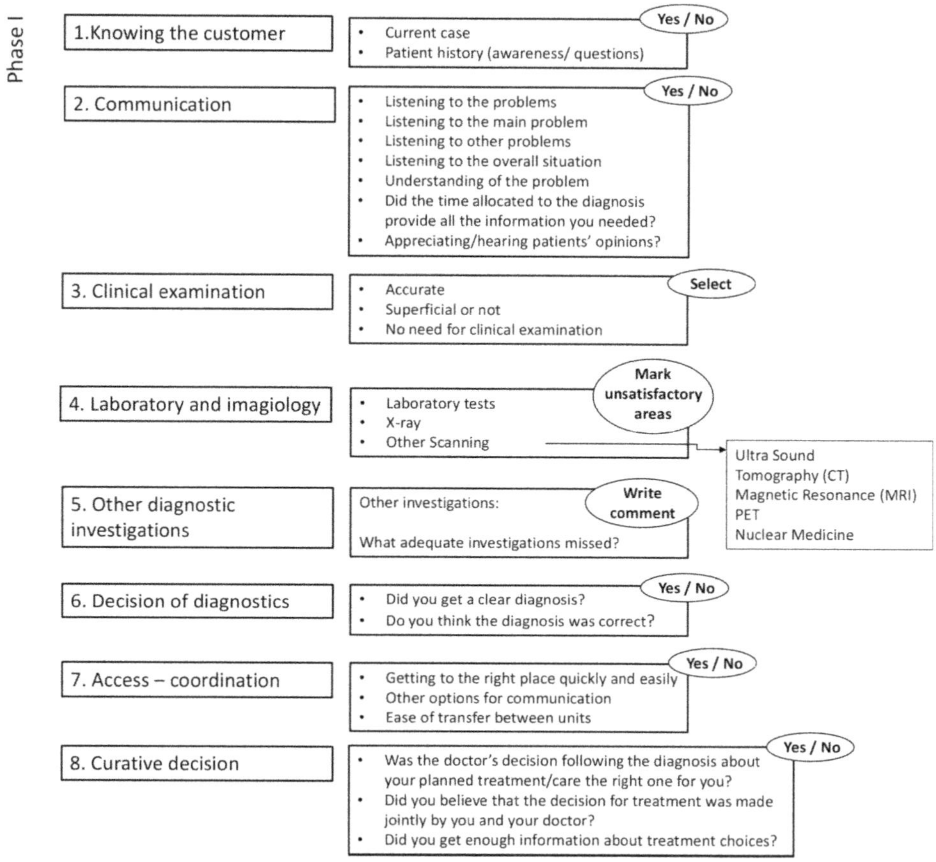

Figure 7.2. Structure of the application. Eight main areas for instant feedback require customers' reaction and marking of unsatisfactory areas. On the right a more advanced level which allows for more detailed feedback.

which the patient believes there are problems), the patient can submit the feedback. It is assumed that, in generally, there are fewer areas for remarks (unsatisfactory areas) than there are acceptable areas. Fractures are examples of cases where there are many misdiagnoses. For example, the patient may believe the session went smoothly but would have liked an x-ray to confirm the diagnosis. In this case, the person marks this subdivision as unsatisfactory. If the patient also feels that the clinical examination was superficial, he or she marks this area as an 'unsatisfactory clinical examination.' Thus, the answer requires two entries.

As in all questionnaires, some patients are willing to spend more time giving feedback. In that case, it is helpful to provide two levels of detail for answers. The input could be presented in a more detailed way (i.e., 'advanced level') (see figure 7.2). Each feedback point could be opened in the advanced state, where it is possible to provide a more specific description of the response. For example, in the 'Laboratory and imagiology' section, the patient may specifically indicate which areas received less attention (laboratory examinations or certain imaging types).

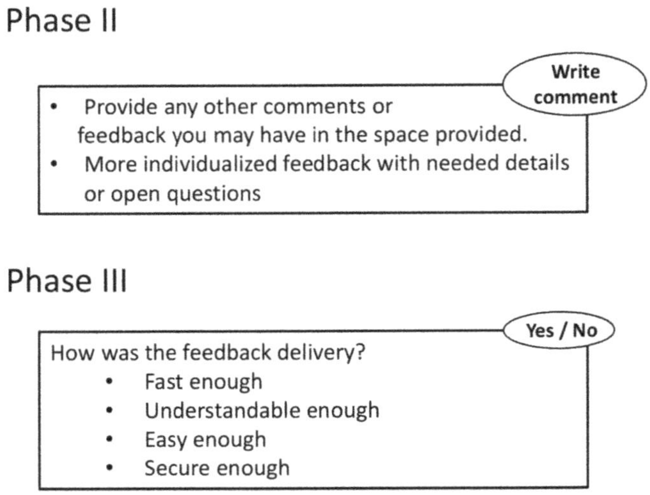

Figure 7.3. Phases II and III are aimed to provide more detailed information.

Similarly, the communication section allows the patient to identify an unsatisfactory area if desired. Suppose the patient feels that they did not receive appropriate or sufficient cause of the problem or a clear diagnosis. In that case, they may mark the section 'Decision of diagnostics?' as 'unsatisfactory' and if they want, they can proceed to the advanced level and select 'no' to the question 'did you get a clear diagnosis?'

A general review of the eight most important sections of the model provides informative knowledge about the quality and the patient's perspective of the diagnostic process. In addition, it is possible to get a picture of the feedback for a specific doctor. Some patients wish to give individual feedback and share their experiences, possibly in a more detailed way. Therefore, open-text feedback is a beneficial part of any feedback format used as a standard tool.

7.8.4 Meaning of the fixed format phase of the model—phase 1

Diagnostics is a demanding area in a care process. For a patient, feedback delivery from this part is not always straightforward. Therefore, structured formats are useful in this area. Patients are nowadays intensively searching for information about their own health condition and especially about issues connected to their own possible diagnosis. Thanks to patient self-diagnostic applications or other gained knowledge, the patient may already have an idea of a possible diagnosis when they arrive at the doctor's consultation. For this reason, it is important that, within the consultancy period, it is already possible to also discuss the healthcare client's own views on the diagnostic decision. Especially challenging are situations in which the patient experiences symptoms and does not feel healthy, but the test results performed do not show a deviation from normal values. In addition, multi-problem groups, such as the elderly, may be a challenging group in a diagnostic sense. Especially in such cases, it is important that the patient has the opportunity to give his or her own views through a formal feedback channel. In such cases, the patient may have the impression that more intensive investigation of the matter could bring more clarity to the problem and a client may have doubts about too low investigation intensity in their case. With a structured model, the care provider gains a clear understanding of clients' views and cues of possible areas of too low care intensity in diagnostics and can thus re-evaluate the diagnostic process or inform the client.

7.8.5 Meaning and management of the free format phase—phase 2

AI provides more efficient possibilities for processing free text. Free text feedback is especially useful in complex cases where, for example, the patient feels that his or her own diagnosis is prolonged. This may be due to poorly coordinated co-operation between different sites. Poor coordination causes situations that may threaten patient safety and increase healthcare costs [85, 86]. As speech recognition and processing systems have also evolved, it makes sense that the patient can also give free-form feedback on their phone interactively with the help of a robot as flexibly as possible.

Unstructured data can be challenging to organize and analyze. This kind of data is typically in text, such as open-ended text responses. In the case of hospitals, the volume of free-text data can be massive. Analyzing handwritten responses or large volumes of text data is time-consuming, expensive, and subject to human error [87, 88]. Big data is defined as 'a collection of a very large amount of data with a wide range of types, making it hard to process using conventional database management systems' [88]. This is why AI-based text analysis and automated knowledge representation and reasoning capabilities can be extremely helpful [87].

Customer feedback may be in the form of PDF documents, photos, or other images, scanned documents, or printed or handwritten documents. Optical Character Recognition (OCR) is the best tool for converting text to digital format in all of these cases (figure 7.4). Most OCR tools provide 98% to 99% accuracy [89]. This level of accuracy would be sufficient in most cases; however, accuracy may suffer in handwritten documents, blurry pictures, and languages other than English.

Handwriting Recognition (HWR), also known as Handwritten Text Recognition (HTR), is an active research area that can deliver a 4.0% Word Error Rate (WER) and 1.6% Character Error Rate (CER) when using deep learning techniques, like bidirectional, long short-term memory networks (BLSTMs) [90].

Another option is feedback in the form of audio. Tools are available to transform spoken audio into digital text. In many European hospitals, doctors' assessments are recorded and converted to text. Digital scribes (speech-processing and natural language processing (NLP) modules) can also convert the audio to text, and to extract salient information from the text [49]. There are many speech-to-text platforms available. They are standard tools, similar to OCR or translating tools. Most of the applications have sufficient accuracy to be usable.

Once open-ended responses are gathered (free-text phase) in digitized text, the material is ready for text analysis. Text analyzing techniques use machine learning algorithms to find quantitative or qualitative data in the text. In free-text form, data is ordinarily unstructured. From this data, it is possible to obtain some qualitative

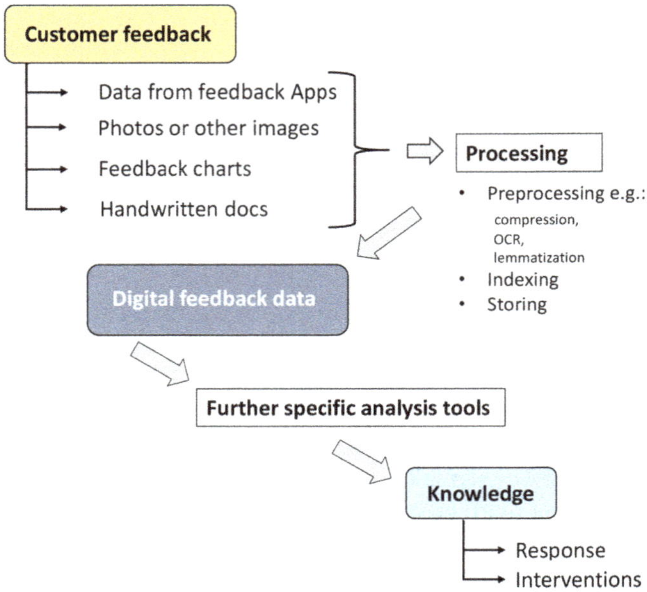

Figure 7.4. Collecting feedback data from patients. Illustration of steps in how to process gained information towards knowledge.

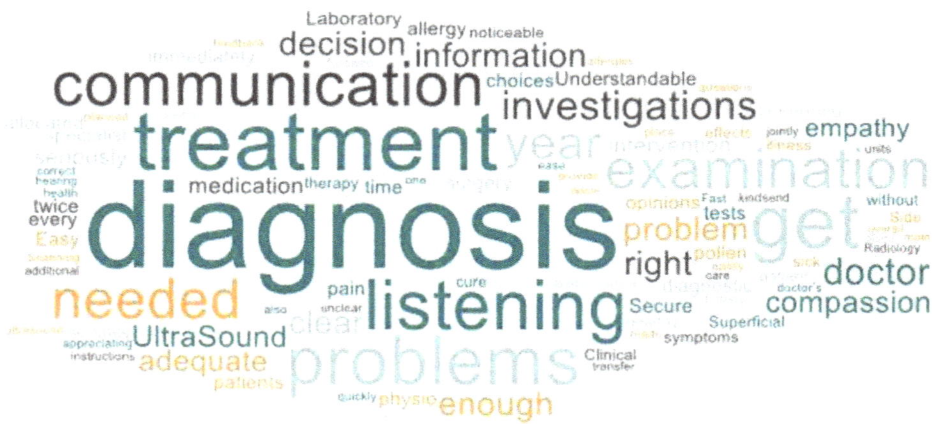

Figure 7.5. Word cloud sample picture of a generic feedback consisting of 240 answers. Picture generated with a free Word Add-in Tool [91].

information beside quantitative information. Two practical tools are word clouds and sentiment analysis.

An easy way to get information from text data and give it some visual appearance at the same time is a data analysis method called 'word cloud'. Word cloud technique provides a visual representation of text by counting word frequencies and showing more frequent words in a visualization. Figure 7.5 is an example of how the word cloud raises those words that exist most frequently in the text phrase.

When examining the open-text feedback, it is essential to understand the customer's undertones or patients' emotions. It is possible to use a set of techniques called sentiment analysis [92]. Sentiment analysis uses machine learning, and it can be supervised or unsupervised. Advanced sentiment analysis even understands irony and sarcasm. We can also run aspect-based sentiment analyses to find the reasons behind the positive or negative responses. The simplest way is to review: positive, negative, or neutral. This is called free-text classification based on polarities and high accuracy rates can be found also by this method [93]. Split or stratified classifications could give even more information to support improvements [93].

7.8.6 Clients' opinions of the feedback delivery system—phase 3

It is noticeable that health consumers can give responses and ideas of usability aspects of feedback systems. User acceptance issues deal typically with flexibility of feedback delivery systems. It is important that feedback delivery is fast enough, the system and its guidelines and outlook are understandable enough, and system use is easy enough for all kinds of users. Aspects of patient privacy are such issues that require special attention because patients are not eager to use applications if they have doubts and questions in this area. Feedback gives material in evolving the system better 'fit for use'.

7.9 Client feedback as a translational development challenge

7.9.1 Enhancing process synergy in organizations

Using an accurate but reasonably simple application, the patient can quickly and simply provide clear and informative feedback on the diagnostic process they experience. Moreover, the open format (open format-narrative phase) allows for individual feedback. It is essential that the patient accurately identifies those aspects they perceived to be deficient in the diagnostic process for their doctor's particular area of practice. The model provides the physician with a better understanding of the patient's experience than is typically possible during a limited consultancy session. The physician also gains an understanding of the patient's view on how the diagnostic process is progressing.

At the organizational level, it is possible to obtain information on the issues that present the most significant challenges in the patient's view. This assists human resource training leaders to focus on issues that are relevant to quality assurance. Up-to-date information on a specific physician helps to target individual counseling assistance. It is also essential to get feedback from system users about the usability of the system. This information is useful for the further maturation procedures of diagnostic-focused feedback systems.

Perceiving entities is essential in systems thinking and in translational design approach. Proper functioning depends on how successfully the parts of the process work, integrate, and form a seamless whole [94]. The overall process should be sufficiently elastic, even in exceptional situations and periods of change. The diagnostic process must be seen as a whole, requiring multi-faceted communication and collaboration to face current challenges. Efficient patient feedback in this area can improve the synergy of the process. The feedback delivery process must be accessible to all customer groups. Accordingly, particular attention should be paid to the needs of older patients when designing user interfaces.

7.9.2 Maturing and validating patient-targeted feedback systems

Well-functioning patient feedback systems in diagnostics are an essential tool for healthcare organizations to improve their image quality. Easy-to-use feedback systems can assure patients that their voice is heard at the most critical stage of the healthcare process. Healthcare organizations can thus increase their image quality value in a remarkable way through intensive and flexible feedback possibilities.

In the area of product quality, patient-targeted feedback systems should focus particularly on privacy, ease of use, and credibility. Customers are only interested in giving feedback if they believe it will be helpful. To ensure customer quality, feedback on the functionality of the diagnostic process is essential. Because doctors are also users of the feedback system, they should also be consulted on how well a feedback system serves them in assessing the diagnostic process's quality.

Diagnostics-focused feedback systems should provide hospital administrators with information on the current state of patient satisfaction about diagnostics and how feedback systems can be improved. This information will provide additional input and material for physician training to enhance the diagnostic process. Patient targeted diagnostics focused feedback system aims to improve the diagnostic process's safety and reliability and thus improve overall process quality.

Patient-targeted feedback systems need their maturation stages to reach acceptable levels of innovation quality. AI brings new opportunities to the field of product design. Systems must evolve through the feedback they receive about their usefulness to ensure that all patients can benefit from the feedback system. System development should not cease at the first well-functioning state in the field of application design.

7.10 Conclusion

The correctness of diagnostics in healthcare is a key area of concern for patients. To ensure patient legal protection, it is important to develop feedback systems that are well-suited to providing feedback on the accuracy of diagnostics. Feedback delivery should be easy for the client and provide care planners and caregivers with sufficiently informative information about the patient's perspective. Narrative feedback defends its place because it gives the patient a free hand to give feedback. The transformation of free-form text into informative and usable data has evolved in part thanks to artificial intelligence applications. However, giving feedback on the diagnostic portion is not easy for the patient in all cases. For this reason, the chapter also presents a format model representing structured feedback that promotes the patient's ability to provide useful and sufficiently informative feedback. Because patients' willingness to use the time required for feedback naturally varies, it is important to consider different levels of time use when developing feedback systems that allow for rapid or more intensive feedback. In the presented model, the quick feedback level response also provides sufficient information as a basis for the quality assessment of the area.

References

[1] Li C, Chen E, Savova G, Fraser H and Eickhoff C 2020 Mining misdiagnosis patterns from biomedical literature *AMIA Jt. Summits Trans. Sci. Proc.* **2020** 360–6

[2] Committee on Diagnostic Error in Health Care, Board on Health Care Services, Institute of Medicine, and The National Academies of Sciences, Engineering, and Medicine 2015 *Improving Diagnosis in Health Care* ed E P Balogh, B T Miller and J R Ball (Washington DC: National Academies Press)

[3] Ozeke O, Ozeke V, Coskun O and Budakoglu I I 2019 Second victims in health care: current perspectives *Adv. Med. Educ. Pract.* **10** 593

[4] Hautz W, Kämmer J E, Hautz S, Sauter T, Zwaan L, Exadaktylos A, Birrenbach T N, Maier V, Müller M and Schauber S K 2019 Diagnostic error increases mortality and length of hospital stay in patients presenting through the emergency room *Scand. J. Trauma Resuscitation Emerg. Med.* **27** 54

[5] Rodziewicz T L and Hipskind J E 2018 *Medical Error Prevention* (Treasure Island, FL: StatPearls Publishing)

[6] Giardina T D, Haskell H, Menon S, Hallisy J, Southwick F S, Sarkar U, Royse K E and Singh H 2018 Learning from patients' experiences related to diagnostic errors is essential for progress in patient safety *Health Affairs* **37** 1821–7

[7] Clark B W, Derakhshan A and Desai S V 2018 Diagnostic errors and the bedside clinical examination *Med. Clin.* **102** 453–64

[8] Robertson J J and Long B 2018 Suffering in silence: medical error and its impact on health care providers *J. Emerg. Medicine* **54** 402–9

[9] Fernholm R, Wachtler C, Malm-Willadsen K, Holzmann M J, Carlsson A C, Nilsson G H and Pukk Härenstam K 2020 Validation and initial results of surveys exploring perspectives on risks and solutions for diagnostic and medication errors in primary care in Sweden *Scand. J. Prim. Health Care* **38** 381–90

[10] Panesar S S, Desilva D, Carson-Stevens A, Cresswell K M, Salvilla S A, Slight S P, Javad S, Netuveli G, Larizgoitia I and Donaldson L J 2016 How safe is primary care? A systematic review *BMJ Qual. Saf.* **25** 544–53

[11] Sari A B, Cracknell A and Sheldon T A 2008 Incidence, preventability and consequences of adverse events in older people: results of a retrospective case-note review *Age Ageing* **37** 265–9

[12] Pukk K, Lundberg J, Penaloza-Pesantes R V, Brommels M and Gaffney F A 2003 Do women simply complain more? National patient injury claims data show gender and age differences *Qual. Manage. Healthcare* **12** 225–31

[13] Sánchez A M and Campos R M 2011 Detection of prescribing related problems at the community pharmacy *Int. J. Clin. Pharm.* **1** 66–9

[14] Royce C S, Hayes M M and Schwartzstein R M 2019 Teaching critical thinking: a case for instruction in cognitive biases to reduce diagnostic errors and improve patient safety *Acad. Med.* **94** 187–94

[15] Newman-Toker D E, Wang Z, Zhu Y, Nassery N, Tehrani A S S, Schaffer A C, Yu-Moe C W, Clemens G D, Fanai M and Siegal D 2020 Rate of diagnostic errors and serious

misdiagnosis-related harms for major vascular events, infections, and cancers: toward a national incidence estimate using the 'Big Three' *Diagnosis* **8** 67–84
[16] Fernholm R, Pukk Härenstam K, Wachtler C, Nilsson G H, Holzmann M J and Carlsson A C 2019 Diagnostic errors reported in primary healthcare and emergency departments: a retrospective and descriptive cohort study of 4830 reported cases of preventable harm in Sweden *Eur. J. Gen. Pract.* **25** 128–35
[17] Omron R, Kotwal S, Garibaldi B T and Newman-Toker D E 2018 The diagnostic performance feedback 'calibration gap': why clinical experience alone is not enough to prevent serious diagnostic errors *AEM Educ. Train.* **2** 339–42
[18] Schiff G D, Hasan O, Kim S, Abrams R, Cosby K, Lambert B L, Elstein A S, Hasler S, Kabongo M L and Krosnjar N 2009 Diagnostic error in medicine: analysis of 583 physician-reported errors *Arch. Intern. Med.* **169** 1881–7
[19] Chimowitz M I, Logigian E L and Caplan L R 1990 The accuracy of bedside neurological diagnoses *Ann. Neurol.* **28** 78–85
[20] Dhaliwal G 2017 *Premature Closure? Not So Fast* (London: BMJ Publishing Group Ltd)
[21] Mahajan P *et al* 2021 An operational framework to study diagnostic errors in emergency departments: findings from a consensus panel *J. Patient Saf.* (published ahead of print)
[22] European Society of Radiology 2010 The future role of radiology in healthcare *Insights Imag.* **1** 2–11
[23] Lexa F J 2021 Duty hour limits for radiologists: It's about time *J. Am. Coll. Radiol.* **18** 208–10
[24] Bruno M A, Walker E A and Abujudeh H H 2015 Understanding and confronting our mistakes: the epidemiology of error in radiology and strategies for error reduction *Radiographics* **35** 1668–76
[25] Oestmann J W, Greene R, Kushner D C, Bourgouin P M, Linetsky L and Llewellyn H J 1988 Lung lesions: correlation between viewing time and detection *Radiology* **166** 451–3
[26] Heher Y K 2020 *Reduction of Diagnostic Error: Following Cytopathology's Lead* (New York: Wiley Online Library)
[27] Kohn L T, Corrigan J and Donaldson M S 2000 *To Err Is Human: Building a Safer Health System* vol 6 (Washington DC: National Academy Press)
[28] Verna R, Velazquez A B and Laposata M 2019 Reducing diagnostic errors worldwide through diagnostic management teams *Ann. Lab. Med.* **39** 121–4
[29] Blease C, Torous J and Hägglund M 2020 Does patient access to clinical notes change documentation? *Front. Public Health* **8** 578
[30] Astier A, Carlet J, Hoppe-Tichy T, Jacklin A, Jeanes A, McManus S, Pletz M W, Seifert H and Fitzpatrick R 2020 What is the role of technology in improving patient safety? A French, German and UK healthcare professional perspective *J. Patient Saf. Risk Manage.* **25** 219–24
[31] Mello M M, Studdert D M and Kachalia A 2014 The medical liability climate and prospects for reform *Jama* **312** 2146–55
[32] Marcusson J, Nord M, Dong H-J and Lyth J 2020 Clinically useful prediction of hospital admissions in an older population *BMC Geriatr.* **20** 1–9
[33] Boumendil A, Aegerter P, Guidet B and Network C-R 2005 Treatment intensity and outcome of patients aged 80 and older in intensive care units: a multicenter matched-cohort study *J. Am. Geriatr. Soc.* **53** 88–93
[34] Ehni H-J and Wahl H-W 2020 Six propositions against ageism in the COVID-19 pandemic *J. Aging Soc. Policy* **32** 515–25

[35] Adams W L, McIlvain H E, Lacy N L, Magsi H, Crabtree B F, Yenny S K and Sitorius M A 2002 Primary care for elderly people: why do doctors find it so hard? *Gerontologist* **42** 835–42

[36] Schofield P 2018 The assessment of pain in older people: UK national guidelines *Age Age.* **47** i1–22

[37] Johansson M M, Barbero M, Peolsson A, Falla D, Cescon C, Folli A and Dong H-J 2021 Pain characteristics and quality of life in older people at high risk of future hospitalization *Int. J. Environ. Res. Public Health* **18** 958

[38] Oh D K, Na W, Park Y R, Hong S-B, Lim C-M, Koh Y and Huh J-W 2019 Medical resource utilization patterns and mortality rates according to age among critically ill patients admitted to a medical intensive care unit *Medicine* **98** e15835

[39] Audisio R 2008 Shall we operate? Preoperative assessment in elderly cancer patients (PACE) can help: A SIOG surgical task force prospective study *Crit. Rev. Oncol. /Hematol.* **65** 156–63

[40] Decavèle M, Dreyfus A, Gatulle N, Weiss N and Houillier C *et al* 2021 Clinical features and outcome of patients with primary central nervous system lymphoma admitted to the intensive care unit: a French national expert center experience *J. Neurol.* 1–10

[41] Wou F, Gladman J R, Bradshaw L, Franklin M, Edmans J and Conroy S P 2013 The predictive properties of frailty-rating scales in the acute medical unit *Age Age.* **42** 776–81

[42] McCabe J J and Kennelly S P 2015 Acute care of older patients in the emergency department: strategies to improve patient outcomes *Open Access Emerg. Med.: OAEM* **7** 45

[43] Edmans J, Bradshaw L, Gladman J R, Franklin M, Berdunov V, Elliott R and Conroy S P 2013 The Identification of Seniors at Risk (ISAR) score to predict clinical outcomes and health service costs in older people discharged from UK acute medical units *Age Age.* **42** 747–53

[44] Seegmiller A C *et al* 2013 Optimizing personalized bone marrow testing using an evidence-based, interdisciplinary team approach *Am. J. Clin. Pathol.* **140** 643–50

[45] van Veen J 2020 Job Criteria for Successful Use of AI (University of Twente)

[46] Rissanen M 2020 Translational health technology and system schemes: enhancing the dynamics of health informatics *Health Inf. Sci. Syst.* **8** 39

[47] Shafqat S, Fayyaz M, Khattak H A, Bilal M, Khan S, Ishtiaq O, Abbasi A, Shafqat F, Alnumay W S and Chatterjee P 2021 Leveraging deep learning for designing healthcare analytics heuristic for diagnostics *Neural Process. Lett.* **53** 1–27

[48] Rong G, Mendez A, Assi E B, Zhao B and Sawan M 2020 Artificial intelligence in healthcare: review and prediction case studies *Engineering* **6** 291–301

[49] Quiroz J C, Laranjo L, Kocaballi A B, Berkovsky S, Rezazadegan D and Coiera E 2019 Challenges of developing a digital scribe to reduce clinical documentation burden *NPJ Digital Med.* **2** 1–6

[50] Jaspan O, Wysocka A, Sanchez C and Schweitzer A D 2021 Improving the relationship between confidence and competence: implications for diagnostic radiology training from the psychology and medical literature *Acad. Radiol.* (in press)

[51] Meyer A N, Payne V L, Meeks D W, Rao R and Singh H 2013 Physicians' diagnostic accuracy, confidence, and resource requests: a vignette study *JAMA Intern. Med.* **173** 1952–8

[52] Graber M L, Trowbridge R, Myers J S, Umscheid C A, Strull W and Kanter M H 2014 The next organizational challenge: finding and addressing diagnostic error *Jt. Comm. J. Qual. Patient Saf.* **40** 102–10

[53] Schiff G D 2008 Minimizing diagnostic error: the importance of follow-up and feedback *Am. J. Med.* **121** S38–42

[54] Berner E S and Graber M L 2008 Overconfidence as a cause of diagnostic error in medicine *Am. J. Med.* **121** S2–23

[55] Sarkar U, Simchowitz B, Bonacum D, Strull W, Lopez A, Rotteau L and Shojania K G 2014 A qualitative analysis of physician perspectives on missed and delayed outpatient diagnosis: the focus on system-related factors *Jt. Comm. J. Qual. Patient Saf.* **40** 461–AP1

[56] Meyer A N, Upadhyay D K, Collins C A, Fitzpatrick M H, Kobylinski M, Bansal A B, Torretti D and Singh H 2020 A program to provide clinicians with feedback on their diagnostic performance in a learning health system *Jt. Comm. J. Qual. Patient Saf.* **47** 120–6

[57] Lalani M, Baines R, Bryce M, Marshall M, Mead S, Barasi S, Archer J and de Bere S R 2019 Patient and public involvement in medical performance processes: a systematic review *Health Expectat.* **22** 149–61

[58] Carr S 2020 Feedback, on the learning curve to improved diagnosis *Soc. Improve Diagnosis Med.* **1** 2020 https://www.improvediagnosis.org/improvedx-march-2020/feedback-on-the-learning-curve-to-improved-diagnosis/

[59] Alolayyan M N, Alyahya M S, Alalawin A H, Shoukat A and Nusairat F T 2020 Health information technology and hospital performance the role of health information quality in teaching hospitals *Heliyon* **6** e05040

[60] Reinders M E, Blankenstein A H, Knol D L, de Vet H C and van Marwijk H W 2009 Validity aspects of the patient feedback questionnaire on consultation skills (PFC), a promising learning instrument in medical education *Patient Educ. Counsel.* **76** 202–6

[61] El-Kareh R, Hasan O and Schiff G D 2013 Use of health information technology to reduce diagnostic errors *BMJ Qual. Saf.* **22** ii40–51

[62] Graber I by M L 2020 2019 2019 John M. Eisenberg patient safety and quality awards: an interview with Gordon D. Schiff *Jt. Comm. J. Qual. Patient Saf.* **46** 371–80

[63] Benson T and Potts H W 2014 A short generic patient experience questionnaire: how Rwe development and validation *BMC Health Serv. Res.* **14** 1–10

[64] Ahmed F, Burt J and Roland M 2014 Measuring patient experience: concepts and methods *Patient-Patient-Centered Outcomes Res.* **7** 235–41

[65] Gertler S A, Coralic Z, López A, Stein J C and Sarkar U 2016 Root cause analysis of ambulatory adverse drug events that present to the emergency department *J. Patient Saf.* **12** 119–24

[66] Baker R, Smith A, Tarrant C, McKinley R K and Taub N 2011 Patient feedback in revalidation: an exploratory study using the consultation satisfaction questionnaire *Br. J. Gen. Prac.* **61** e638–44

[67] McDonald K M 2014 The diagnostic field's players and interactions: from the inside out *Diagnosis* **1** 55–8

[68] Haskell H W 2014 What's in a story? Lessons from patients who have suffered diagnostic failure *Diagnosis* **1** 53–4

[69] McDonald K M, Bryce C L and Graber M L 2013 The patient is in: patient involvement strategies for diagnostic error mitigation *BMJ Qual. & Saf.* **22** ii33–9

[70] Baines R, Regan de Bere S, Stevens S, Read J, Marshall M, Lalani M, Bryce M and Archer J 2018 The impact of patient feedback on the medical performance of qualified doctors: a systematic review *BMC Med. Educ.* **18** 173

[71] Welling D 2014 The Friends and Family Test Review (NHS England)

[72] Robert G and Cornwell J 2013 *Rethinking Policy Approaches to Measuring and Improving Patient Experience* (London: SAGE Publications)

[73] Davis F D 1989 Perceived usefulness, perceived ease of use, and user acceptance of information technology *MIS Quart.* **13** 319–40
[74] Yan Z, Kantola R and Zhang P 2011 A research model for human-computer trust interaction *2011 IEEE 10th Int. Conf. on Trust, Security and Privacy in Computing and Communications* (Piscataway, NJ: IEEE) pp 274–81
[75] Gabel M, Foege J N and Nüesch S 2019 The (in)effectiveness of incentives-a field experiment on the adoption of personal electronic health records *ICIS* pp 1–7
[76] Alexander P A and Murphy P K 1998 The research base for APA's learner-centered psychological principles *How Students Learn: Reforming Schools through Learner-Centered Education* (Washington DC: American Psychological Association) pp 25–60
[77] Malik M J, Ahmad M, Kamran M R, Aliza K and Elahi M Z 2020 Student use of social media, academic performance, and creativity: the mediating role of intrinsic motivation *Interact. Technol. Smart Educ.* **17** 403–15
[78] Pintrich P R, Marx R W and Boyle R A 1993 Beyond cold conceptual change: The role of motivational beliefs and classroom contextual factors in the process of conceptual change *Rev. Educ. Res.* **63** 167–99
[79] Heinze K, Suwanabol P A, Vitous C A, Abrahamse P, Gibson K, Lansing B and Mody L 2020 A survey of patient perspectives on approach to health care: focus on physician competency and compassion *J. Patient Exp.* **7** 1044–53
[80] Sibbald M, de Bruin A B and van Merrienboer J J 2013 Checklists improve experts' diagnostic decisions *Med. Educ.* **47** 301–8
[81] Schiff G D *et al* 2005 *Diagnosing Diagnosis Errors: Lessons From A Multi-Institutional Collaborative Project* (Rockville, MD: Agency for Healthcare Research and Quality)
[82] Gandhi J S 2000 Re: William Osler: a life in medicine *BMJ* **321** 1087
[83] Kugler J and Verghese A 2010 The physical exam and other forms of fiction *J. Gen. Intern. Med.* **25** 756
[84] Greco M, Powell R and Sweeney K 2003 The improving oractice questionnaire (IPQ): a practical tool for general practices seeking patient views *Educ. Prim. Care* **14** 440–8
[85] Crowson M G and Chan T C 2020 Machine learning as a catalyst for value-based health care *J. Med. Syst.* **44** 1–3
[86] Greenwood-Lee J, Jewett L, Woodhouse L and Marshall D A 2018 A categorisation of problems and solutions to improve patient referrals from primary to specialty care *BMC Health Serv. Res.* **18** 1–16
[87] Neves J, Vicente H, Esteves M, Ferraz F, Abelha A, Machado J, Machado J, Neves J, Ribeiro J and Sampaio L 2018 A deep-big data approach to health care in the AI age *Mob. Netw. App.* **23** 1123–8
[88] Raja R, Mukherjee I and Sarkar B K 2020 A systematic review of healthcare big data *Sci. Program.* **2020** 5471849
[89] Council G 2018 Using OCR: how accurate is your data? | Transforming data with intelligence. https://tdwi.org/articles/2018/03/05/diq-all-how-accurate-is-your-data.aspx
[90] Carbune V, Gonnet P, Deselaers T, Rowley H A and Daryin A *et al* 2020 Fast multi-language LSTM-based online handwriting recognition *Int. J. Doc. Analy. Recogn. (IJDAR)* **23** 89–102
[91] Anon 2021 Pro word cloud *Pro Word Cloud* https://appsource.microsoft.com/en-us/product/office/wa104038830?tab=overview

[92] Singh J, Singh G and Singh R 2017 Optimization of sentiment analysis using machine learning classifiers *Hum. Cent. Comput. Inf. Sci.* **7** 32
[93] Sajid A, Awais M, Mehmood M A, Batool S, Shahzad A and Zafar A 2020 Patient's feedback platform for quality of services via 'Free Text Analysis' in healthcare industry *EMITTER Int. J. Eng. Technol.* **8** 316–25
[94] Meadows D 1991 System dynamics meets the press, an excerpt from the global citizen *The Global Citizen, Meadows, D.* (Washington, DC: Island Press) pp 1–12

Chapter 8

Soft computing techniques for efficient processing of large medical data

Hussain Ahmed Choudhury and Nidul Sinha

During the last era, the usage of digital photography methodologies in radiology has grown substantially due to the recent developments in digital image processing and storage technology. About 90% of hospitals only take digital radiographs, including computed tomography (CT), magnetic resonance imaging (MRI), ultrasound (US), nuclear medicine (NM), and digital angiography subtraction (DSA). Also, traditional chest or skeletal x-rays, which make up another 70% of the radiographs, can be converted into digital signals for subsequent computed radiography processing (CR). The reason for this interest in digital images is clear: the representation of images in digital form facilitates the transmission of images and allows the transformation of visual diagnostic information in useful and novel ways. There is one possible problem with digital images, despite these benefits, namely, the large number of bits needed for their representation. The amount of data generated by these methods is immense, and when transmitting the data over a network, this may be a problem. In the field of medicine, image compression has been implemented to resolve this problem. Some examples of different biomedical image forms are x-ray images, CT scans, MRI images, Ultrasound images, Mammography images, Optical imaging. So the huge amount of data generated by different tests, videography of medical processes, and medical imaging are compressed to store and process the data efficiently with limited hardware resources. Various software and hardware standards are available for making video and image compression cost-effective and time-efficient. This chapter discusses the various soft computing techniques which are applied in the field of video compression to make the process faster by accelerating the motion estimation.

8.1 Introduction

In medical practice, medical imaging has become an essential medium that reduces the mortality rates, and the requirement of investigative operations and also leads to

doi:10.1088/978-0-7503-3815-8ch8

a decrease in hospital admissions and increases in life expectancy [1]. Study shows that in the US during the year 2003, medical imaging was found out to be about 12.8% for patients with more than 65 years of age [2]. Earlier, the medical imaging checks had been taken on radiological film, but nowadays all are processed digitally.

There was an exponential growth in the amount of data generated by the healthcare sector and the use of digital data in the form of images and videos become an integral part of the medical field also. This has led to an increase in research interest for the processing of medical data and to inform public policy. Customized and specially developed software are required to store and process those huge data and these approaches and methods can be useful in other areas including research on the cardiovascular area. Patient genetic and historic health record information can benefit reducing *cardiovascular risk*, whereas crowed sourced environmental data helps in *cardiovascular epidemiology*.

European Organization published a report on Nuclear Research (CERN) in 2013 that revealed that a data center stored 100 petabytes of medical data in the last two decades, but in just the last 3–4 years, 75% of total data was recorded and generated by the Large Hadron Collider [1]. Biological sciences and medical data are one of the major sources of such a huge amount of data. Fifty thousand sequenced genomes are available in the online database and less than $1000 are charged for whole-exome sequencing and per patient almost 700–800 GBs of uncompressed data [2, 3]. In today's scenario, a test done by a CT scanner can generate 600 MB to a few GBs of data with higher in-plane resolution. In many hospitals, the medical data and related huge data sets are stored, retrieved, processed, and managed by Picture Archiving and Communication Systems (PACS). Wherever the amount of data becomes huge, data/image compression becomes essential for efficiently managing those data with limited resources. Since the beginning of PACS, various new compression techniques were developed even before the standard compression methodologies were adopted [3]. However, designing of exclusive compression methods significantly increases the expense and the work needed to integrate and shift data between divergent sources and systems, and interoperability and compatibility of these schemes require the usage of standards for compression in a communication system [4]. The outsized genomic datasets were known for a long time, and solutions were also proposed to store these huge data and how to interrogate them for disease association studies [15]. High-resolution equipment such as MRIs produces progressively detailed images that support the diagnosis but needs vast and increasing amounts of storage and computational power to do the analysis.

Image compression decreases the bit budget of a graphics file in bytes without degrading the image quality to an undesirable level. The reduction of file size makes it possible to store more images in a given amount of disk or memory space. The time taken for the so compressed photographs to be transmitted over the Internet or downloaded from websites is also reduced. Several different methods are used in which it is possible to compress image files. The two most popular formats are JPEG and GIF formats for Internet use. For photos, the JPEG approach is more widely used, whereas the GIF approach is generally used for line art and other images containing geometric shapes. The images have spatial redundancies and videos have both temporal and spatial redundancies. The role of data compression in medical imaging is not limited to only images but it covers video and audio signals too. Advanced medical exercise uses many physiological signals (e.g., electrocardiogram (ECG), electroencephalogram (EEG), and electromyogram (EMG)) which must be processed in clinical rehearsal. Data compression is essential in storing and processing such data. To compress the videos which are a collection of images and compress images, motion estimation (ME) plays a key role. An efficient ME technique not only reduces the time of compression but also plays a vital role in keeping the quality of images/videos which is of utmost importance for medical analysis.

In this chapter, the focus will be on those modern image compression standards that are not covered by many researchers. The best and most appropriate approaches to achieve video compression through accurate and efficient estimation of the motion vector. So, various block-based ME techniques are also discussed in detail which is the most useful and widely accepted approach for doing ME efficiently, which in turn makes the video compression efficient. Various experimental results will be presented based on various research works done recently on video compression of large data along with the development and implementation of various soft computing techniques for achieving optimized video compression.

8.2 Understanding the concept: video compression

Video compression represents the technique for reducing the bit requirement to encode digital video content, which leads to faster processing, less storage requirement, and lower transmission bandwidth requirement. The key idea behind video compression involves the removal of any kind of noise, redundant and irrelevant information which are not critical to watching the video contents. A video compression codec (format) is regarded as an efficient one if it can achieve the above benefits without causing much hardware overhead and without compromising the visual experience of the contents of the video. Higher and efficient data compression is possible for digital video data than that of analog video data. Lossless and lossy are the two techniques for data compression, where with the first type there is no loss of video information and the same information can be decoded as the in the original, while in the second type the loss of video information happens due to the removal of less important or irrelevant information. Balancing the quality, speed, resource utilization and power consumption are the challenges in video compression techniques. To efficiently process the video data, videos must be encoded through a compression process.

As the videos are a collection of images or frames, the encoding of videos will include the encoding of each of the frames. But there is a difference in encoding still images and video sequences. The images or frames only have spatial redundancy, whereas the signals in video vary in space as well as in time and they have both spatial and temporal redundant information. The spatial redundancy is due to the correlation that exists between the nearby pixel values and the temporal redundancy exists between the signals that vary in the time since the frames are captured very fast. This can be well understood by the fact that the videos are captured by high-quality cameras and at very high speed represented by the frame rate of videos like 30 fps (i.e., 30 frames per second) meaning that within a second, 30 different frames are being captured, that is, to capture 1 frame, 33 milliseconds are required. It is a well-known fact that the variation in video information is owing to the physical displacement of the object from one frame to another, so, it can be argued that there will a considerable amount of redundant information popularly referred to as temporal redundancy between two successive frames of a video as the physical movement of the objects within a span of 33 milliseconds will be very limited. The best example is that for a news anchor briefing the news in a news-room/studio, there will be no change in the background, chair, desk, etc due to non-movement of the objects, which is the reason for spatial redundancy between the frames of a video, whereas there will be a change of movement of lips, hands, head, shoulders, and eyes but to a very limited extent. So, this type of very low degree of movement leads to temporal redundancy. To encode and compress all such videos, both spatial and temporal redundancies should be exploited.

8.3 Image compression standards

During the latter part of the last century, the emergence and development of digital imagery led to increasing demand for digital transmission and storage of images. Identifying the necessity of suitability and interoperability between various image communications and loading devices, several standardization efforts for image compression have been initiated over the past few years by agencies of international standard such as the International Standards Organization (ISO), the International Telecommunications Union (ITU) and the International Electro-technical Commission (IEC). In promoting the growth of digital photography, these principles have played a major role. Various image compression standards are discussed in this section.

8.3.1 JPEG

JPEG refers to 'Joint Photographic Experts Group' and specifies the working group WG1 of the ISO/IEC Joint Technical Committee 1, Study Committee 29 (ISO/IEC JTC1/SC29/WG1). The WG1 committee had developed many image compression standards at the international level.

8.3.2 JPEG2000

The standardization process to improvise the standard of JPEG Compression, WG1 committee initiated the process in the latter part of 1990. The improved standardized features include 16 bits deep samples being supported, superior bit-rate performance (especially at low bit-rates), support for samples of up to 16 bits deep, advanced transmission, and single architecture supporting both lossless and lossy compression.

8.3.3 JPEG-LS

The standard denoted by JPEG-LS summarizes lossless and near-lossless compression procedures for compressing grayscale, bi-level, and color images [51]. Several significant improvements including ease of implementation, lower memory requirement, and lesser complexity are possessed by JPEG-LS. The compression attained by JPEG-LS is very comparative with the methods that are based on more computationally challenging coding practices, like arithmetic coding, despite the simplicity of the coding procedures. Since JPEG-LS provides state-of-the-art lossless compression efficiency, for some medical applications requiring lossless compression, it is especially suitable.

8.3.4 JPEG-XR

To compress continuous-tone images like photographic images, the JPEG-XR standard was introduced [62]. Two features of JPEG-XR are the key features that are very important for medical image compression, namely the JPEG-XR standard that supports depths up to 32 bits for the input image. Second, both lossy and lossless compression is provided by JPEG-XR standard with the identical signal flow path.

8.3.5 H.265

The Joint Collaborative Team on Video Coding (JCT-VC) suggested another name High-Efficiency Video Coding (HEVC) to H.265 video coding standard which is jointly recognized by the ITU-T Video Coding Experts Group (VCEG) and the ISO/IEC Moving Picture Expert Group (MPEG) [67]. In the case of efficiency in the coding of materials/images captured by the camera, HEVC/H.265 shows better results than the existing coding standard up to 50% reduced bit-rate while keeping the same perceptual quality [67]. In 1993, a new and improvised video coding standard, namely Digital Imaging and Communications in Medicine (DICOM), was released. This standard is a very well-accepted standard for medical image data processing. It has transformed radiology exercises to digitally equipped data from the film-based workflow.

Three-dimensional information is available in a video signal which is modeled in spatial and temporal domains. The compression of videos is done by eliminating the redundant information available in both domains. Experimental evidence revealed that transform domain coding techniques are suitable to exploit spatial redundancies much better than predictive coding techniques, whereas the temporal redundancies can be exploited using predictive coding like Differential Pulse Code Modulation (DPCM) and Adaptive Differential Pulse Code Modulation (ADPCM). Since videos have both types of redundancies, we need to exploit both by using a Hybrid Video Codec where firstly the temporal redundant information is exploited using predictive coding techniques. Since the inception of coding standards says MPEG, Hybrid Video Codec architecture is being used. The Hybrid Video Codec structure is displayed in figure 8.1.

The Codec consists of two halves—encoder and decoder part. In the encoder, the prediction error of the residual signal is calculated by subtracting the input video

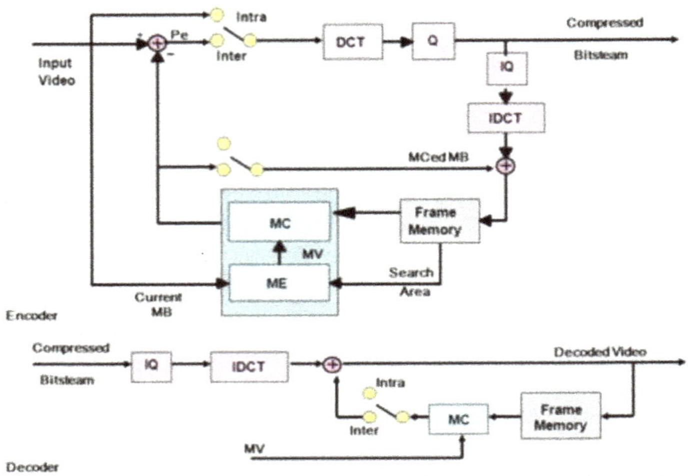

Figure 8.1. Encoder and decoder sections of hybrid video codec.

from the predicted video, and then the residual signal is encoded using DCT which is followed by quantizer and entropy coding. The encoder encodes the bit-stream of the residual signal but not the original signal itself. The decoder part of the codec regenerates the error frame which has some difference from the original one due to quantization that was done at the encoder side. Taking the earlier or upcoming frame as a reference, the motion estimator block of the encoder predicts the next frame or past frame and calculates the coordinate displacement vector also called a motion vector (MV) using a practice called motion esitmation (ME). The received signal is entropy decoded, de-quantized and inverse transform domain coding, that is, inverse DCT (IDCT) is used at the decoder terminal. Then the predicted video is added to the error to get the input video which is not the replica of the input video/ frames because, at the input end, the lossy compression is used.

8.3.6 Types of coding and frames

When the videos are taken and stored for processing, the frames must be encoded using some reference frames, either past or future frames. But as we know when we capture the first frame, there is no past frame nor future frame to refer to. In such cases, such images/frames are treated as still images and only spatial redundancy will exist which will be directly encoded by a process called Intra-frame coding and the frame is called I-frame. Temporal redundancies will not exist in such cases. Here the information is high and the bit requirement will be high. There is another way to encode a frame that uses the previous or coming frame as a reference called the predictive frame (P-frame), and the process is called inter-frame coding or predictive coding. The frames for which both the past frames and the future frames are used as a reference for coding them are known as B-frame and the process is called Bi-Directional prediction, which is also a part of inter-frame prediction. These types of frames are depicted in figure 8.2.

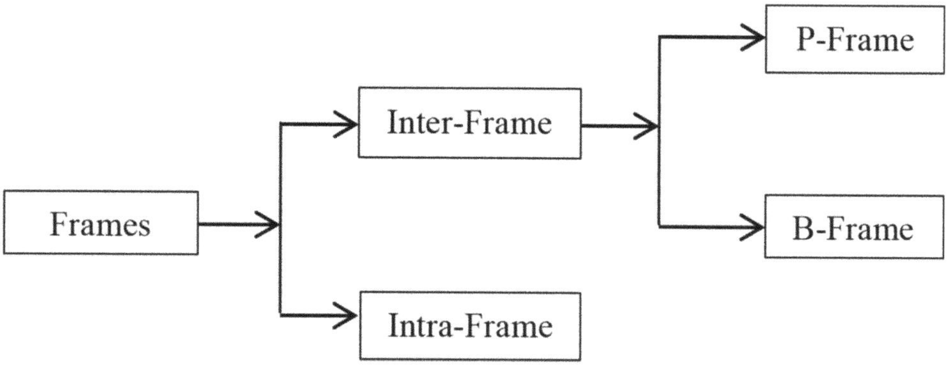

Figure 8.2. Different frame types.

8.4 Motion estimation and the necessity of it in video coding?

ME is the vital component of video compression. ME with motion compensation is used for the elision of temporal redundancy. Since a video is a collection of frames and there is little difference between two closely located frames, there is no need to encode every frame of a video. Rather we can intra-code the first frame and encode the change in information amongst the frames which are represented by MV and pass the same to the decoder side. The ME block of codec determines the displacement of objects in a video in terms of coordinate difference known as MV which is used by a decoder to regenerate the original video. The process of finding the MV is known as ME and this is the most complex part of video compression. The encoding of only the difference of frames, that is, MV will greatly reduce the bit budget to represent the video as the bits required to encode the whole frame are higher in comparison to the bits required to encode only MV. The efficiency of the compression process heavily depends on the complexity of ME process. So, the target of the research work is always to design such a methodology that the whole ME becomes fast and accurate. There are many approaches available for ME but due to the simplicity and speed, the block matching approach is widely accepted and research is ongoing to make the ME process more easy, accurate, and fast by developing new Block Matching Algorithms (BMAs). The methodology of BMA for achieving ME and its components are shown in figure 8.3.

8.4.1 Forward and backward motion estimation

In the video coding techniques, while removing temporal redundancies, frames are encoded concerning some other past or future frame. This type of coding is known as inter-frame coding or predictive coding. The frames that correspond to this type of coding are known as P-frame. In the encoding process, if the frame k (current frame) is encoded using the past frame say $(k-1)$th frame (previous frame) to predict what frame number k is going to be, we term it as forwarding prediction (FP) as future prediction is done for the kth frame by calculating MV. The process of FP is shown in figure 8.4.

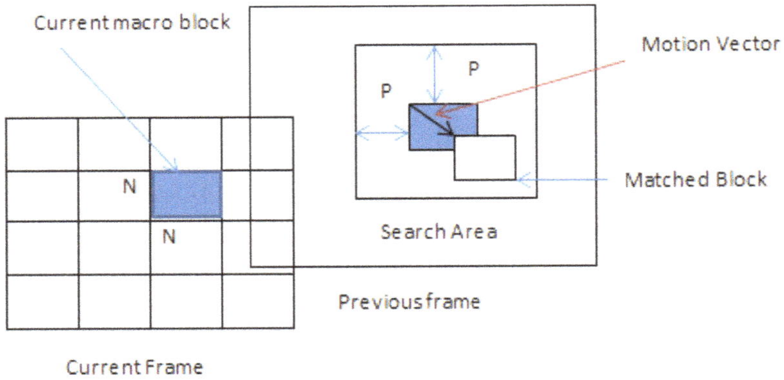

Figure 8.3. Components of motion estimation.

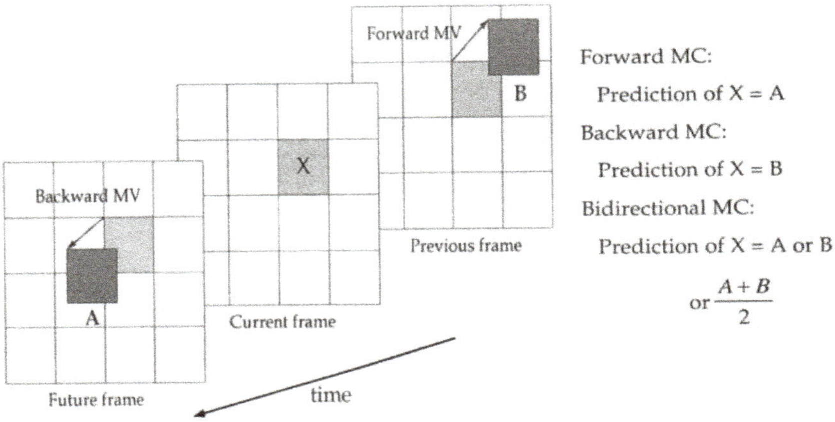

Figure 8.4. Forward and back prediction of frames.

As the past frame is used to predict the future of a frame by finding out MV, we can term it as backward ME. Conversely, when an upcoming frame is utilized to forecast the past position of the current MB in the target frame, it is designated as a backward prediction (BP) and is shown in figure 8.4 and as we go ahead in time to predict the past, this is referred to as forward ME.

8.4.2 Block matching concept

The concept behind the BM is to partition the images into a non-overlapping block called macro-blocks (MBs) of pixels assuming that all pixels within the MB undergo the same amount of displacement and to perform ME efficiently by finding out MV, that is, coordinate difference between the anchor MB and the most similar MB in the target frame based on certain matching measures. The goal of all BMAs is to evaluate the matching measures within a predefined search range (denoted by 'p') to determine the most correlated MB in the target frame, and the efficiency, speed, and accuracy of BMAs are vital for faster and accurate video compression. The efficiency

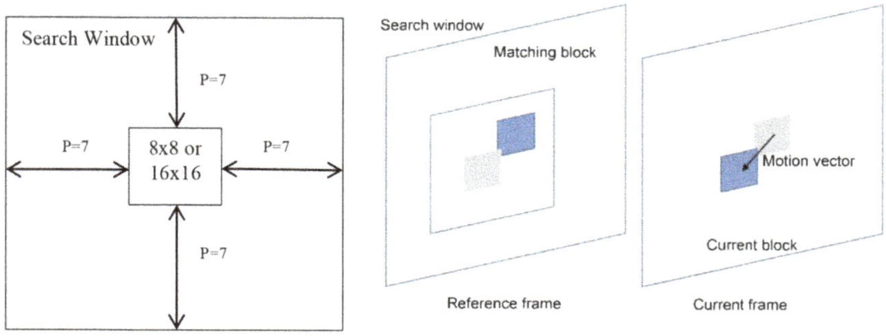

(a) Search range and search parameter

(b) Searching process of BMA

Figure 8.5. Search range and process of block matching within the search range.

of the BMA is judged by the computational complexity involved in finding out the best similar MB and the quality of the regenerated image. The concept of BMA, search range and its process can be well understood from figures 8.5(a) and (b).

The evaluation matrices used for finding the best match are:

i. Sum of absolute difference (SAD)
ii. Mean square error (MSE)
iii. Sum of absolute difference (MAD)
iv. Vector matching criteria (VMC)
v. Total absolute difference from mean (TADM)

8.5 What is soft computing: techniques and differences

Computation is a method of transforming the data of one type to another anticipated form using specific controls that are applied. According to computation, the antecedent is called the input, and the consequent is called the output. A mapping function is used to transform the prescribed input into an acceptable output. Computing is primarily applicable to the field of engineering. There exist two kinds of information processing; hard computing, and soft computing (SC). Some problems are solved by using existing mathematical algorithms which are programmed through hard computing which results in precise output value. Numerical problems are a clear example of hard computing.

Professor Zadeh defined SC as [1]: *'SC is not a single methodology. Rather, it is a partnership in which each of the partners contributes a distinct methodology for addressing problems in its domain. In this perspective, the principal constituent methodologies in SC are complementary rather than competitive. Furthermore, soft computing may be viewed as a foundation component for the emerging field of conceptual intelligence. The principal partners at this juncture are fuzzy logic (FL), neuro-computing (NC), and probabilistic (PR), with the latter subsuming genetic algorithms, chaotic systems, belief networks, and parts of learning theory'.*

The following are the characteristics of soft computing.

- Problems can be solved without any proper mathematical modeling.

- It generates diverse results when a problem is solved for one input from time to time.
- It uses nature-inspired algorithms like evolution, genetics, the intelligence of swarm particles, etc.
- These techniques can easily adapt in nature.

8.6 Standard techniques for motion estimation

BMAs are often divided into three groups. Pattern-Based BMAs (PBBMAs) are the first group because they are based on various search point patterns such as rectangular-shaped, square-shaped, hexagon, or diamond-shaped, etc Three-Step Search (TSS) [2], New TSS (NTSS) [3], Quick TSS [4], Reduced Three-Step Logarithmic Search (RTSLS) [5], 4-Step Search (4 s) [6, 7], Diamond Search (DS), [8, 9], Cross Diamond Search (CDS) [10], New CDS (NCDS) [10], Hexagon shaped BMA (HEXBMA) [11], Simple and Effective Search (SES) [12], etc. The Second Category considers and uses the similarity among the current MB and the adjacent MBs to estimate current the MB's movement, for example, Adaptive Rood Pattern Search (ARPS) [12–14], Inter-block correlation-based BMA [15], Correlation Search Algorithm (CSA) [16], Correlation Based Rood Pattern Search (CBRPS) [17], etc. The third group consists of all BMAs that are based on the concept and behavior of natural genetics or natural intelligence events which are called soft computing based BMAs. These are also referred to as BMAs inspired by Nature, such as the ME using Genetic Algorithm [18–27], Particle Swarm Optimization based BMAs [28–38], Artificial Bee Colony (ABC-BM) [39] based BMA, etc.

8.7 Soft computing techniques for motion estimation

The practice of achieving a better solution, that is, better than the current best solution of a problem is known as optimization and is the method followed to make the algorithm operate as meritoriously or as efficiently as possible. In recent times, Nature-inspired algorithms (NIAs), evolutionary algorithms, swarm intelligence, SC techniques, etc have become buzzwords in the field of optimization. Many computer science field problems together with other engineering disciplines are using SC techniques for finding optimal solutions for real-life problems. The optimization approach adopted by them to implement the concept and process of design to solve everyday problems motivated the researchers to explore the field further. Out of all biological or Nature-mimicked algorithms, Swarm Intelligence Algorithms (SIAs) [40] have the highest acceptance in the field of optimization. Besides being a non-deterministic algorithm, an algorithm for stochastic optimization may be heuristic or meta-heuristic type by nature.

To a large extent, the success of NIAs in overcoming the problems faced by Pattern Based BMA (PBBMA) in Video Compression influenced the researchers to conduct comprehensive research to apply more and more NIAs, especially swarm intelligence techniques for ME. There has been a decent amount of research and many improved versions of simple particle swarm optimization (PSO) have been suggested for ME, such as pattern-based PSO [32], clonal PSO [33], memetic PSO [35], etc. The problem with all these BMAs, however, remains that with a low convergence rate, high dependency on parameters, every algorithm may get stuck at local minima, causing a lack of population diversity, preventing them from achieving the global goal they need.

8.8 Conceptual terms used in different SC techniques

8.8.1 Chromosomes and genes

The chromosome is the collection of genes and it is treated as a string of values, that is, a function, say $F(x;y;z)$,, having three variables if needed to be maximized when 10 binary bits are required to represent one variable, then 30 bits will be required to represent a chromosome consisting of three genes.

8.8.2 Chromosome representation

A chromosome consists of genes namely object genes and strategy genes and it represents data for x and y coordinates.

8.8.3 Cross-over

The generation of new offspring (new solution) by mixing up portions of chromosome (solutions) with other corresponding portions of another chromosome is termed as cross-over.

8.8.4 Mutation

To generate a better version of offspring or to produce a better solution, mutation may change the gene value representing the problem solution completely from one generation to the next generation.

8.8.5 Weighting function and PBME

The function of search points having minimum value, that is, least search locations for the best match in all directions on a plane is represented by a Weighting function (WF) and is vital in determining the performance of BMAs. The best BMAs are associated with the least value of WF.

8.9 Some well-established soft computing based BMA

8.9.1 Genetic algorithm-BMA

An efficient optimization algorithm founded on biological genetics and Darwin's theory of natural selection is named Genetic Algorithm (GA) [24, 57]. The optimization of the ME process using GA starts with the encoding of parameters of BMA and an appropriate fitness function is selected to find the maximum matching MB, that is, corresponding MV. In search space, positions of search are encoded by chromosome with a finite length alphabet. In a population, an individual

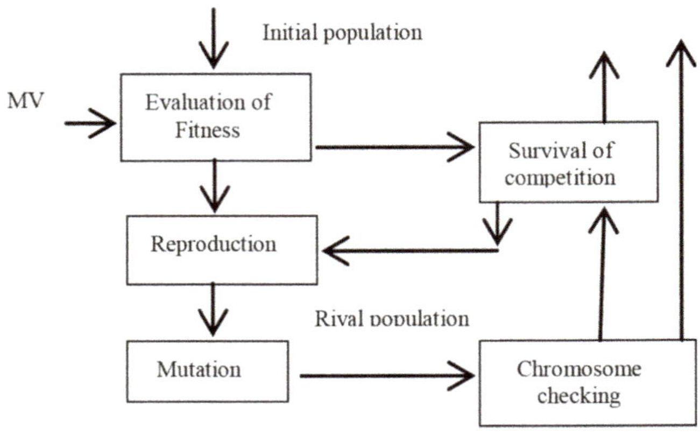

Figure 8.6. Search pattern of genetic algorithm for ME.

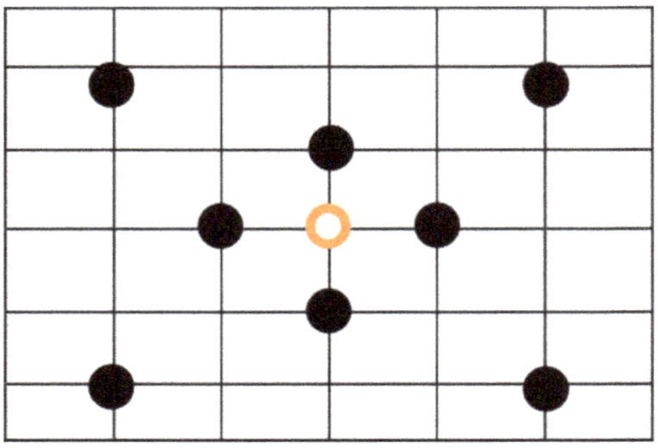

Figure 8.7. Block diagram of GA-BM.

is represented by one chromosome. An initial population of size M chromosomes is taken which will generate offspring generations of the same size in an iterative way.

Figures 8.6 and 8.7 depict the GA based BM [25–32]. The limitations of PBBMAs are overcome by the use of GA, but the implementation couldn't be possible properly due to higher computational complexity.

Steps of GA-BMA

1. The initial population and pattern used in BM using GA are displayed in figure 8.7.
2. The fitness of each chromosome is calculated, and the mean fitness value of the generation is selected.
3. The finest fitness value will replace the copy of the chromosome as per the rules mentioned above.
4. Until the stopping criteria is not matched, the search will continue with steps 2 and 3 or else stop.
5. The chromosome with the highest fitness is converted to the search location and the corresponding MV is noted.

8.9.2 Inter-block/inter-frame fuzzy search algorithm

The Inter-Block/Inter-Frame Fuzzy Search (IIFS) was proposed by Roan *et al* [35]. It uses the inter-block and inter-frame fuzzy prediction to determine the motion vectors of image blocks efficiently. It beats the common and famous BMAs like FS, TSS, DS, SES, 4 s, 2DLS, and a few others in terms of the following measures: (1) Avg. of prediction error for absolute prediction per pixel, (2) Avg. block distortion measure (e.g., MAD), (3) Avg. PSNR value, (4) Avg. Euclidean distance between actual MV and predicted MV, (5) Avg. probability to select the actual MV, (6) computational cost, and (7) bit requirement for the encoding of MV.

8.9.3 Basic block-matching using particle swarm optimization

Kennedy and Eberhart [43] proposed PSO which is inspired by nature and optimizing in nature. This algorithm became popular due to its optimizing ability and speed of convergence. This PSO algorithm is also used in the field of video compression to optimize the ME process. This algorithm is easier to use in practice than GA as it doesn't use mutation and cross-over to regenerate the offspring. Moreover, PSO is based on the nature of bird flocking and doesn't have a gradient, and is self-adaptive. Du *et al* [44] had used PSO for the first time to optimize the ME which overcomes the problem of local optima.

A solution in a search window or solution space in PSO is denoted by a particle that searches through the solution space for the best match location by adjusting the velocity dynamically. The particle position in a solution space which represents the position of a particle with the highest fitness value becomes the best matching location and it gives the required MV. Using the experience of a flying swarm and its knowledge, a particle updates the velocity. In a D-dimensional space, particles are represented as volume less point. $Xp_{(best)}$ represents the personal best coordinates location having the highest fitness value, whereas $Xg_{(best)}$ denotes the best location within the population.

$Si = (S_{i1}, S_{i2}, \ldots, S_{id})$ denotes '*i*'th particle in PSO and
$Pi = (P_{i1}, P_{i2}, \ldots, P_{id})$ represents the $Xp_{(best)}$ position of that particle.

Each particle updates its velocity vector '*V*' and position vector '*X*' according to equations (8.1) and (8.2).

$$\begin{aligned} VId(t+1) = w * Vid(t) + C1 \times rand1\,(.\,) \times (Pid - Xid) \\ + C2 \times rand2\,(.\,) \times (Pid - Xid) \end{aligned} \tag{8.1}$$

$$Xid(t+1) = Xid(t) + Vid(t+1),\ 1 \leqslant i \leqslant N,\ 1 \leqslant d \leqslant D \tag{8.2}$$

N = No. of Particles, D = Dimensionality

$Vi = (V_{i1}, V_{i2}, \ldots, V_{id})$, $V_{id} \in [-V_{max}, V_{max}]$: '*i*th' particle's velocity vector

$Xi = (Xi1, Xi2, \ldots, Xid)$, $Xid \in [-X_{max}, X_{max}]$: '*i*th' particle's position vector, w = inertia weight, C_1 and C_2 are constants known as acceleration constants and taken as 2.0; r_1 and r_2 are random numbers between [0,1], Pg and Pi are global best and local best. The steps of PSO based BMA [45–54] are briefed below.

PSO-BM Algorithm

1. Eight particle locations are selected in a different direction and initialized with random velocities.
2. Calculate the fitness values, that is, *SAD* for each particle.
3. Personal best (P_{best}) and Global best (G_{best}) are updated using equation (8.3) by the PSO algorithm based on a particle's fitness value.

$$Yi(t+1) = \begin{cases} Y_i(t) & \text{if } f(X_i(t+1)) \geqslant f(Y_i(t)) \\ X_i(t+1) & \text{if } f(X_i(t+1)) < f(Y_i(t)) \end{cases} \tag{8.3}$$

   X_i is the position vector of the particle '*i*' $f(X_i(t+1))$ is the '*i*'th particle's fitness value at $X_i(t+1)$ position $Yi(t)$ gives the current P_{best} of the particle '*i*'
4. Position vector and velocity vectors of the particle are updated using equations (8.1) and (8.2).
5. Until the stopping conditions are met, the above steps are followed.
6. The matching MB location and its MV will be the G_{best} position.

8.9.4 Harmony search block matching algorithm

Geem *et al* [56] had suggested a new population-based optimization approach called Harmony Search (HS) which mimics the process of continuously polishing the pitches for getting better harmony by a musician. Fitness approximation model attached with HS to get the best MV to get better harmony in music. Figure 8.8 is the block level diagram of HS-BM. The time of execution is greatly saved in doing ME accurately because of the integration of the fitness calculation strategy for finding out the MV.

The solution is also known as 'Harmony' in HS and is represented by *n*-dimensional real vectors. Harmony Memory (HM) is the initial memory in HS where harmony vectors are stored which are generated randomly. A new Harmony candidate is produced or created by applying pitch modification strategy or randomized re-initialization. The newly generated Harmony candidate is matched with the poorest harmony and HM is updated. Until the limiting condition is not met, a better candidate harmony vector replaces the poorest harmony vector.

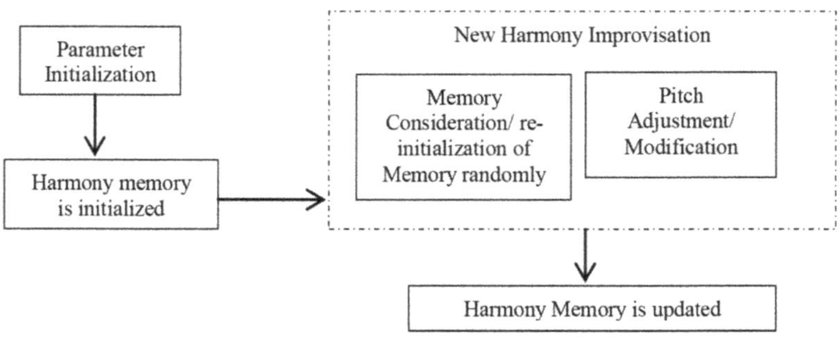

Figure 8.8. HS-BM algorithm.

The x and y components of 2-dimensional MV in search space S are represented by u and v in HS. In the search space, a particle is signified as equation (8.4).

$$p_i = \{\hat{u}_i, \hat{v}_i | -W \leqslant \hat{u}_i, \hat{v}_i \leqslant W\} \tag{8.4}$$

Where 'i' is a particle and it represents a possible location. The phases of the HS algorithm are:

a. Initialization of the problem and its parameters.
b. HM initialization.
c. Improvisation of New Harmony vector.

Harmonic Memory (HM) update

Some of the parameters, namely HM size (HMS), that is, the number of solution vectors present in HM, HM Consideration Rate (HMCR), the pitch adjusting rate (PAR), the distance bandwidth (BW), and a total number of iterations denoted by no. of improvisations (NI) are to be tuned for better performance.

This BMA combines the fitness approximation method with HS and overcomes the problem of fixed search patterns, better and accurate results are shown by the proposed BM when compared with popular BMAs and this balances the number of search point locations and the efficiency of coding.

8.9.5 Cat swarm optimization (CSO-BMA)

Hadi *et al* [56] suggested a novel Nature-inspired SC technique for ME called Cat Swarm Optimization (CSO-BM). The CSO-BM is an evolutionary technique. Since the algorithm doesn't follow any definite search pattern, the chances of getting the global minimum accurately will be more and with a better quality solution. The optimization technique mimics the cat's behavior.

A cat's approach can be seen in two phases. The cat is accustomed to observing its target very closely while pretending to be at rest, which can be referred to and framed as seeking model. The next phase of the cat's approach is framed as a tracing model where the cat goes behind the target. A matching MB is denoted by a cat in the search area in reference or current frame. In each iteration the position of the cat is modified using CSO strategy till a position with minimum cost function, that is, best match is found.

CSO Movement = Seeking model + tracing Model.

The working procedure of CSO-BM is briefed below and shown in figure 8.9.

Algorithm: Steps of CSO-BM algorithm

Step 1: Nine virtual cat's locations are taken as initial population, that is, 9 MB.

Step 2: Cat starts searching for the best MB for each MB in M dimensional space in different directions with some initial velocities within the maximum limit. A few of the cats are in tracing mode and others are taken as seeking mode as per mixture ratio (MR) which shows the joining of seeking mode with tracing mode.MR = 20% (tracing mode) and MR = 80% (seeking mode).

(Continued)

Step 3: Cats' positions are used in fitness function, that is, BDM is computed for every cat. The position of the cat with the best solution (x_{best}) is stored in memory, which is the best solution calculated till now.
Step 4: Based on flag value, cats make a move. Let's say cat_i is observing, then the seeking model or the tracing mode process is used for cat_i.
Step 5: Based on MR values of cats, they are selected, and tracing mode is applied to them and the remaining cats will be in seeking mode.
Step 6: If the limiting condition is met, end the algorithm and the best cat position with the lowest BMD will be selected. Otherwise, steps 3 to 5 are repeated.

8.9.6 CUCKOO search based BMA (CS-BMA)

The features of Brood Parasitism of cuckoo species and Levy flight that is found in some fruit flies and birds are the basis of Cuckoo search which is applied in ME optimization and is suggested by Bhattacharjee *et al* [60]. The important concept and steps used here are briefed below.

a. ***Nest selection:***
   Every nest contains an egg and each egg denotes a solution. So, a group of eggs, that is, nests are chosen as the initial population.

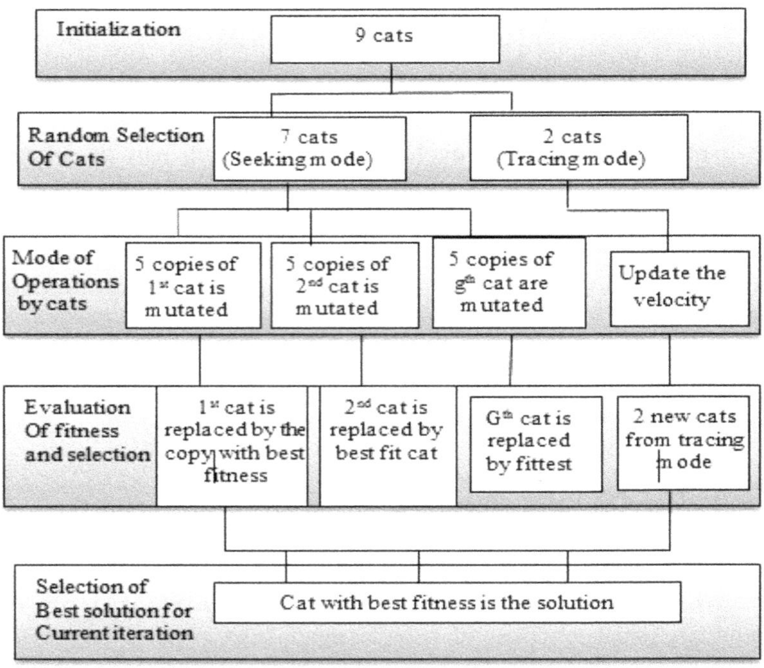

Figure 8.9. Strategy adopted in CSO-BM.

b. ***Laying of eggs by Cuckoos:***
Levy flight method given by equation (8.5) is used by the Cuckoo to generate a new solution S_{new} from the current solution S.

$$S_{\text{new}} = S + \alpha \oplus \text{Levy}(\lambda) \tag{8.5}$$

where step size = $\alpha > 0$, $\oplus$ = entry-wise multiplication Levy(λ) produces a random walk where exploration is controlled by Levy distribution and exploitation of search space is determined by producing step length randomly in the range $1 < \lambda \leqslant 3$.

c. ***New generation selection***
The host bird replaces the host eggs with cuckoo eggs to denote the updating of the old solution with better solutions. If the better cuckoo egg is found, it will signify the worst solution which will be neglected by the host bird and the bird will build a new host. This process of building a new host represents the production of the new solution. The host bird finds the cuckoo eggs with a probability of ρ_a which plays a major role in search space by denoting both local and global search, that is, $\rho_a = 0.25$ corresponds to 25% exploitation and 75% denotes exploration.

Steps of CS-BMA

1. Initialize the parameters: $\rho_a = 0.25$, $D = 2$ dimension, $P = 8$, Max_generation = 4, generation = 1, *MB size* = 16 × 16.
2. First population NP = 5 where search space is $(2P + 1) \times (2P + 1)$.
3. Calculate MAD between the candidate MB and the MBs in the reference frame, Bi such that $i \in 1$ to NP.
4. While (generations<Max_generation) do
5. The new population of size NP, using Levy flight method V_i is generated which uses equation (8.5).
6. By using the fitness approximation approach, MAD is calculated for each V_i by and check the following For $i = 1$ to $NP = 5$

            error measure for least value is checked
            i.e. if $MAD(V_i) < MAD(B_i)$
        Bi=Vi
      end if
   end for
7. ρ_a a fraction of the worst solution is swapped with modified solutions obtained by using randomly selected walks.
8. Generation is incremented by 1.
9. end while
10. The lowest value of MAD corresponding to some position in search space is selected for MV calculation.
11. end.

8.9.7 The ABC-BM algorithm

Another iterative technique based on a natural phenomenon and using swarm intelligence for optimization is called Artificial Bee Colony optimization. The random food sources, that is, locations, are used as starting population. Three key operations listed below are implemented for the optimization process till limiting conditions are met. These are:

- send the employee bees;
- food sources are picked up by Onlooker bees;
- scout bees are specified.

The ABC optimization is implemented successfully for efficient ME and steps of ABC-BMA [41] are shown using the block diagram in figure 8.10.

8.9.8 ABC-DE

Warasucheep *et al* [58] amalgamated the concept of Differential evolution with Artificial Bee Colony Optimization to propose the algorithm called DE-ABC algorithm. Converse to that, ABC optimization is merged with DE based on some other criteria for ME which is known as ABC-DE and is suggested by Bhattacharjee *et al* [60]. This BMA is designed 'for an optimal solution of BM corresponding to the least no. of MAD calculation'. In this BMA, mutation, and cross-over operations of DE override the process to produce new food sources, that is, bee phase and onlooker bee phase, which is shown in figure 8.11.

This hybrid BMA has become advantageous as it picks up the exploration feature in the search space of DE and the exploitation feature of ABC.

8.9.9 HS-DE based BMA

DE-HS is a hybrid algorithm designed by Chakraborty *et al* [59] which uses the mutation operator of DE instead of the pitch tuning approach of the HS algorithm to perturb the target vector. Bhattacharjee *et al* [60] came up with a concept reverse to this algorithm known as HS-DE which uses cross-over operation instead of mutation operator of DE so that more variation can be added in the perturb vector, and figure 8.12 demonstrates the workflow of the HS-DE algorithm.

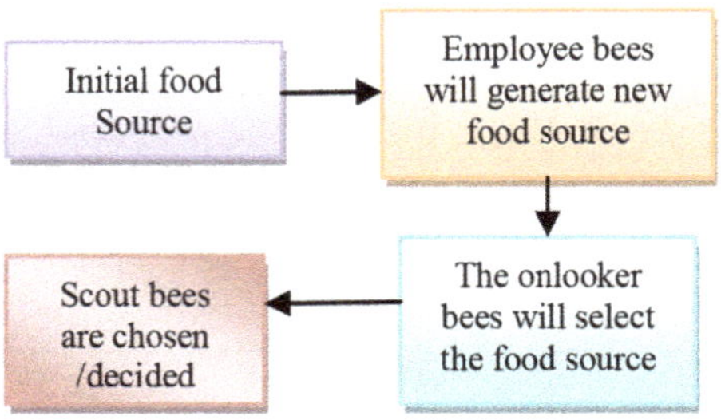

Figure 8.10. Block diagram of ABC-BMA.

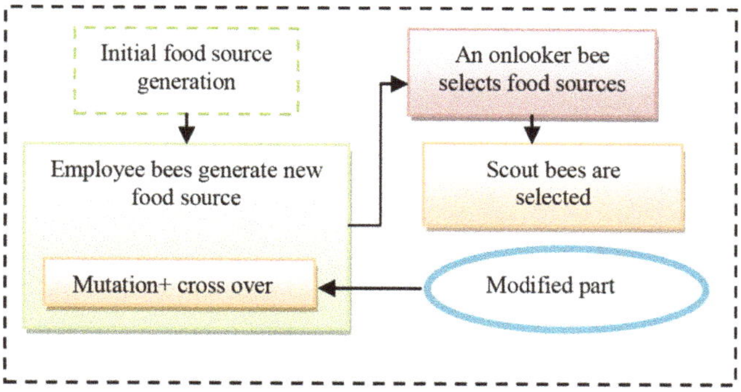

Figure 8.11. ABC-DE algorithm for BM block diagram.

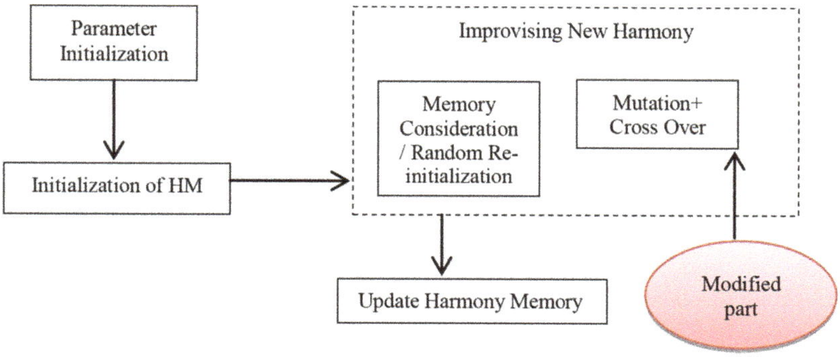

Figure 8.12. Working model of HS-DE base BMA.

The early convergence issue of HS and the difficulties of DE is successfully addressed by this hybrid HS-DE by implementing the concept of cross-over and mutation operator instead of the pitch tuning concept of HS.

8.9.10 'Deterministically starting-GA' (GA_{Det})

More *et al* [64] postulated a BMA called 'Deterministically Starting-GA' (GA_{det}) based on the property of adaptive convergence and early deterministic population of GA. This BMA is fruitful for x265 standard type video codec and it adopts the concept of survival of the fittest. The reduction of search points for the best matching MB is the motto of this BMA. Predicted and bi-directional frames are taken to have three reference frames. The early population that is created is taken to be at different spatio-temporal positions in the frames and at pre-specified HEX locations and all are a function of pre-encoded coding units. The newly designed BMA is beneficial for deployment of x256 video codec standard structure. In x265 CODEC's framework, GA_{Det} reduces the search point at selected classes of videos which are used for experiment (figure 8.13).

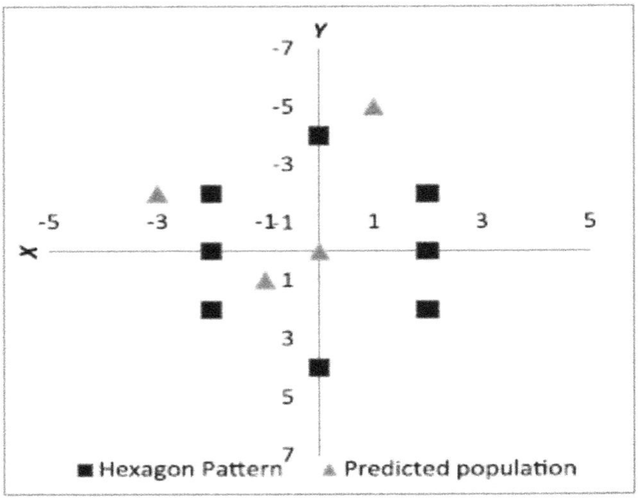

Figure 8.13. Initial population of GA_{det}.

Steps of $GA_{det\text{-}}$ BMA

---

i. The size of the window is 8×8, No. of generations, that is iterations = 10. Initial population size = 12 as displayed in figure 8.13 and probability of deciding the candidate MB is considered to be 0 with Roulette Wheel.
ii. A deterministic approach is used for encoding.
iii. Fitness function values are calculated.
iv. Probabilities and cumulative distribution function of cost values are calculated.
v. A new set of the population is generated.
a. The final population is updated as per values found in the Roulette Wheel approach and selects the best coordinates for the new population known as the mating pool.
b. if, iterations < 5; crossover operation is selected else.
c. If, iteration = 5; mutation is applied.
vi. Limiting criteria:
a. If (last iteration's minimum SAD – current minimum SAD) < 0.1% of their average; jump to step b else if the iteration number <10; go-to step ii.
b. New SAD values are updated and go to sub-pel ME.

8.9.11 Enhanced Grey-wolf optimizer-BMA (EGWO-BMA)

Betka *et al* [65] suggested a Grey wolf optimizer (GWO) algorithm for solving the problem of ME using the unique learning automata (LA) concept. By doing so, that is, adding the concept of LA, the exploration and exploitation facility of GWO are refined, and also the identification of objective function is done if unimodal or multi-model. Full exploitation of possible regions within the search window is required by a unimodal function. The exploration feature is useful for the multi-model objective function.

The structure found employing LA is then used in appropriate areas to produce new results. In the formation process, two methods are needed. In the first one, the function is updated by exploiting a Gaussian distribution for unimodal function; in the second one, the distribution is randomly explored to support exploration in multimodal function. Then block-based ME is improved by applying EGWO. The EGWO seeks better solutions to all benchmarks than regular GWO. And, six test videos are evaluated by the EGWO algorithm which is compared with many efficient methods. The results highlight that the EGWO experiences only deterioration in efficiency of nearly −0.71 relating to PSNR, which is better than most of the BMAs. Moreover, it achieves a better degree of efficiency with very few search points, that is, tests 10.34 MBs in the target frame per candidate MBs in the candidate frame and displays the appropriateness of EGWO for accurate optimization with complications.

8.9.12 Chessboard search pattern strategy

In a video sequence, MB with temporal and spatial correlations is shown in figure 8.14. A variety of BMAs is suggested by several people who use the knowledge about the movements of nearby objects to adapt their search strategies. Based on his technological breakthrough Amirpour *et al* [66] have proposed the Chessboard Search Pattern strategy (CSP) method. Similar to the chessboard pattern, MBs in a frame are categorized in two sets of black MB set and white MBs shown in figure 8.15, and a different search strategy is employed for each search type. Because of this approach, the number of collocated neighboring blocks will increase for each current MB and it guides us to an improved prediction of MV for each MB.

A few BMAs like ARPS, CSA, etc consider only four contiguous MBs for defining a category in their design. They neglected to use spatial knowledge about eight spatially neighboring individuals MBs. Also, since CSP calculates LUC information of eight neighboring MBs, it produces better performance. The CSP works as follows:

- Some random MVs are allotted initially to all black MBs while searching for best-matched MBs in the search space. Three spatially located MBs: top left, top right, temporal, and MB with (0,0) are taken as starting SP while finding

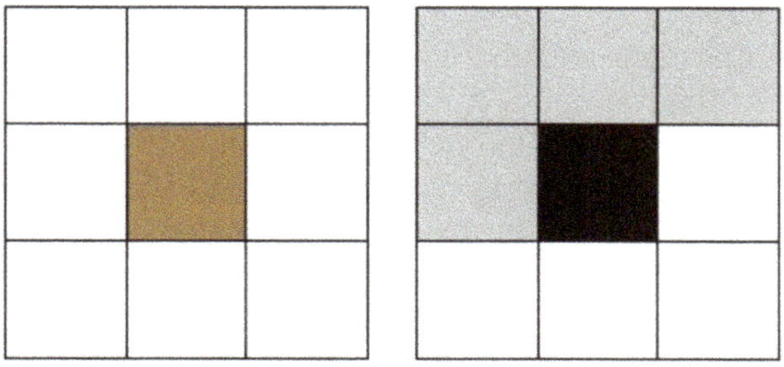

(a) Corresponding MB in the referenc frame (temporal neighbor) (b) MB of the current frame (current MB= ■ Spatial neighbor=)

Figure 8.14. Neighboring MBs of the candidate MB.

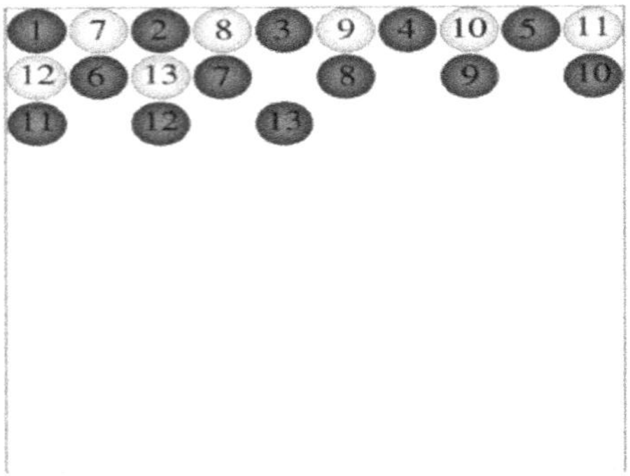

Figure 8.15. Black MBs and white-colored MBs like a chess board.

matching MBs for black colored MBs only. After finding the MVs of black MBs, MVs of white-colored MBs are computed.

- With the beginning of checking seven nearby MBs: left, top left, top, top right, right, bottom, bottom right, bottom left along with temporally collocated MBs data are used as a forecaster.

CSP achieved comparable results with FS in terms of PSNR while achieving a great improvement in the case of time and search point requirement over a few other existing BMAs by applying the information of eight neighboring MBs.

8.10 Results and discussion

The chapter discusses the few BMAs which are inspired and based on the concept of natural phenomena, and they are found to be efficient in the field of ME also. There are many more Nature-inspired SC techniques used for block matching that could not be explained in the chapter such as: Four-step GA-BMA (4SGA), Genetic Rhombus pattern Search (GRPS), Memetic PSO-BMA, Clonal PSO-BMA, Efficient Fuzzy Search (EFS), Momentum-directed GRPS (MD-GRPS), Pattern-Based PSO-BMA, Mutation and simplex integrated PSO-BMA, Simulated Annealing-BMA, etc. The available research studies have proven that the rigidity of regular BMAs for the ME process is addressed very effectively by the SC techniques used for ME. The problem of local optimum and the fixed pattern search is dealt with in all these algorithms by using the concept of dynamic initial velocity, random locations, early detection, mutation, cross-over, and many such biological events.

The various SC techniques that have been used as BMA for ME are surveyed and many of them are implemented on many video sequences. The results reported in other research studies and results obtained in the experiments are listed in table 8.1. The average search points that are required to check for the best match and the average PSNR values are shown in the said table. The overall results and performance show that the application of SC techniques greatly enhances the process of ME and these will speed up the video compression process.

Table 8.1. Comparative result analysis between various soft computing techniques for BMA.

Sl. No.	BMAs	Computational complexity	PSNR	Methodology
1.	Genetic algorithm for ME (GA-ME) [23–28]	37.7	29.2	– It is based on the natural selection theory of Darwin. – New populations are regenerated using mutation and crossover operators.
2.	4-step GA (4SGA) [32]	26.5	32.32	– 4 s and GA are merged to get the advantages of both in ME.
3.	Lightweight Genetic Algorithm (LGSA) [34]	18.1	29.64	– Random values are produced in the reproduction stage. – LGSA skips the cross-over operation.
4.	Inter-block/inter-frame fuzzy search (IIFS) [35]	10.2	26.82	– Current MB's motion vectors are found by using inter-block and inter-frame fuzzy prediction.
5.	Efficient Fuzzy Search (EFS) [36]	10.32	27.7	– The similarity between candidate MB and its neighboring MBs is used here and MV of current MB is decided by using Fuzzy reasoning.
6.	Genetic Rhombus pattern search (GRPS) [37–40]	9.1	34.68	– The algorithm works in such a way that the WF is the lowest in all its positions.
7.	Clonal PSO-BM (CPSO-BM) [41]	8.2	34.51	– PSO-based ME is integrated with the clonal features of the natural immune system to give the added advantage of exploration.
8.	Momentum Directed GRPS (MD-GRPS) [42]	39.45	34.17	– This algorithm updated the WF called Refined Weighting Function which models the search locations in ME process.
9.	PSO-BM (PSO-BM) [44, 48]	21.96	27.1	– The global minimum is found using bird flocking nature in this BMA.

(*Continued*)

Table 8.1. (*Continued*)

Sl. No.	BMAs	Computational complexity	PSNR	Methodology
10.	Memetic PSO-BM (MPSO-BM) [49]	14.417	32.01	– Dynamic inertia weight is used.
11.	PSO with Mutation and Simplex Method (MSPSO) [50, 51]	7.79	43.5	– The exploration feature of PSO and exploitation feature of the Simplex method is merged for finding the best matching MB.
12.	Simulated Annealing —BMA (SAA) [52]	10.38	35.512	– The global minimum is searched and found using the probabilistic method. – It uses the concept of the formation of pure crystalline solid by the slow process of cooling liquids.
13.	Differential Evolution-BMA (DE-BMA) [53]	12.675	33.85	– cross over, mutation, and selection operation is implemented.
14.	Artificial Bee colony-based Block Matching (ABC-BMA) [54]	11.57	33.265	– Nearest neighbor interpolation (NNI) is utilized for calculating fitness functions.
15.	PSO Based Parallel ME algorithm (PSO-PME) [55]	15.825	28.41	– The best matching MB is searched for a candidate MB in a frame. – At the same moment, PSO is used to all MBs in a frame parallel and results are synchronized to modify the MV which exploit the high similarity between the MBs
16.	Harmony Search-BMA (HS-BMA) [56].	12.35	34.01	– Tuning of Music is the key to the improvisation of the population-based Harmony Search algorithm integrated with a fitness approximation approach for finding the most suited MB.
17.	Cat Swarm Optimization based BMA (CSO-BMA) [58, 59]	16.54	32.88	– It doesn't use a fixed pattern in searching and also uses the global search feature of Cat Swarm Optimization (CSO) for motion estimation.

18.	CUCKOO search-BMA (CSBMA) [60]	6.95	33.4	– It amalgamates the Breeding facility of cuckoo and levy flight feature of some fruit flies for finding the best match.
19.	ABC-Differential Evolution based BM (ABC-DE) [61, 63]	17.56	37.835	– Food source generation of ABC is exchanged with Mutation and cross-over operation of the DE algorithm.
20.	Harmony Search and Differential Evolution (HS-DE for BM) [62, 63]	5.312	36.85	– Cross-over operator is applied in Harmonic Search.
21.	'Deterministically Starting'-GA (GA Det) [64]	13.26	32.51	– The deterministic starting population used in GA is the concept behind this BMA.
22.	Enhanced Grey Wolf Optimizer (EGWO-BMA) [65]	9.21	30.43	– The objective function is tested if uni-model or multi-model using Learning automata and exploitation is done by applying Gaussian Distribution.
23.	Chessboard search Pattern—BMA (CSP) [66]	5.45	31.75	– Current MB's coordinates, that is, MV is predicted using the MVs of eight neighboring MBs. – Raster scan is not applied. – MBs of a frame is segmented into the white and black set and different search technique is used in each set.

Acknowledgment

The authors would like to thank the Department of IT of CVR College of Engineering for providing the necessary facility to carry out the research. The authors would also like to thank Ms Nasima A Laskar for continuous motivation, NIT Silchar for necessary technical support in carrying out the work.

References

[1] Jain J and Jain A 1981 Displacement measurement and its application in interframe image coding *IEEE Trans. Commun.* **29** 1799–808

[2] Chan M H, Yu Y B and Constantinides A G 1990 Variable size block matching motion compensation with applications to video coding *Proc. IEEE (Communications, Speech, and Vision)* pp 205–12

[3] Koga T 1981 Motion-compensated interframe coding for video-conferencing Proc. National Telecommunication Conf. *(New Orleans, LA)* G5.3.1–5

[4] Li R, Zeng B and Liou M L 1994 A new three-step search algorithm for block motion estimation *IEEE Trans. Circuits Syst. Video Technol.* **4** 438–42

[5] Po L M and Ma W C 1996 A novel four-step search algorithm for fast block motion estimation *IEEE Trans. Circuits Syst. Video Technol.* **6** 313–7

[6] Zhu S and Ma K K A 2000 A new diamond search algorithm for fast block-matching motion estimation *IEEE Trans. Image Process.* **9** 287–90

[7] Zhu C, Lin X and Chau L P 2002 Hexagon-based search pattern for fast block motion estimation *IEEE Trans. Circuits Syst. Video Technol.* **12** 349–55

[8] Cheung C H and Po L M 2002 A novel cross-diamond search algorithm for fast block motion estimation *IEEE Trans. Circuits Syst. Video Technol.* **12** 1168–77

[9] Jia H and Zhang L 2004 A new cross diamond search algorithm for block motion estimation *Proc. IEEE Int. Conf. Acoustics, Speech, and Signal Processing* pp iii-357–60

[10] Cheung C-H and Lai-Man P A 2002 Novel small-cross-diamond search algorithm for fast video coding and videoconferencing applications *Proc. Int. Conf. Image Process.* pp 681–4

[11] Choi W I, Jeon B and Jeong J 2003 Fast motion estimation with the modified diamond search for variable motion block sizes *Proc. Int. Conf. Image Process.* pp II-371–4

[12] Barjatya A 2004 Block matching algorithms for motion estimation *IEEE Trans. Evol. Comput* 225–39

[13] Cheung C-H and Po L-M 2005 Novel cross-diamond-hexagonal search algorithms for fast block motion estimation *IEEE Trans. Multimedia* **7** 16–22

[14] Hashad A, Sadek R and Mandour S 2010 A novel reduced diamond search algorithm with early termination for fast motion estimation *Int. J. Video Image Process. Netw. Sec. (IJVIPNS)* **10** 14–22

[15] Hsieh C H, Lu P C, Shyn J S and Lu E H 1990 Motion estimation algorithm using inter-block correlation *Electron. Lett.* **26** 276–7

[16] Tsai J C, Hsieh C H, Weng S K and Lai M F 1998 Block-matching motion estimation using a correlation search algorithm *Signal Process. Image Commun.* **13** 119–33

[17] Alkanhal M, Turaga D and Chen T 1999 Correlation-based search algorithms for motion estimation *Picture Coding Symp.* pp 99–102

[18] Nie Y and Ma K K 2002 Adaptive rood pattern search for fast block-matching motion estimation *IEEE Trans. Image Process.* **11** 1442–9

[19] Choudhury H A and Saikia M 2013 Comparative study of block matching algorithm for motion estimation *Proc. Int. Conf. Advanced Computer Science and Information Technology* 73–8

[20] Choudhury H A and Saikia M 2015 Block matching algorithms for motion estimation: a performance-based study *Lecture Series on Advances in Communication and Computing* (Berlin: Springer) pp 149–60

[21] Fister I Jr, Yang X S, Fister I, Brest J and Fister D 2013 A brief review of nature-inspired algorithms for optimization, arXiv preprint arXiv:1307.4186 178–87

[22] Siddique N and Adeli H 2015 Nature-inspired computing: an overview and some future directions *Cogn. Comput.* **7** 706–14

[23] Holland J 1975 *Adaption in Natural and Artificial Systems* (Ann Arbor, MI: University of Michigan Press)

[24] Yuelei X, Duyan B and Baixin M 2000 A genetic search algorithm for motion estimation *Proc. 5th Int. Conf. Signal Processing Proc. and 16th World Computer Congress* pp 1058–61

[25] Chow K H-K and Liou, M L 1993 Genetic motion search algorithm for video compression *IEEE Trans. Circuits Syst. Video Technol.* **3** 440–5

[26] Moscheni F and Vesin. J-M 1995 A genetic algorithm for motion estimation,15° Colloquesur le traitement du signal et des images, FRA, GRETSI, Grouped' Etudes du Traitement du Signal et des Images

[27] El Ouaazizi A, Zaim M and Benslimane R 2011 A genetic algorithm for motion estimation *Int. J. Comput. Sci. Netw. Sec. (IJCSNS)* **11** 165–72

[28] Lin C-H and Wu J-L 1996 Genetic block matching algorithm for video coding *Proc. Multimedia* 544–7

[29] Davis T E and Principe C J 1991 A simulated annealing-like convergence theory for the simple genetic algorithm *Belez and Booker* 174–81

[30] Michalewiez Z 1992 *Genetic Algorithms + Data Structure = Evolution Programs* (Berlin: Springer)

[31] Gorpuni P 2009 Development of fast motion estimation algorithms for video compression *MTech Thesis* National Institute of Technology, Rourkela

[32] So M F and Wu A 1998 Four-step genetic search for block motion estimation *Proc. IEEE Int. Conf. on Acoustics, Speech and Signal Processing* pp 1393–6

[33] Immanuel S and Pandian A *et al* 2011 A study on block matching algorithms for motion estimation *IJCSE* **3** 34–44

[34] Lin C-I and Ja-Ling W 1998 A lightweight genetic block-matching algorithm for video coding *IEEE Trans. Circuits Syst. Video Technol.* **8** 386–92

[35] Roan Y-T and Chen P-Y 2000 A fuzzy search algorithm for the estimation of motion vectors *IEEE Trans. Broadcast.* **46** 121–7

[36] Chen P-Y and Jou J M 2001 An efficient blocking-matching algorithm based on fuzzy reasoning *IEEE Trans. Syst. Man Cybern., B (Cybern)* **31** 53–9

[37] Tsai J J and Hang H M 2007 A genetic rhombus pattern search for block motion estimation *Proc. IEEE Int. Symp. on Circuits Syst.* pp 3655–8

[38] Tsai J J and Hang H M 2010 On the design of pattern-based block motion estimation algorithms *IEEE Trans. Circuits Syst. Video Technol.* **20** 136–43

[39] Po L-M, Ting C-W, Wong K-M and Ng K-H 2007 Novel point oriented inner searches for fast block motion estimation *IEEE Trans. Multimedia* **9** 9–15

[40] Tsai J J and Hang H M 2007 On adaptive pattern selection for block motion estimation algorithms *Proc. IEEE Int. Conf. on Acoustics, Speech and Signal Processing, ICASSP* pp I-1173–6

[41] Tan Y and Xiao Z M 2007 Clonal particle swarm optimization and its applications *Proc. IEEE Congress on Evolutionary Computation* pp 2303–9

[42] Tsai J J and Hang H M 2008 On modeling genetic pattern search for block motion estimation *Proc. 15th IEEE Int. Conf. on Image Processing, ICIP* pp 1980–3

[43] Kennedy J 2011 Particle swarm optimization *Encyclopedia of Machine Learning* (Boston, MA: Springer) pp 760–6

[44] Du G Y, Huang T S, Song L X and Zhao B J 2005 A novel fast motion estimation method based on particle swarm optimization *Proc. Int. Conf. on Machine Learning and Cybernetics* pp 5038–42

[45] Yuan X and Shen X 2008 Block matching algorithm based on particle swarm optimization for motion estimation *Proc. Int. Conf. on Embedded Software and Systems (ICESS)* pp 191–5

[46] Bakwad K M, Pattnaik S S, Sohi B S, Devi S, Gollapudi S V, Sagar C V and Patra P K 2008 Small population-based modified parallel particle swarm optimization for motion estimation *Proc. 16th Int. Conf. on Advanced Computing and Communications (ADCOM)* pp 367–73

[47] Damodharan K and Muthusamy T 2014 Analysis of particle swarm optimization in block matching algorithms for video coding *Sci. J. Circuit Syst. Signal Process.* **3** 17–23

[48] Thamarai M and Shanmugalakshmi R 2010 Video coding using directed particle swarm optimization *CiiT Int. J. Digit. Image Process.* **11** 1404–11

[49] Nagpal P and Baghla S 2011 Video compression by the memetic algorithm *Int. J. Adv. Comput. Sci. App. (IJACSA)* **2** 142–5

[50] Zhang P, Wei P, Yu H Y and Fei C 2011 A novel search algorithm based on particle swarm optimization and simplex method for block motion estimation *Int. J. Digit. Content Technol. App.* **6** 207–16

[51] Zhang P, Wei P, Yu H and Wang Z 2010 Simplex particle swarm optimization for block matching algorithm *Proc. Int. Symp. on Intelligent Signal Processing and Communication Systems (ISPACS)* pp 1–4

[52] Shi Z, Fernando W A C, Kondoz A and Tsuzuki M S G 2012 Simulated annealing for fast motion estimation algorithm in H. 264/AVC *Simulated Annealing-Single and Multiple Objective Problems* (London: IntechOpen) pp 175–94

[53] Cuevas E, Zaldivar D, Pérez-Cisneros M and Oliva D 2013 Block-matching algorithm based on differential evolution for motion estimation *Eng. Appl. Artif. Intell.* **26** 488–98

[54] Cuevas E, Zaldívar D, Pérez-Cisneros M, Sossa H and Osuna V 2013 Block matching algorithm for motion estimation based on Artificial Bee Colony (ABC) *Appl. Soft Comput.* **13** 3047–59

[55] Jalloul M K 2013 A novel parallel computing approach for motion estimation based on particle swarm optimization *Proc. Int. Conf. on Engineering of Recon Figurable Systems and Algorithms (ERSA)*

[56] Cuevas E 2013 Block-matching algorithm based on harmony search optimization for motion estimation *Appl. Intell.* **39** 165–83

[57] Kung C M, Cheng W S and Jeng J H 2014 Application of genetic algorithm to hexagon-based motion estimation *Sci. World J.* **2014** 689294

[58] Hadi I and Sabah M 2014 A novel block matching algorithm based on cat swarm optimization for efficient motion estimation *Int. J. Digit. Content Technol. App.* 33–8

[59] Hadi I and Sabah M 2015 Improvement cat swarm optimization for efficient motion estimation *Int. J. Hybrid Inf. Technol.* **8** 279–94

[60] Bhattacharjee K and Kumar S 2017 A novel block matching algorithm based on Cuckoo search *Proc. 2nd Int. Conf. on Telecommunication and Networks (TEL-NET)* pp 1–5

[61] Worasucheep C 2015 An opposition-based hybrid artificial bee colony with differential evolution *IEEE Congress on Evolutionary Computation (CEC)* pp 2611–8

[62] Chakraborty P, Roy G G, Das S, Jain D and Abraham A 2009 An improved harmony search algorithm with differential mutation operator *Fundam. Inform.* **95** 401–26

[63] Bhattacharjee K, Kumar S, Pandey H M, Pant M, Windridge D and Chaudhary A 2018 An improved block matching algorithm for motion estimation in video sequences and application in robotics *Comput. Electr. Eng.* **68** 92–106

[64] More V N, Prashant P B and Sutaone M S 2018 Accelerating motion estimation by genetic algorithm approach in x265 *J. Electron. Imaging* **27** 1–13

[65] Betka A, Terki N, Toumi A and Dahmani H 2019 Grey wolf optimizer-based learning automata for solving block matching problem *Signal, Image Video Process.* **14** 285–93

[66] Amirpour H, Ghanbari M, Pinheiro A and Pereira M 2019 Motion estimation with chessboard pattern prediction strategy *Multimedia Tools Appl.* **78** 21785–804

[67] Ohm J R, Sullivan G J, Schwarz H, Tan T K and Wiegand T 2012 Comparison of the coding efficiency of video coding standards—including high efficiency video coding (HEVC) *IEEE Trans. Circuits Syst. Video Technol.* **22** 1669–84

Chapter 9

A comparison of Parkinson's disease prediction using ensemble data mining techniques with features selection methods

Dhyan Chandra Yadav and Saurabh Pal

Nerve cells or neurons are very important parts of the human body. The brain manages the control system and blood circulation by nerve cells. So it is necessary to know about symptoms of initial stage neuron disturbance in the body system. The 'main objective of this chapter is to protect the human body by initial knowledge about Parkinson's disease. We used machine learning algorithms and analyzed Parkinson's symptoms.

Machine learning algorithms provide help in prediction of attributes and give maximum accurate results. In this paper, we used Naïve Bayes, Decision Tree, Extra Tree, Random Forest and Bagging ensemble method for better prediction compared with all other performed work in this field or in the medical field. All the selective algorithms are tree based algorithms and they have different and important properties for better prediction on a large dataset. We use Bagging ensemble method with all selective algorithms and provide a unique result of prediction.

After all experiments, we find a better result with Bagging algorithms compared to all other selective algorithms, Naïve Bayes, Decision Tree, Extra Tree and Random Forest. Bagging algorithms evaluated with Kappa (0.958), Overall Fraction Correct (0.98), Mis-classification Rate (0.02), Sensitivity (0.979) and Specificity (0.983).

9.1 Introduction

Parkinson's disease is a very dangerous disease in the human body in which nerve cells become dead in a particular area. The nerve system runs by dopamine chemical in the human brain so dead neurons do not produce dopamine. Parkinson's disease is not observed at random in any human body because it is directly related with dopamine. Dopamine does not finish suddenly in the body.

doi:10.1088/978-0-7503-3815-8ch9

If dopamine production is less in the body then it indicates some symptoms in the human body such as:

- minor tremors felt in hands, legs and head;
- minor stiffness felt in limbs and trunk;
- minor slowness seen in movement;
- seen impaired balance and coordination;
- seen depression and difficulty in speaking;
- seen disruptions in sleeping.

It is critical to correctly diagnose and declare Parkinson's disease. If dopamine production stops in the body then Parkinson's disease will be at a high level.

9.2 Related work

Some researchers have done work on Parkinson's disease by different features selection techniques: GA. PSO, correlation based, filtered based etc [1–5].

Nemmi *et al*, discussed two Parkinsonian syndromes identified by MRI protocol and used pipeline combined with several feature selection and finally found best accuracy (94%). The pipeline evaluated more relative important features of Parkinson's's disease with a different model set. The pipeline performed a good balance between classification accuracy and relative important features [1].

Tejeswinee *et al*, discussed a neuro-degenerative data set by data mining technique. They found a correlation based feature subset selection method gave the highest accuracy (94%) by support vector machine (SVM) and used different classifiers on 111 instances of a Parkinson's dataset in which they found 74 genes unique and 37 different genes different [2].

Behroozi *et al*, discussed Parkinson's disease. They used multiple classifier frameworks KNN, SVM Linear Kernal, SVM (RBF), Naïve Bayes and Discriminants Analysis for speech dataset. They used filter based feature selection and found accuracy K-nearest neighbor (K-NN) ($K = 7$) (77%), SVM Linear Kernal (85%), radial based functional (RBF) (87%), Naïve Bayes (80%) and Discriminants Analysis (82%)[3].

Tubishat M *et al*, analyzed algorithms for features selection. They used 'Salp Swarm Algorithm, Classification, Feature selection Optimization, Machine Learning Algorithm' and 'Opposition Based Learning' on 18 different datasets. They finally selected the optimal subset in wrapper mode and solved the feature selection problem [4].

Xiao B *et al*, predicted hybrid features of Parkinson's disease which was based on QSM, SN and CNN. They observed a dataset from MRI image biomarkers and evaluated area under curve (AUC), sensitivity, specificity and accuracy by NF, convolutional neural networks (CNN) and SVM. SVM evaluated highest accuracy (96%) after features selection [5].

Some authors have predicted on the basis of machine learning algorithmssuch as: SVM, Naïve Bayes, Random Forest' etc [6–10].

Cavallo *et al*, analyzed a feature array as the most significant to discriminate among the different classes and different groups of classification. They compared SVM, Random Forest and Naïve Bayes by various datasets. Finally, they achieved highest accuracy of SVM (97%) [6].

Berus *et al*, analyzed 26 different voice samples of Parkinson's patients. They used 'multiple feed-forward artificial neural networks (ANNs) in the prediction of Parkinson's's disease of tested individuals. Finally, they found highest accuracy (86%) of neural network [7].

Drotar and Zdenek, discussed identification of diseases or differential diagnosis of various types of disorders. They used machine learning algorithms SVM, RF, AdaBoost, Deep Belief Networks, K-NN, Naïve Bayes, LDA and Perceptron. They found better framework for classification and calculated accuracy. Finally, they found classification accuracy of SVM (94%), RF (97%), Ada Boost (93%), Deep Belief Networks (76%), K-NN (96%), Naïve Bayes (96%), LDA (91%) and Perceptron (98%) [8].

Sharma *et al*, predicted Parkinson's disease for identification of symptoms. They presented the Modified Grey Wolf Optimization algorithm for symptom identification of premature stages of Parkinson's disease. They used datasets of voice, handwriting and speech. They used RF, KNN and Decision Tree for better prediction and by measured (94%) accuracy by forward algorithm [9].

Bellino *et al* discussed the relationship between gait parameters and falls incidence. They predicted the risk among older adults of approximately 105 adults older than 65. The entire functional and fundamental assessment fall event was recorded in diaries. J48 algorithm was applied for fall in future prediction with (84%) accuracy [10].

Some authors used ensemble methods for better prediction. They added various algorithms in Bagging, Stacking, Boosting etc ensemble methods [11, 12].

Yadav and Pal discussed thyroid patients and their predictions. They used a thyroid symptoms based dataset and generated an ensemble technique for prediction. They generated techniques (Stacking) and (Bagging + Boosting) applied, and after evaluation they found (97%) ROC of stacking [11].

Yadav and Pal analyzed hormones disorders in thyroid disease. They used J48, Hoeffding and RF for better prediction. Selected machine learning algorithms trained input samples in various forms then found better classification accuracy of the ensemble method [12].

9.3 Methodology

The proposed methodology is divided into three main parts:

1. Predict Parkinson's disease using different machine learning classifiers and analyze the obtained result.
2. Select important features from the feature selection methods Chi square, Extra Tree and Heatmap prepared dataset with high importance.
3. Apply once again selected machine learning classifiers on the prepared dataset (after feature selection) comparing the results from previous predictions.

9.3.1 Data description

The selected dataset contains three voice recording replications of the continued (sustained). The number of instances in the whole dataset is 756 and available numbers of attributes are 21. All the dataset depends upon replication consideration. The examination of dataset depends upon matching a combination of classical concepts of some subject voice recordings. It is a critical problem to identify more similar features from different subjects (table 9.1).

In most of the studies, we find Parkinson's disease identifies by many symptoms. In this chapter we select and predict speech based dataset categories as:

1. Contain the repetition of one term;
2. Consist of different spoken terms.

Dataset is accessible from the UCI machine learning repository. We select a Parkinson's speech dataset with multiple types of sound recording for prediction.

Table 9.1. Parkinson's dataset features and description.

Feature name	Description	
ID	Subjects are required for identification	
Recording	How many times recording is available	
Status	0 = Healthy, 1 = Parkinson's disease	
Gender	0 = Man, 1 = Woman	
RPDE	Recurrence period density entropy in measurement	
DFA	Signal fractal scaling exponent of detrended fluctuation analysis in measurement	
PPE	Pitch (area of play) period entropy in measurement	
GNE	Glottal-to-noise excitation ratio in measurement	
Feature name	**Group**	**Measure**
Jitter	'Local, Absolute, Rap, PPQ5 and DDP'	Frequency
Pulses	'Number of pulses, Period: Number, Mean and Standard Derivation'	Pitch Local Perturbation
Shimmer	'local (Shim_loc), dB (Shim_dB), 3-point (Shim_APQ3), 5-point (Shim_APQ5), 11-point (Shim_APQ11)'.	Amplitude perturbation quotient
Harmonic-to-noise ratio	0–500 Hz (HNR05) 0–1500 Hz (HNR15) 0–2500 Hz (HNR25) 0–3500 Hz (HNR35) 0–3800 Hz (HNR38).	Frequency band
Mel frequency cepstral coefficient	0–12 (MFCC0, MFCC1,..., MFCC12) and (Delta0, Delta1,..., Delta12).	MFCC-based spectral and their derivatives

Some features focused on only identification, recording, status and gender of particular diseases of Parkinson's. Some other features measure signal scaling, area of play, noise and density entropy.

Six features related to all words and voiced features of frequency. The feature Glottal isolates the voiced folds vibrations during large variation in vocal folds.

Jitter measures cycle-to-cycle variations in frequency and Shimmer measures the variations of peak amplitude decibels.

Both Jitter and Shimmer are defined by different points mentioned in the above table.

9.3.2 Whisker plotting

We used whisker plot for Parkinson's data because it easily represents variables location with spread at a glance (figure 9.1). It is required to know the summary about all features of the Parkinson's dataset. Whisker plot checks outlier data (normal/non-normal).

9.3.3 Histogram plotting

We used a histogram for frequency measurement of data in graphical form (figure 9.2). In the histogram is found the distribution of data with data summary in bar. Each bar frequency is represented along with each feature in the dataset.

9.4 Algorithms description

In this chapter we use different data mining tree algorithms with ensemble method for better prediction.

9.4.1 Decision tree

Decision tree is used for prediction of variables of many medical datasets. It is focused on dependable variables or target variable (figure 9.3). It is basically used for

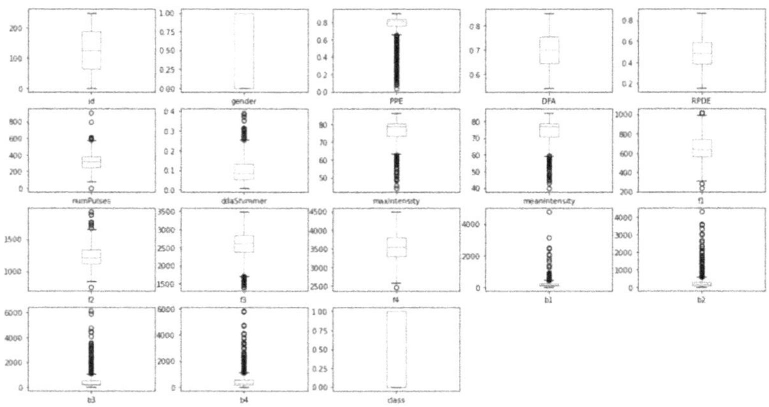

Figure 9.1. Representation of Parkinson's dataset by Whisker plot.

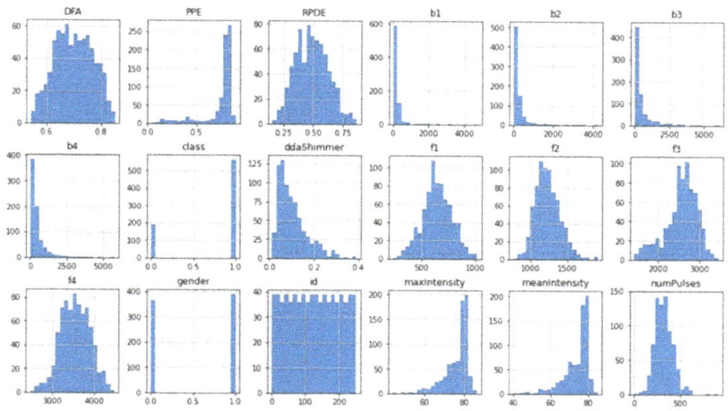

Figure 9.2. Representation of Parkinson's dataset by histogram.

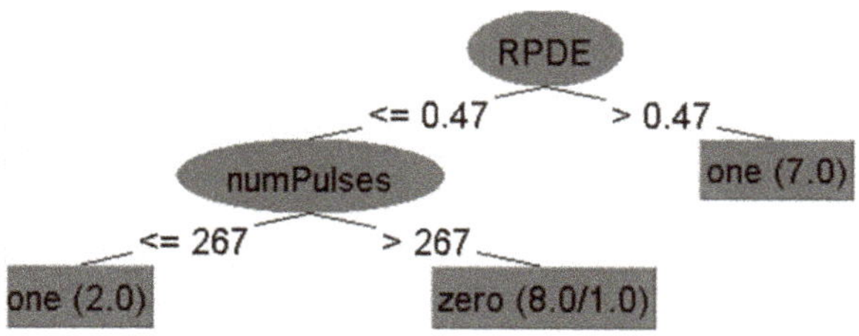

Figure 9.3. Graphical representation of decision tree algorithms.

identifying class within target variable. In this research paper we used decision tree for the prediction of Parkinson's dataset [13].

9.4.2 Naïve Bayes

Naïve Bayes is a very fast predictor. In this chapter we take Parkinson's medical dataset for prediction (figure 9.4). Naïve Bayes performed fast prediction on a class of test data and categories of a numeric medical dataset [14].

9.4.3 Random forest

RF is a uniform split test predictor for a medical dataset. Random tree judges the next and best split of a tree in the selected variables (figure 9.5). RF (TD: Training Data; DT : Decision Tree) compares irrelevant and correlated variables [15].

9.4.4 Extra tree

Extra tree has two different keys compare to random tree:

- split tree without replacement;
- nodes split are not best splits;
- it is used for averaging improved accuracy in prediction;
- It also controls the over-fitting [16].

Attribute	Class one (0.75)	Class zero (0.25)
id		
mean	120.7606	139.4219
std. dev.	71.2196	75.3487
weight sum	564	192
precision	1	1
gender		
mean	0.5691	0.3594
std. dev.	0.4952	0.4798
weight sum	564	192
precision	1	1
....	....	....
....	....	....
apq5Shimmer		
mean	0.0444	0.0356
std. dev.	0.0265	0.0248
weight sum	564	192
precision	0.0118	0.0118
apq11Shimmer		
mean	0.0599	0.0413
std. dev.	0.0352	0.0294
weight sum	564	192
precision	0.014	0.014
ddaShimmer		
mean	0.1084	0.0895
std. dev.	0.0664	0.065
weight sum	564	192
precision	0.0109	0.0109

Figure 9.4. Graphical representation of Naïve Bayes learner.

In this research we also used Extra tree for feature selection.

9.4.5 Bagging ensemble method

Bagging is an ensemble of machine learning algorithms. We can use these machine learning algorithms in a multiple dataset. So we can use it for a Parkinson's medical dataset for a multiple weak model to aggregate the predictions and get the final prediction (figure 9.6). It reduces variance and avoids over-fitting [17].

The main objective of this chapter is to prepare a classification framework which focuses on important features and their consistency values for each test. We evaluated many machine learning classification algorithms. We used Bagging ensemble method as the proposed method. The proposed work is demonstrated by achieved methodology in figure 9.7. All the proposed work is divided in three parts (I, II and III). These are described by following details:

I. Experiment-I evaluated the prediction of a previous Parkinson's dataset and compared Decision Tree, Naïve Bayes, RF, Extra Tree and Bagging Ensemble method.

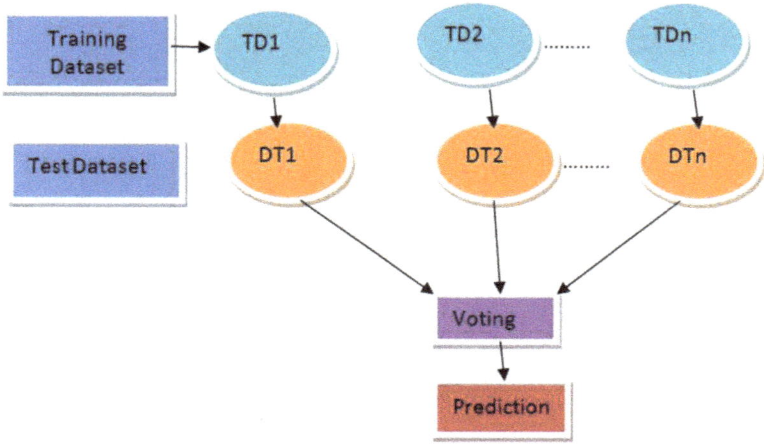

Figure 9.5. Graphical representation of RF for training and testing set.

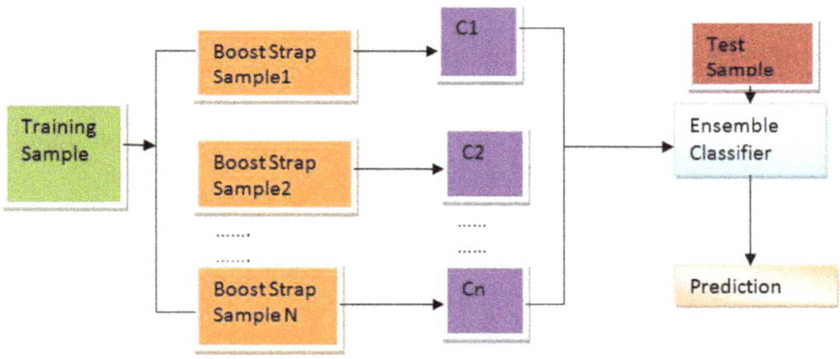

Figure 9.6. Graphical representation of bagging ensemble method.

II. Features importance is the selection process by which we find out the available important features in the whole dataset. We used these important features in prediction by selected machine learning algorithms and improved the outcomes.

9.4.6 Features selection method in Parkinson's disease

- Chi Square method
- Measure Feature Importance by Extra Tree and Measure Feature Selection by Heat Map Matrix

III. Experiment-III evaluated the prediction of newly prepared Parkinson's dataset after features selection and compare Decision Tree, Naïve Bayes, RF, Extra Tree and Bagging Ensemble Method.

9.5 Results

All the predicted results are available in three parts as per the following details:

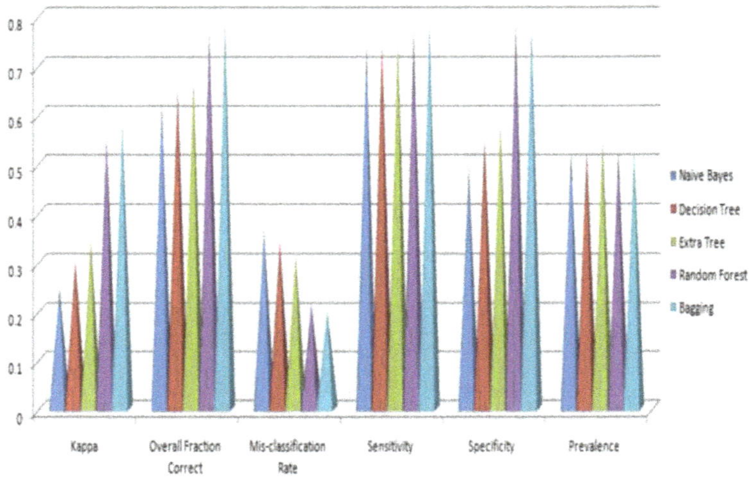

Figure 9.7. Representation of measurement of different algorithms for Parkinson's disease.

9.5.1 Evaluation of result after prediction on Parkinson's dataset

The number of instances in the Parkinson's dataset is 756 and available numbers of attributes are 21. Table 9.2 represents experiment-I; we find the evaluated values of Bagging Ensemble method for Kappa (0.589), Overall Fraction Correct (0.795), Miss-classification Rate (0.205), Sensitivity (0.799), Specificity (0.79) and Prevalence (0.528) is better compared to all other selected algorithms, Naïve Bayes, Decision Tree, Extra Tree and RF.

In figure 9.7, we find the result Kappa (high), Overall Fraction Correct (high), Mis-classification Rate (low) and Sensitivity (high) compare with other algorithms.

9.5.2 Result of features importance methods

Some results are described by various techniques as:

9.5.3 Chi-square test

Chi square test is important to measure the variance between expected frequencies and observed frequency (figure 9.8). This test measured the difference between the frequencies for easily testing the relationship between features on Parkinson's disease.

9.5.4 Extra tree

Extra Tree is an ensemble classifier model. We used Extra Tree method for features importance in a Parkinson's dataset (figure 9.9). One can visualize a better performance for feature selection from weak learner to stronger learner.

	Specs	Score
6	numPeriodsPulses	1864.725328
5	numPulses	1851.130248
0	id	397.462037
20	class	192.000000
1	gender	12.218525
15	locDbShimmer	5.659781
4	RPDE	1.785588
18	apq11Shimmer	0.812435
19	ddaShimmer	0.542172
14	locShimmer	0.540169
3	DFA	0.490823
17	apq5Shimmer	0.300749
16	apq3Shimmer	0.180714
2	PPE	0.154257
13	ddpJitter	0.108102
9	locPctJitter	0.093565
12	ppq5Jitter	0.065695
11	rapJitter	0.036044
7	meanPeriodPulses	0.017692
8	stdDevPeriodPulses	0.005754
10	locAbsJitter	0.000906

Figure 9.8. Representation of top most important features selects best classes.

9.5.5 Heat map

In this study we used Heat Map for observation target variables. Heat Map easily represents how features are correlated and easily finds which features are correlated with target variables (figure 9.10).

9.5.6 Evaluation of results after features selection

Table 9.3 represents experiment-III, we find the results after features selection. The Bagging Ensemble Method for Kappa (0.958), Overall Fraction Correct (0.98), Miss-classification Rate (0.02), Sensitivity (0.979), Specificity (0.983) and Prevalence (0.62) is better compared to all other selected algorithms, 'Naïve Bayes, Decision Tree, Extra Tree and Random Forest'.

In figure 9.11, find the result Kappa (high), Overall Fraction Correct (high), Mis-classification Rate (low) and Sensitivity (high) compared with other algorithms.

9.6 Discussion

After all the experiments and their results we discuss the better performance of classifiers. In table 9.2 and figure 9.8, we find 'Naïve Bayes, Decision Tree, Extra Tree, Random Forest and Bagging Ensemble' have Kappa, 0.248, 0.304, 0.35, 0.563, **0.589;** Overall Fraction Correct, 0.63, 0.656, 0.683, 0.782, **0.795;** Mis-classification Rate, 0.37, 0.344, 0.317, 0.218, **0.205;** Sensitivity, 0.749, 0.749, 0.761, 0.774, **0.799;** Specificity, 0.496, 0.552, 0.585, 0.79, **0.79** and Prevalence, 0.528,

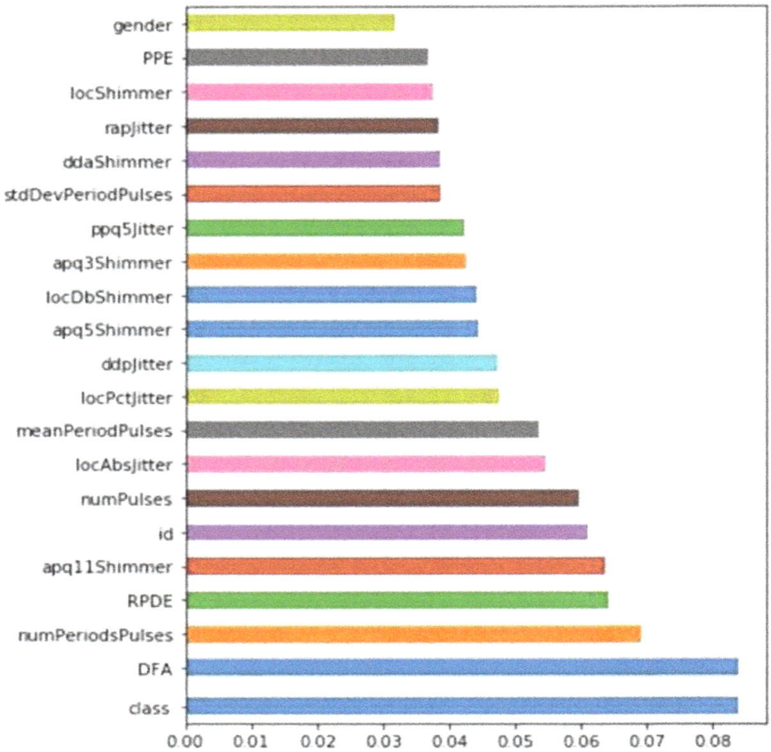

Figure 9.9. Graph visualization by extra tree for feature importance.

Table 9.2. Different tree algorithms performance for Parkinson's dataset.

Statistics	Naïve Bayes	Decision tree	Extra tree	Random forest	Bagging
Kappa	0.248	0.304	0.35	0.563	0.589
Overall fraction correct	0.63	0.656	0.683	0.782	0.795
Mis-classification rate	0.37	0.344	0.317	0.218	0.205
Sensitivity	0.749	0.749	0.761	0.774	0.799
Specificity	0.496	0.552	0.585	0.79	0.79
Prevalence	0.528	0.528	0.554	0.528	0.528

0.528, 0.554, 0.528, **0.528.** In table 9.3 and figure 9.12, we find Naïve Bayes, Decision Tree, Extra Tree, RF and Bagging Ensemble have Kappa, 0.589, 0.667, 0.744, 0.85, **0.958**; Overall Fraction Correct, 0.795, 0.835, 0.874, 0.927, **0.98**; Mis-classification Rate, 0.205, 0.165, 0.126, 0.073, **0.02**; Sensitivity, 0.799, 0.814, 0.883, 0.893, **0.979**; Specificity, 0.79, 0.862, 0.862, 0.983, **0.983** and Prevalence, 0.528, 0.567, 0.567, 0.62, **0.62.**

After all the observations, we find (tables 9.2 and 9.3, figures 9.8 and 9.12) the better predicted performance is represented by the Bagging Ensemble Method.

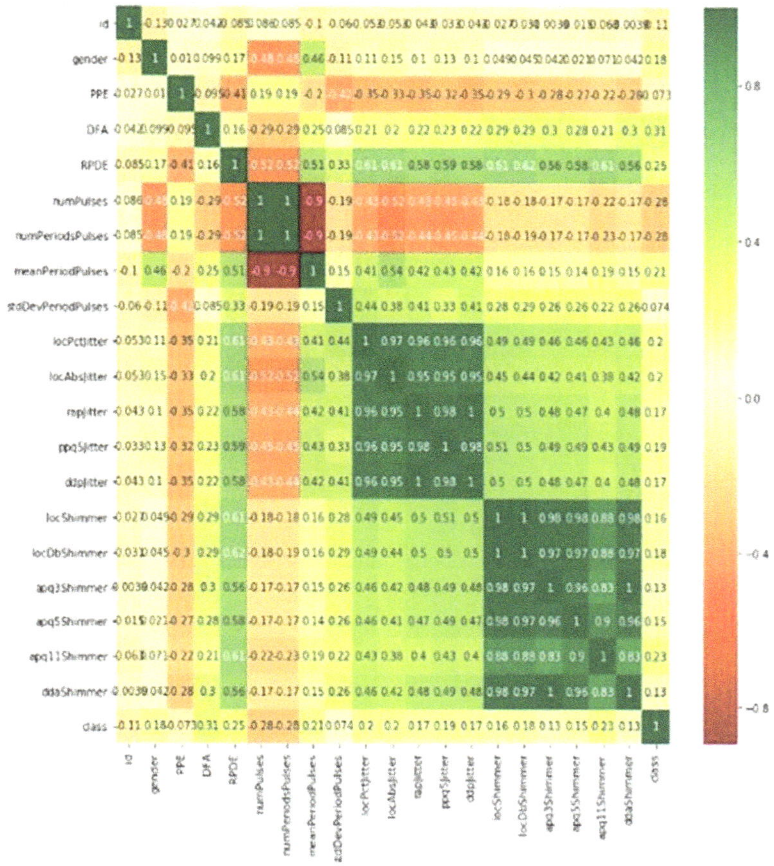

Figure 9.10. Representation of heat map matrix visualization for feature importance.

Table 9.3. Representation of different tree algorithms performance after features selection.

Statistics	Naïve Bayes	Decision tree	Extra tree	Random forest	Bagging
Kappa	0.589	0.667	0.744	0.85	0.958
Overall fraction correct	0.795	0.835	0.874	0.927	0.98
Mis-classification rate	0.205	0.165	0.126	0.073	0.02
Sensitivity	0.799	0.814	0.883	0.893	0.979
Specificity	0.79	0.862	0.862	0.983	0.983
Prevalence	0.528	0.567	0.567	0.62	0.62

We find a major gap between different classifiers' performance. The prediction of all selected classifiers depends upon more related features. If the relation between features is high then classification accuracy is always high. Figure 9.12 represents the improvement of accuracy is continuous for each classifier after features selection.

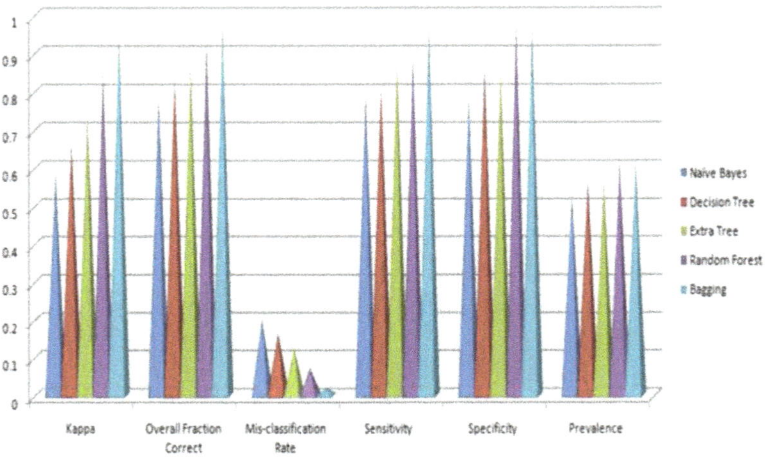

Figure 9.11. Representation of different algorithms for Parkinson's disease after features selection.

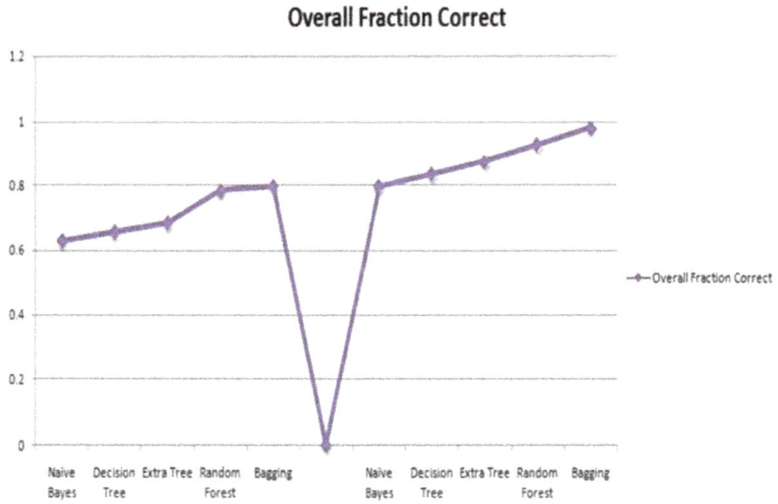

Figure 9.12. The prediction of different classifiers in Parkinson's disease.

Parkinson's is a very dangerous disease and many research works on this disease have already been done using machine learning algorithms. Some research papers are mentioned on Parkinson's Disease using machine learning. The research areas, using techniques and their performance are listed in table 9.4. On the basis of our previous analysis of Yadav and Pal [26–29], we calculated high accuracy on the basis of the ensemble method and majority of voting. In this chapter, we try to predict better performance by some selected classifiers and finally find better classification accuracy compared to all other listed research papers. The highest accuracy of any previous research paper is (97%) by RF but in our research we find (98%) classification accuracy of Bagging Ensemble Method.

Table 9.4. Representation of previous years' paper performance.

Author's name	Area of application	Methods	Accuracy
Khoury *et al* [18]	Disease of Parkinson's	K-NN	90
		CART	86
		RF	83
		NB	80
		SVM	76
		K-Means	75
		GMM	69
Pérez *et al*[19]	Disease of Parkinson's	RBF	85
		Linear	84
		MLP	81
		Quadratic	79
Tejeswinee *et al* [2]	Disease of Parkinson's	RF	85
		K-NN	82
		SVM	94
Cavallo *et al* [6]	Disease of Parkinson's	RF	79
		SVM	80
Mostafa *et al* [20]	Disease of Parkinson's	DT	86
		NB	74
		NB	88
		RF	87
		SVM	86
Turker *et al* [21]	Disease of Parkinson's	KNN	97
		Linear SVM	84
		RBF SVM	87
		Log-Reg	85
Ricciardi *et al* [22]	Disease of Parkinson's	RF	86
Betrouni *et al* [23]	Disease of Parkinson's	SVM	84
		KNN	88
Oh *et al* [24]	Disease of Parkinson's	Convolutional NN	85
Cigdem *et al* [25]	Disease of Parkinson's	SVM	94

9.7 Conclusion

The achieved UCI dataset contains three voice recording replications and their continuity. In a Parkinson's disease dataset, we take 756 instances and 21 attributes with target variable. All the predictions were completed and prepared a better result by features selection techniques. After the prediction, we found improvement of all selected classifiers but Bagging Ensemble Method predicted better performance from the previous to the final experiment. In future, we can use other ensemble techniques for other large datasets and select more features selection techniques for better prediction results in machine learning.

Acknowledgments

The author is grateful to Veer Bahadur Singh Purvanchal University Jaunpur, Uttar Pradesh, for providing financial support to work as Post-Doctoral Research Fellowship.

References

[1] Nemmi F, Pavy-Le Traon A, Phillips O R, Galitzky M, Meissner W G, Rascol O and Péran P 2019 A totally data-driven whole-brain multimodal pipeline for the discrimination of Parkinson's disease, multiple system atrophy and healthy control *NeuroImage: Clin.* **23** 101858

[2] Tejeswinee K, Shomona G J and Athilakshmi R 2017 Feature selection techniques for prediction of neuro-degenerative disorders: a case-study with Alzheimer's and Parkinson's disease *Procedia Comput. Sci.* **115** 188–94

[3] Behroozi M and Sami A 2016 A multiple-classifier framework for Parkinson's's disease detection based on various vocal tests *Int. J. Telemed. App.* **2016** 6837498

[4] Tubishat M, Idris N, Shuib L, Abushariah M A and Mirjalili S 2019 Improved salp swarm algorithm based on opposition based learning and novel local search algorithm for feature selection *Expert Syst. App.* **145** 113122

[5] Xiao B, He N, Wang Q, Cheng Z, Jiao Y, Haacke E M, Yan F and Shi F 2019 Quantitative susceptibility mapping based hybrid feature extraction for diagnosis of Parkinson's disease *NeuroImage: Clin* **24** 102070

[6] Cavallo F, Moschetti A, Esposito D, Maremmani C and Rovini E 2019 Upper limb motor pre-clinical assessment in Parkinson's disease using machine learning *Park. Relat. Disord.* **63** 11–116

[7] Berus L, Klancnik S, Brezocnik M and Ficko M 2019 Classifying Parkinson's disease based on acoustic measures using artificial neural networks *Sensors.* **19**

[8] Drotar P and Zdenek S M 2014 Comparative study of machine learning techniques for supervised classification of biomedical data *Acta Electrotechn. Inform* **14** 5–10

[9] Sharma P, Sundaram S, Sharma M, Sharma A and Gupta D 2019 Diagnosis of Parkinson's disease using modified grey wolf optimization *Cogn. Syst. Res* **54** 100–15

[10] Bellino G M, Schiaffino L, Battisti M, Guerrero J and Rosado-Muñoz A 2019 Optimization of the KNN supervised classification algorithm as a support tool for the implantation of deep brain stimulators in patients with Parkinson's disease *Entropy.* **21** 346

[11] Yadav D C and Pal S 2019 To generate an ensemble model for women thyroid prediction using data mining techniques *Asian Pac. J. Cancer Prev* **20** 1275–81

[12] Yadav D C and Pal S 2019 Decision tree ensemble techniques to predict thyroid disease *Int. J. Recent Technol. Eng. (IJRTE)* **8** 8242–6

[13] Che D, Liu Q, Rasheed K and Tao X 2011 Decision tree and ensemble learning algorithms with their applications in bioinformatics *Software Tools and Algorithms for Biological Systems* (New York: Springer) pp 191–9

[14] Zhou Y, Howroyd J, Danicic S and Bishop J M 2015 Extending naive bayes classifier with hierarchy feature level information for record linkage *Workshop on Advanced Methodologies for Bayesian Networks* (Cham: Springer) pp 93–104

[15] Sachin R, Sowmya V, Govind D and Soman K P 2017 Dependency of various color and intensity planes on CNN based image classification *Int. Symp. on Signal Processing and Intelligent Recognition Systems* (Cham: Springer) pp 167–77

[16] Cutler A, Cutler D R and Stevens J R 2012 Random forests *Ensemble Machine Learning* (Boston, MA: Springer) pp 157–75

[17] Bühlmann P 2012 Bagging, boosting and ensemble methods *Handbook of Computational Statistics* (Berlin, Heidelberg: Springer) pp 985–1022

[18] Khoury N, Attal F, Amirat Y, Oukhellou L and Mohammed S 2019 Data-driven based approach to aid Parkinson's's disease diagnosis *Sensors.* **19** 242

[19] Pérez C J, Campos-Roca Y, Naranjo L and Martín J 2016 Diagnosis and tracking of Parkinson's disease by using automatically extracted acoustic features *J. Alzheimers Dis. Park* **6** 2161–0460

[20] Mostafa S A, Mustapha A, Mohammed M A, Hamed R I, Arunkumar N, Ghani M K, Jaber M M and Khaleefah S H 2019 Examining multiple feature evaluation and classification methods for improving the diagnosis of Parkinson's disease *Cogn. Syst. Res.* **54** 90–9

[21] Tuncer T, Dogan S and Acharya U R 2020 Automated detection of Parkinson's disease using minimum average maximum tree and singular value decomposition method with vowels *Biocybern. Biomed. Eng.* **40** 211–20

[22] Ricciardi C *et al* 2019 Using gait analysis' parameters to classify Parkinsonism: a data mining approach *Comput. Methods Programs Biomed* **180** 105033

[23] Betrouni N, Delval A, Chaton L, Defebvre L, Duits A, moonen A, Leentjens A F and Dujardin K 2019 Electroencephalography-based machine learning for cognitive profiling in Parkinson's disease: preliminary results *Movement Disord* **34** 210–7

[24] Oh S L, Hagiwara Y, Raghavendra U, Yuvaraj R, Arunkumar N, Murugappan M and Acharya U R 2018 A deep learning approach for Parkinson's disease diagnosis from EEG signals *Neural Comput. App.* **32** 10927–33

[25] Cigdem O, Beheshti I and Demirel H 2018 Effects of different covariates and contrasts on classification of Parkinson's disease using structural MRI *Comput. Biol. Med.* **99** 173–81

[26] Yadav D C and Pal S 2021 Analysis of heart disease using parallel and sequential ensemble methods with feature selection techniques: heart disease prediction *Int. J. Big Data Analyt. Healthcare (IJBDAH)* **6** 40–56

[27] Yadav D C and Pal S 2020 *Analysis of Heart Patients Using a Tree Based Ensemble Model* (Bristol: IOP Publishing Ltd) pp 10-1–23

[28] Yadav D C and Pal S 2019 Thyroid prediction using ensemble data mining techniques *Int. J. Inform. Technol.* https://doi.org/10.1007/s41870-019-00395-7

[29] Yadav D C and Pal S 2020 Prediction of heart disease using feature selection and random forest ensemble method *Int. J. Pharm. Res.* **12** 56–66

IOP Publishing

Chapter 10

A comparative analysis of image enhancement techniques for detection of microcalcification in screening mammogram

Gaurav Makwana, Ram Narayan Yadav and Lalita Gupta

Breast cancer is the main source of cancer-related death in women of all ages. Among various imaging techniques, mammography is the most reliable and cost-effective technique for the diagnosis of breast malignancy. Radiologists investigate the presence of microcalcification and the pattern of its spread and interpret the information. However, diagnosis of the abnormality is completely subjective and depends upon the experience and expertise of the radiologists. There is always a possibility of human error due to poor contrast and noise that might cause the misleading diagnosis of abnormalities like calcification, masses, etc. Therefore, it is beneficial to use image processing techniques for mammogram image enhancement to improve the image quality for better interpretation of the image. In this chapter image enhancement techniques are applied to reduce the different types of noises like impulse noise, Gaussian noise, and speckle noise to increase the contrast of the mammogram images. The performance comparison of various image enhancement techniques like spatial domain filtering, frequency domain filtering and machine learning technique is shown. A quantitative measure of performance comparison is provided in terms of the parameters like Mean Square Error (MSE), Peak Signal-to-Noise Ratio (PSNR), Signal-to-Noise Ratio (SNR), mean, variance, etc. The test results indicate that the median filter can reduce impulse noise with the lowest MSE of 0.0206, whereas CNN is a better option to remove Gaussian and speckle noise with MSE of 0.0026 and 0.0017, respectively. We have also seen that these methods increase the contrast that helps in improving the diagnostic efficiency of mammograms.

10.1 Introduction

Cancer refers to the uncontrolled growth of epithelial cells in a particular location of the body. Malignant growths can be characterized by the kind of influenced cells or

doi:10.1088/978-0-7503-3815-8ch10

organs where this starts. There are roughly 100 sorts of cancer. It is an intricate and diverse illness since malignant development can happen in any part of the body. Breast malignancy is the uncontrolled development of epithelial cells in the breast. It is the second most common malignancy in women, however, it can affect men also. Additionally, it is the second leading reason for cancer death in women after lung malignancy because many times breast disease does not cause any agony or uneasiness until it has spread to close-by tissue [1]. Invasive ductal carcinoma (IDC) is the most widely recognized sort of breast disease in women of all ages and having a low survival rate [2].

Breast cancer is recognized by various names, contingent upon where it begins in the woman's breast. Bleeding from the nipple or pain in the armpit and a lump can indicate malignancy, and change in the size or shape of the breast is also an indication of abnormality. Breast tumors may be of two types benign and malignant. Non-cancerous (benign) tumors comprise connective tissue, adenoma, fibro-adenoma. Fibro-adenoma is the most common benign mass due to the combination of connective tissue and epithelial cells in the breast. Two main types of breast cancer are non-invasive breast cancer and invasive breast cancer. In non-invasive cancer, normal epithelial cells are replaced by malignant cells lining the ducts or lobules in the breast tissue. Non-invasive breast cancers stay within the milk ducts or lobules, called carcinoma *in situ* (CIS). Invasive breast cancer is the most common type of breast cancer, it starts from the milk duct but spreads into the surrounding normal tissue inside the breast. The most common screening method for the identification of breast cancer is mammography. It is used for the early detection of suspicious areas in breast cancer. Doctors detect, diagnose, and evaluate breast cancer by screening mammography. The advantage of using mammography is that it can scan a very small lump. However, mammography still has some disadvantages such as being challenging to diagnose irregularity in the dense breast tissue diagnosis in young patients [3, 4].

Mammographic screening can recognize a few malignant growths that are not detectable, while a few malignancies are detectable, but not distinguishable on the mammogram [5]. Screening mammography is more unlikely to identify early breast malignant growth at a treatable stage. To begin with, because in younger women breast thickness is commonly high [6, 7] and due to higher breast density, screening mammography brings about more false-positive tests, with the related anxiety and superfluous biopsies. Since women younger than 50 are more unlikely to have malignant breast growth, fewer women benefit from screening and the lower frequency of malignant breast growth increases the cost of mammography screening for a lifetime [8].

Early recognition is essential to the possibility of fruitful treatment since the malignant growth might be intrusive and spread to any part of the body. This recognition can be too troublesome since the principal indications of breast cancer are regularly symptomatic. This is the reason x-ray mammography is broadly used to screen for breast malignant growth. The mammogram can show small breast tissue changes, which may demonstrate too small tumors to be distinguished either by the radiologist or by a specialist doctor. There is an expanded breast malignant growth chance related to the fact that other realized hazard variables might affect breast tissue, which causes long and momentary changes to appear on the mammogram. In mammography, it is believed that connective tissue, fat, and epithelial components can be dysplasia, and the ductal pattern represents periductal fibrosis [9]. A few specialists have discovered that the mammogram's general measure of radiographic thickness is related to risk [10–12].

Imaging techniques such as MRI, x-ray, ultrasound, mammogram, etc, cannot differentiate cancerous cells from non-cancerous cells [13, 14]. Experienced radiologists identify useful information and interpret that information, but many times false diagnosis might be possible. To improve evaluation skills and diagnosis consistency to the doctor and reduce the subjective error, image processing techniques can be used to identify breast calcification types. Calcifications in the breast are small calcium deposits that appear as high-intensity regions in the mammogram. Calcifications are of two types, micro-calcifications, and macro-calcifications. Macro-calcifications are benign lesions that appear as coarse, scattered calcium deposits, whereas micro-calcifications are isolated calcium deposits that usually appear in clusters.

A micro-calcification cluster in the mammographic image may have breast cancer. The radiologist uses different shapes, sizes, and distribution of micro-calcification to identify malignant or benign. Malignant is a small dot-like structure that varies in size, shape, and density, whereas benign is a large, rounded shape structure homogeneous in shape [15]. These medical images help doctors in the detection of the abnormality in breast tissue. Analysis of the image in the early stage is complicated due to uncertainty in the tumor's location. In the early-stage healthy and unhealthy cells are overlaid so it becomes very difficult to detect different intensity [16, 17]. Noise can also affect the image's quality and a noisy image requires more computational time [18, 19].

Computer-aided tools that can compare the results with radiologist data are advantageous [20, 21]. Image processing techniques can be used to identify the area of interest including: filter selection for noise removal, image resizing, contrast enhancement, and removal of noise from the image to distinguish between cancerous and non-cancerous cells. The Otsu thresholding method minimizes the interclass variance of thresholded black and white pixels. Laplacian subband [22] is also a solution for removing unstructured, spurious artifacts from the image. Shukla *et al* [23] proposed an algorithm based on the K operator with Riesz kernel for image denoising. Adam *et al* [24] combine averaging and nonlinear Gaussian filtering to reduce speckle reduction and additive random noise reduction. Chen *et al* [25] suggested median filtering to eliminate impulsive noise. Adaptive median filters [26] can also be used for noise reduction, which replaces the pixel value with the local neighborhood's weighted median. Still, it has some demerits; image smoothing also removes some sufficient detail in the image [27]. There is another possibility of wrong diagnosis due to blood vessels, and tissues.

The contrast enhancement method increases the contrast of the image over a threshold [28] but it has some drawbacks, like it may cause some regions to be under enhanced or over enhanced, which may result in information loss [29]. Pixel modification may also be used for contrast enhancement [30, 31]. This can be achieved by increasing the contrast ratio of the image. Another way for image enhancement is local histogram modification like histogram equalization, contrast stretching, and local histogram processing in an image's local area [32, 33]. This local enhancement method distorts the image quality to some extent because these transformations are not monotonic mapping. Dong *et al* [34] propose a non-local concentrated sparse representation (NCSR) denoising method by combining sparse coding coefficient (SCC) and sparsity. NCSR constructs an overcomplete dictionary by learning the prior blocks and using non-local redundancy sparseness of the image to reduce the noise. Another stacked sparse denoising auto-encoder (SSDA) model is proposed by Xie *et al* [35] based on sparse coding with neural networks that require manual parameter adjustment during the training phase. Another approach for image denoising is image transformation. A Gaussian scale mixture (GSM) model can be very useful for finding an effective description of local image statistics [36]. Markov random fields (MRFs) can also be used to capture statistical regularities of pixel intensities.

This chapter aims to discuss the various image enhancement and noise-reducing methods for the analysis of mammogram images for better diagnosis of breast microcalcification. In the following section we discuss the various spatial domain method for image enhancement like histogram modeling, histogram equalization, histogram matching, average filtering, Gaussian filter, median filter, etc, and frequency domain methods such as Butterworth, Gaussian low pass filtering, Homomorphic filtering, wavelet transform, and finally convolutional neural network. We have shown an improvement in the image quality after applying these methods for the analysis of the image corrupted by speckle, Gaussian, and impulse noise. Finally, the conclusion summarizes the chapter.

10.2 Image enhancement in spatial domain

Several spatial domain techniques manipulate the pixel values of an image for better representation. The following section deals with some methods for image enhancement.

10.2.1 Histogram modeling

A histogram of an image is a plot between the numbers of occurrence of a gray level to the number of gray level values. If [0, L-1] is the gray level of an image then the histogram can be defined as $h(r_i) = n_i$ where r_i is the ith intensity value and n_i is the number of pixel of intensity r_i. The histogram provides more insight into image contrast and brightness [37, 38]. A normalized histogram of an image is defined as

$$P(r_i) = \frac{n_i}{\text{Total number of Pixels}} \tag{10.1}$$

Contrast enhancement methods based on histogram modeling are very simple in comparison to the frequency-domain methods. It gives a high contrast image with a wide dynamic range of the intensity scale. This method can also be used to increase the brightness of an image by changing the histogram of an image.

10.2.2 Histogram equalization

Histogram equalization (HE) improves the contrast of an image by stretching out the gray level range of the image, as shown in figure 10.1. This technique increases the global contrast of an image by stretching out the intensity range of the image, but it is not always true there may be some cases when it decreases the contrast [37, 38].

10.2.3 Histogram matching

Histogram matching is another histogram-based contrast enhancement method; it specifies the shape of the histogram by mapping gray levels of the original image into a desirable level. This method is used to generate a processed image that has a predetermined histogram [37]. Figure 10.2 shows that the brightness of the output image is very high and may cause information loss.

10.2.4 Averaging filter

It replaces each pixel in an image with the average value of all its neighbors. Mean filtering is like a convolution filter based around a kernel. This kernel controls the shape and size of the neighborhood that represents the amount of filtering [37, 38]. Results of average filtering for contrast enhancement of a mammogram image are given in figure 10.3. An increase in Mask size causes blurring to the original image.

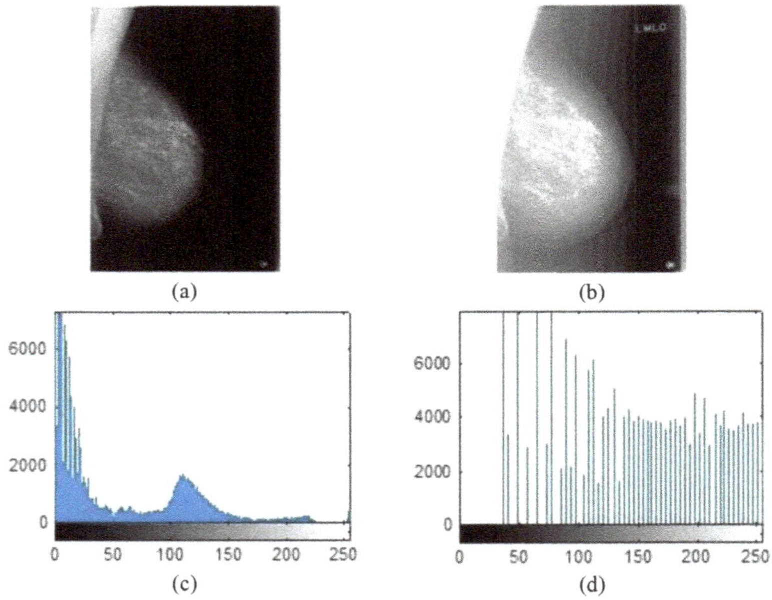

Figure 10.1. Contrast enhancement by using HE:(a) A DDSM database Mammographic Image, (b) image after HE, (c) histogram of image, (d) histogram of HE image.

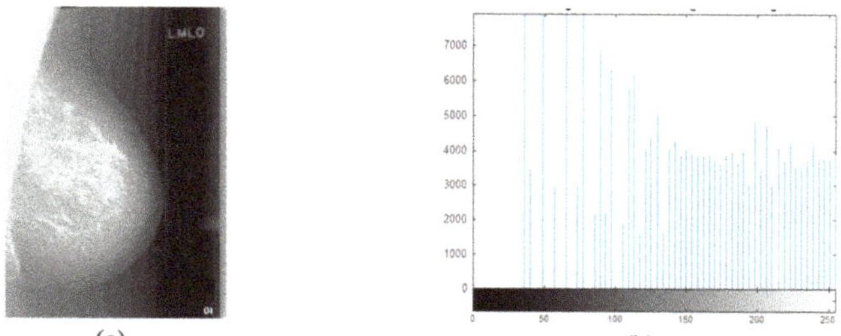

(a) (b)

Figure 10.2. Contrast enhancement by using histogram matching: (a) implementation of histogram matching, (b) histogram of image.

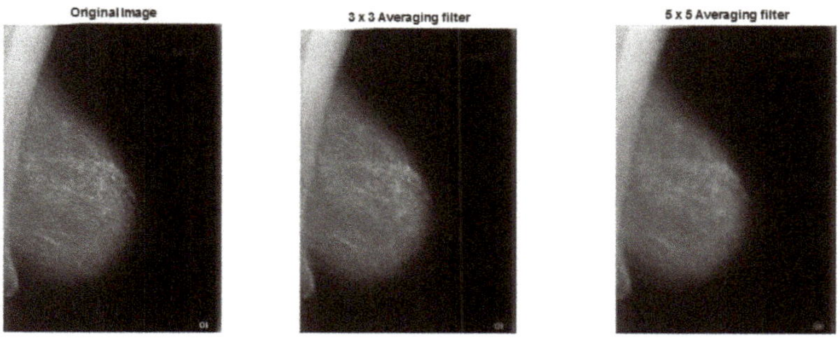

(a) (b) (c)

Figure 10.3. Output of averaging filtering. (a) Input mammogram image, (b) 3 × 3 averaging filter output, (c) 5 × 5 averaging filter output.

10.2.5 Gaussian filter

It is another linear smoothing filter. The weight of the Gaussian filter is chosen according to the shape of the Gaussian function. It is defined as [37, 38]

$$h(x, y) = \frac{1}{\sqrt{2\pi}\sigma} e^{-\frac{x^2+y^2}{2\sigma^2}} \tag{10.2}$$

The above function shows that the Gaussian filter is separable. Figure 10.4 shows that amount of smoothing depends upon the standard σ. Mathematically, a Gaussian filter modifies the image by convolving with a Gaussian function.

10.2.6 Median filter

Median filter is a nonlinear statistical filter that smoothens the image by replacing the value of the center pixel by the median of the neighborhood pixel. In median filtering, first all pixels within the mask are sorted in ascending or descending order, then median value is replaced with the centre pixel value [37, 38]. The output of the median filtering is shown in figure 10.5.

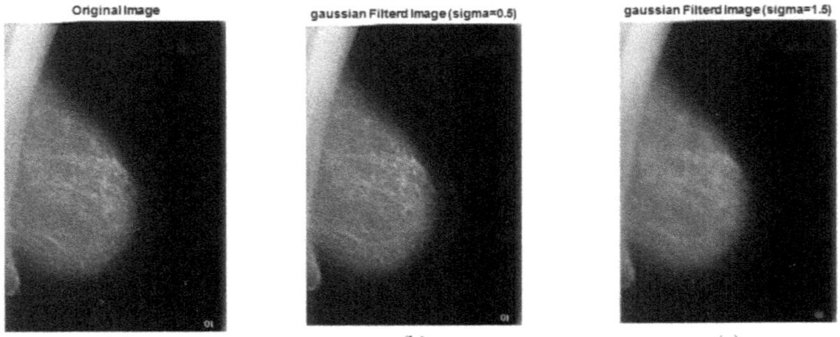

(a) (b) (c)

Figure 10.4. Output of Gaussian filtering. (a) Input mammogram image, (b) Gaussian filter output for $\sigma = 0.5$, (c) Gaussian filter output for $\sigma = 1.5$.

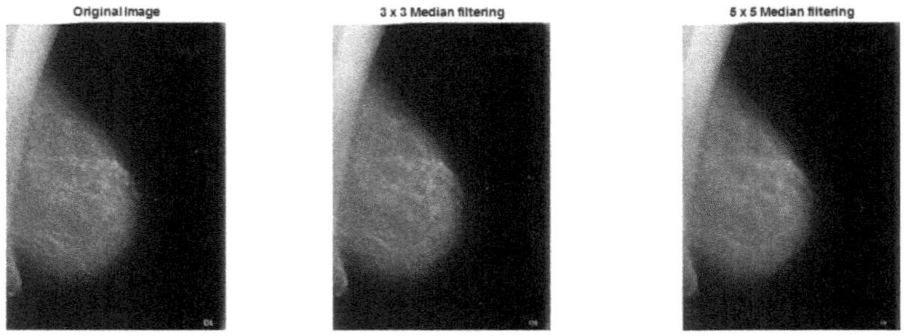

(a) (b) (c)

Figure 10.5. Output of median filtering. (a) Input mammogram image, (b) 3×3 median filter output, (c) 5×5 median filter output.

10.3 Image enhancement in frequency domain

The concept of filtering is easier to visualize in the frequency domain. Therefore, an enhancement of image $f(x, y)$ can be done in the frequency domain, based on its Fourier transform [37, 38]. The advantage of using the frequency domain method is that we can regain the same image by applying inverse transmission technique and by choosing the proper weighting function, modification or attenuation of certain frequency components are possible.

Let $h(x, y)$ and $f(x, y)$ be the weighting function and original image, respectively. Filtering of image $f(x, y)$ is done by convolution in spatial domain as follows.

$$g(x, y) = h(x, y) * f(x, y) \tag{10.3}$$

Where * is a convolution operator. In frequency domain method it is corresponding to the multiplication of image spectrum $F(u, v)$ with the Fourier transform of the weighting function $H(u, v)$ as follows

$$G(u, v) = H(u, v)F(u, v) \tag{10.4}$$

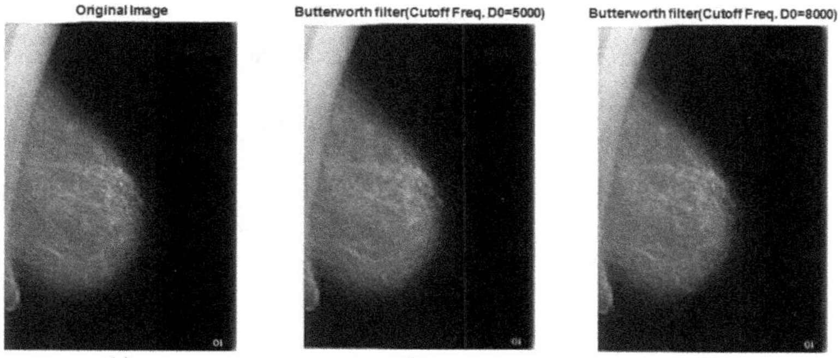

(a) (b) (c)

Figure 10.6. Output of Butterworth filtering. (a) Input mammogram image, (b) Butterworth filter output for cutoff frequency at radii = 5000 pixels, (c) Butterworth filter output for cutoff frequency at radii = 8000 pixels.

10.3.1 Butterworth filtering

Butterworth filter of order n and cutoff frequency D_0 is defined as [37].

$$H(u, v) = \left[\frac{1}{1 + [D(u, v)/D_0]^{2n}}\right] \tag{10.5}$$

It gives smooth transition from low frequency region to high frequency region. By increasing the order of the filter, we can control the sharpening of an image. The outputs corresponding to different cutoff frequency are illustrated in figure 10.6.

10.3.2 Gaussian low-pass filter

The Gaussian low-pass filter (GLPF) can be defined as below.

$$H(u, v) = e^{-D^2(u, v)/2\sigma^2} \tag{10.6}$$

where, $D(u, v)$ is the distance from the center of the frequency rectangle. Figure 10.7 shows the result of applying a Gaussian low-pass filter on a noisy mammogram image. The output result of the GLPF is less smooth than the Butterworth filter.

10.3.3 Homomorphic filtering

It involves transforming multiplicative noise into additive noise and then applying a linear operation. Although, due to poor illumination, some regions of the image might appear brighter or some other regions might appear dark, a homomorphic filter can correct this nonuniform illumination in the image. For a linear filter to be applied to images corrupted by speckle noise, the speckle noise needs to be transformed to additive noise using a logarithmic transformation before the convolution operation is applied [38]. Homomorphic filtering techniques use illumination and reflectance model to enhance or restore the degraded image.

Let image $f(x, y)$ be defined as

$$f(x, y) = i(x, y) \times r(x, y) \tag{10.7}$$

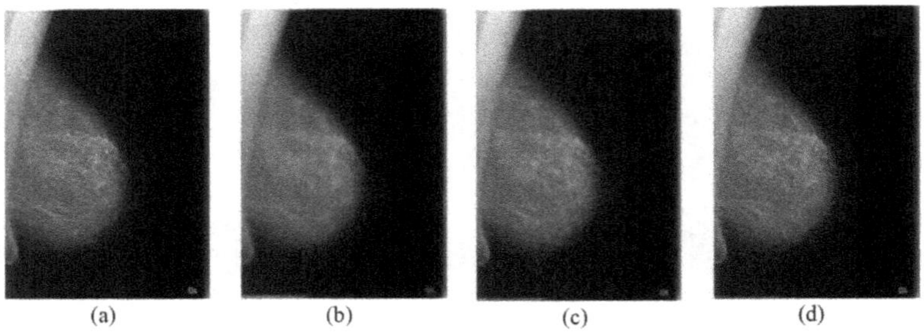

Figure 10.7. Output of GLPF. (a) Input mammogram image (b) GLPF output for $\sigma = 25$, (c) GLPF output for $\sigma = 50$, (d) GLPF output for $\sigma = 100$.

where, $i(x, y)$ is illumination and $r(x, y)$ is reflectance. Here, $i(x, y)$ is a lower frequency component than $r(x, y)$. Homomorphic filtering reduces the low-frequency component of an image in spatial domain to have a high-pass filtering $f(x, y)$ that transforms to the frequency domain by first converting the product term to addition. It can be achieved by using the logarithm of both sides then applying Fourier transform as shown below [35, 36].

$$\ln[f(x, y)] = \ln[i(x, y)] + \ln[r(x, y)] \tag{10.8}$$

$$\Im[\ln[f(x, y)]] = \Im[\ln[i(x, y)]] + \Im[\ln[r(x, y)]] \tag{10.9}$$

Let

$$\Im(u, v) = I(u, v) + R(u, v) \tag{10.10}$$

Next, to have better illumination high pass filtering is required.

$$G(u, v) = H(u, v) \cdot \Im(u, v) \tag{10.11}$$

Now, filtered image $G(u, v)$ is transferred to spatial domain using inverse Fourier transform.

$$g(x, y) = \Im^{-1}[G(u, v)] \tag{10.12}$$

$g(x, y)$ is not in its original form, therefore, to eliminate the logarithm, an exponential function is used. Figure 10.8 shows the result of applying homomorphic filtering.

10.3.4 Discrete wavelet transform

In discrete wavelet transform (DWT), the signal is filtered through a set of digital filters at different scale. It decomposes the image into a sequence of different frequency components. In an image N level of decomposition can be performed that results in $3N + 1$ different frequency bands such as, LL, LH, HL and HH. Low-low (LL) frequency components give average information of an image and other frequency components give directional information like low–high (LH), high–low (HL), and high–high (HH) gives horizontal, vertical, and diagonal coefficients, respectively [39, 40].

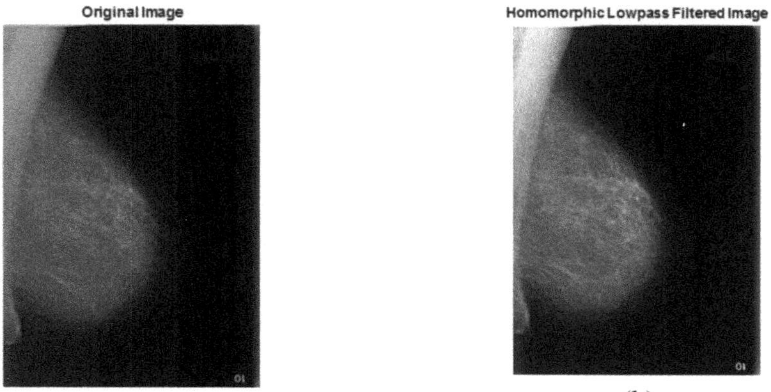

(a) (b)

Figure 10.8. Output of homomorphic filtering. (a) Input mammogram image, (b) homomorphic filter output result.

2-D scaling function $\varphi(x, y)$ and 2-D wavelet function $\xi^H(x, y)$, $\xi^V(x, y)$ & $\xi^D(x, y)$ are separable in nature [41]. A function and wavelet function are said to be separable if it can be expressed as

$$\varphi(x, y) = \varphi(x)\,\varphi(y) \tag{10.13}$$

$$\xi^H(x, y) = \xi(x)\varphi(y) \tag{10.14}$$

$$\xi^V(x, y) = \phi(x)\xi(y) \tag{10.15}$$

$$\xi^D(x, y) = \xi(x)\,\xi(y) \tag{10.16}$$

$\phi(x, y)$ gives coefficient of image approximation and intensity variation in different directions found by $\xi^H(x, y)$, $\xi^V(x, y)$ and $\xi^D(x, y)$

Scaled and translated basis function can be defined as

$$\phi_{j,m,n}(x, y) = 2^{j/2}\phi(2^j x - m, 2^j y - n) \tag{10.17}$$

$$\psi^i_{j,m,n}(x, y) = 2^{j/2}\psi^i(2^j x - m, 2^j y - n) \tag{10.18}$$

$$i = \{H, V, D\} \tag{10.19}$$

The DWT of an $M \times N$ dimensional image $f(x, y)$ can be represented as

$$W_\varphi(j_0, m, n) = \frac{1}{\sqrt{MN}} \sum_{x=0}^{M-1} \sum_{y=0}^{N-1} f(x, y)\,\varphi_{j_0,m,n}(x, y) \tag{10.20}$$

$$W^i_\xi(j, m, n) = \frac{1}{\sqrt{MN}} \sum_{x=0}^{M-1} \sum_{y=0}^{N-1} f(x, y)\,\xi^i_{j,m,n}(x, y) \tag{10.21}$$

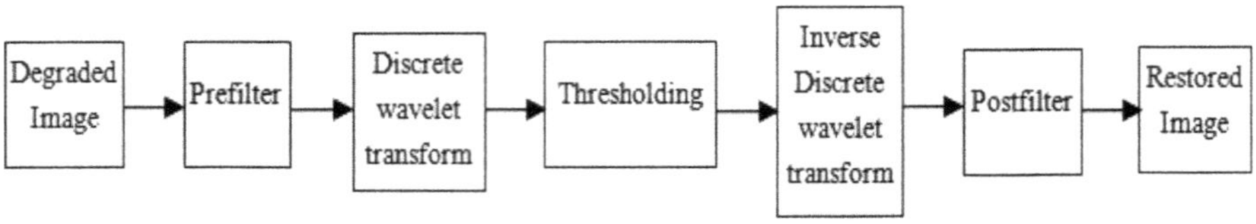

Figure 10.9. Wavelet based image denoising.

where $i = \{H, V, D\}$ refer to the decomposition direction of the wavelet and j_0 is an arbitrary start scale. $W_\phi(j_0, m, n)$ represent approximation of image $f(x, y)$ at scale of j_0 and $W_\xi^i(j, m, n)$ denotes the horizontal, vertical and diagonal coefficient at scale $j \geqslant j_0$. DWT is very important in resolution enhancement as well as preserving the high frequency component.

Figure 10.9 shows the image denoising process using a wavelet transform. Thresholding is a very important process in image denoising. A proper selection of thresholding can denoise the image because many times small value thresholding cannot remove noise and a larger value may cause loss of image detail as well.

Image thresholding can segment an image to obtain the specific feature. It is very difficult to identify the microcalcification in a mammogram using thresholding technique because of its low contrast. Thresholding can also be used for noise attenuation in the spatial domain as well as in frequency domain [42]. Thresholding can be of two types, hard thresholding and soft thresholding.

In hard thresholding pixel value below some threshold is set to zero. It is used to obtain the binary image from the grayscale image. It is defined as

$$f'(m, n) = \begin{cases} f(m, n), & \text{if } |f(m, n)| > t \\ 0, & \text{otherwise} \end{cases} \tag{10.22}$$

Hard thresholding causes ringing effect in the denoised image, soft thresholding method can be a solution to this problem. In soft thresholding, values for both positive and negative coefficients are being shrunk towards zero. It is defined as

$$f'(m, n) = \begin{cases} f(m, n) - t, & \text{if } |f(m, n)| > t \\ f(m, n) + t, & \text{if } |f(m, n)| < -t \\ 0 & \text{if } |f(m, n)| \leqslant t \end{cases} \tag{10.23}$$

Generally, soft thresholding is a better option to minimize the MSE. These wavelet thresholding techniques filter each wavelet coefficient from the detailed sub-bands by using the threshold function to get the modified wavelet coefficients.

10.4 Convolutional neural network

Convolution neural network (CNN) is a deep learning tunable architecture that is a feed-forward neural network consisting of multiple trainable nonlinear transformation stages. It extracts the feature vector in every stage, which represents the input and output vector, respectively. CNN includes the feature extractor in the training process, which modifies the weights during the training process.

CNN consists of two networks one that extracts a feature of the input image and the second classifies the extracted feature [43]. CNN has three types of network layers, which are convolution, pooling, and fully connected layers. The convolution kernel $h(m, n)$ is also known as the convolution filter passing over the image $x(m, n)$ and feature map values are calculated as follows.

$$G(m, n) = x(m, n) \times h(m, n) = \sum_{j}\sum_{k} h(i, j)x(m - j, n - k) \quad (10.24)$$

where 'm' and 'n' are the pixel coordinate and * is a convolution operator.

Convolution is a proficient method of feature extraction with minimum data set redundancy. The convolution kernel is a feature identifier that filters the important feature of the image and produces a convolution map about the distribution of these features. The neurons figure out how to assemble the data to gain a higher-order feature of the image in the next convolutional layers [44]. Since convolution operation shrinks the image, when the kernel moves through the image, the impact of the outskirts pixels on the feature map is very small compared to the center pixels, it might decrease the spatial resolution of the image. CNN uses image padding to minimize this problem. Another method to reduce the feature map size is stride. The stride function is just like a sliding window, that controls the amount of movement of the convolution kernel to the input image. Usually, we shift the kernel by one pixel, but step size can be increased if a small feature map or less overlapping of the receptive field is required. The second layer of CNN is the pooling layer. It reduces the feature map size of the input matrix. There are two pooling mechanisms used in practice which are max pooling and average pooling.

The convolutional layer typically includes a non-linear activation function. Non-linearity is important to model the complex function. Rectified linear unit (ReLU) activation function is generally used because it shows a better convergence rate as compared to the other activation function. It is defined as

$$R(x) = \max(0, x) \quad (10.25)$$

The last hidden layer of CNN is known as fully connected layers [45]. The output of this layer is a column vector, and each row of the column vector is corresponding to a different class. Classification of these different classes depends on the probability estimation of each class. Practically, input to the fully connected layer must be as small as possible, whereas pooling and stride reduce the size of the data matrix of fully-connected layers. During the training process, we calculate the MSE between the restored image and degraded image to optimize the output. In this training model, stochastic gradient descent (SGD) is used for parameter optimization. This can be represented as in [46]

$$w_n^{(i+1)} = w^{(i)} - \beta \cdot \frac{\delta\xi}{\mathrm{dw}} \qquad \forall\, i = 1, 2, 3.... \quad (10.26)$$

where $w_n^{(i)}$, β and ξ are the iteration parameters, learning rate and loss function, respectively. Now, if g_{mn} is the pixel at (m, n) position and y_{mn} is the expected output then the loss function is defined as

$$\xi(w, m, n) = h(N(f(w_g, g_{mn})), y_{mn}) \tag{10.27}$$

where $f(.)$ is output of CNN network.

10.5 Evaluation criteria

We have defined some criteria of image performance to validate the efficiency of our method. Commonly used performance indications are MSE, PSNR, SNR, Mean, and Variance.

10.5.1 Mean square error

The mean square error (MSE) is measured by cumulatively squaring the error between the restored image and the degraded image [47, 48]. Mathematically, MSE is calculated as follows.

$$\mathrm{MSE} = \frac{1}{mn}\sum_{x=0}^{m-1}\sum_{y=0}^{n-1}[g(x, y) - \bar{g}(x, y)]^2 \tag{10.28}$$

Where $g(x, y)$ and $\bar{g}(x, y)$ are degraded and filtered (restored) image, respectively. 'm' and 'n' are the dimensions of the image.

10.5.2 Peak signal-to-noise ratio

The peak signal-to-noise ratio (PSNR) of an image is calculated as the ratio of square of the maximum possible pixel values to the MSE of the image [49, 50]. The high-quality image has a high PSNR.

Mathematically, PSNR is represented as

$$\mathrm{PSNR} = 10\log_{10}\left(\frac{\mathrm{MAX}^2}{\mathrm{MSE}}\right) \tag{10.29}$$

10.5.3 SNR

SNR is defined as the ratio of signal power to noise power. It is represented as

$$\mathrm{SNR} = 10\log_{10}\left[\frac{\sum_{x=0}^{m-1}\sum_{y=0}^{n-1}[g(x, y)]^2}{\sum_{x=0}^{m-1}\sum_{y=0}^{n-1}[g(x, y) - \bar{g}(x, y)]^2}\right] \tag{10.30}$$

10.5.4 Mean

Mean gives an average gray level to get an idea about intensity profile [37]. It can be expressed as

$$\mu = \frac{1}{n}\sum_{i=0}^{n-1} g_i \tag{10.31}$$

where 'n' is number of signals.

10.5.5 Variance

Histogram width is the measure of the amount of grey level in an image [37]. Variance measures the deviation of that gray level from the mean value. It can be given as

$$\sigma^2 = \frac{1}{n}\sum_{i=0}^{n-1} (g_i - \mu)^2 \tag{10.32}$$

10.6 Results and discussion

There are many reasons for an image to be noisy, like imperfect instruments, wrong image acquisition steps, power line interference, patient discomfort, image transmission, compression, etc. It is required to denoise the image before image data analysis. In medical imaging, signal backscattered from the background soft tissue causes speckle noise that affects image quality, making diagnosis more difficult, so it becomes imperative to remove the noise to improve tissue structures and image quality. Another noise that affects the image quality is Gaussian noise. The cause of Gaussian noise is low sensor illumination, temperature, and electronic interference during transmission due to poor sensor connection. Impulse noise (salt and pepper) is another form of noise that affects an image's diagnosis accuracy. It occurs due to the sharp disturbance in an image because of a defect of the camera sensor, system software, or hardware failure during image acquisition and data transmission. In this chapter, our focus is to filter these noises from the affected mammogram images. Here, we have used different filtering techniques like average filtering, median filtering, Gaussian filtering, Butterworth, second-level wavelet decomposition, and CNN to remove noises. Analysis of these filtering techniques is based on some performance measures such as MSE, PSNR, SNR, mean, and variance to validate the efficiency.

Figure 10.10 shows the breast mammogram image. Figure 10.11(a) shows the image with speckle noise. Figure 10.11(b) and (c) is the result obtained by the averaging filtering method with 3 × 3 and 5 × 5 filter masks, respectively. Figure 10.11(d) and (e) are the results obtained after applying the median filter of 3 × 3 and 5 × 5 filter masks, respectively. Figure 10.11(f) is the result obtained after applying the convolutional neural network algorithm for noise reduction. Figures 10.11(g)–(j) are the result obtained after applying the second level

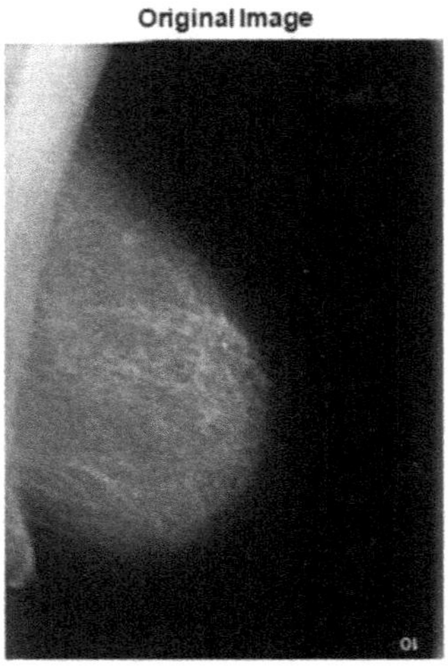

Figure 10.10. Breast mammogram image.

decomposition of the wavelet transform. To evaluate the performance of the methods MSE, SNR, PSNR, mean, and variance are calculated. From table 10.1 we can easily evaluate that the CNN gives better performance for speckle noise reduction. Butterworth filter adds image smoothing, i.e., it also removes some high-frequency pixel (edge) while filtering, second-level wavelet decomposition over enhances the mammographic image but CNN gives better subjective analysis and statistical data shows that CNN has minimum MSE, high SNR, and PSNR. This shows that CNN is a better method for speckle noise reduction.

Figure 10.12(a) shows the image with Gaussian noise, figures 10.12(b) and (c) is the result obtained by the averaging filtering method with 3 × 3 and 5 × 5 filter masks, respectively. Figures 10.12(d) and (e) are the results obtained after applying the median filter of 3 × 3 and 5 × 5 filter masks, respectively. Figures 10.12(f) and (g) are the result of the Gaussian and Butterworth filter, respectively. Figures 10.12(h)–(k) are the result obtained after applying the second level decomposition of the wavelet transform. Figure 10.12(l) is the result obtained after applying the CNN algorithm for noise reduction. Statistical analysis for Gaussian noise reduction is shown in table 10.2. CNN shows better performance for Gaussian noise reduction. Statistical data verify that it has minimum MSE, and high PSNR and SNR. The subjective analysis also shows that CNN enhances the image better as compared to all other filtering techniques and the result.

Figure 10.13(a) shows the image with impulse noise. Figures 10.13(b) and (c) are the result obtained by the averaging filtering method with 3 × 3 and 5 × 5 filter masks, respectively. Figures 10.13(d) and (e) are the results obtained after applying the median filter of 3 × 3 and 5 × 5 filter masks, respectively. Figures 10.13(f) and (g) are the result of the Gaussian and Butterworth filter, respectively. Figures 10.13(h)–(k) are the result obtained after applying the second level decomposition of the wavelet transform. Figure 10.13(l) is the result obtained after applying the CNN algorithm for noise reduction. Statistical analysis for impulse noise reduction is shown in table 10.3

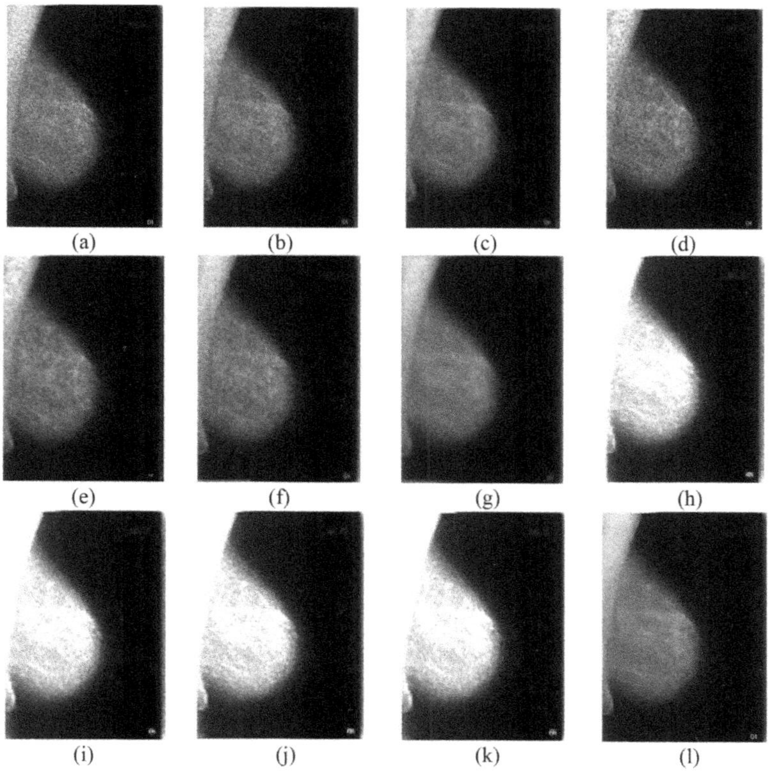

Figure 10.11. (a) Image with speckle noise, (b) 3 × 3 averaging filter output, (c) 5 × 5 averaging filter output, (d) 3 × 3 median filter output, (e) 5 × 5 median filter output, (f) Gaussian, (g) Butterworth, (h) wavelet-HL, (i) wavelet LH, (j) wavelet-HH, (k) wavelet-LH-HH, (l) CNN.

Table 10.1. Performance evaluation for Speckle noise.

		MSE	SNR	PSNR	Mean	Variance
Mean filter	3 × 3	65.125	−0.1382	10.3439	50.9442	18.259
	5 × 5	61.756	−0.0444	10.4326	50.6045	15.762
Median	3 × 3	0.0052	60.489	70.9821	0.1996	0.231
	5 × 5	0.0060	59.9077	70.3608	0.1988	0.0224
Gaussian		66.412	−0.2044	10.2508	51.6158	16.251
Butterworth		62.880	−0.0698	10.4271	51.4107	13.259
Wavelet	HL	0.0972	47.6616	58.2529	−0.0103	0.0079
	LH	0.0970	47.6711	58.2624	−0.0107	0.0060
	HH	0.0973	47.6585	58.2498	−0.0111	0.0071
	LH-HH	0.0968	47.6805	58.2718	−0.0107	0.0047
CNN		0.0017	65.2186	75.8051	0.2025	0.0218

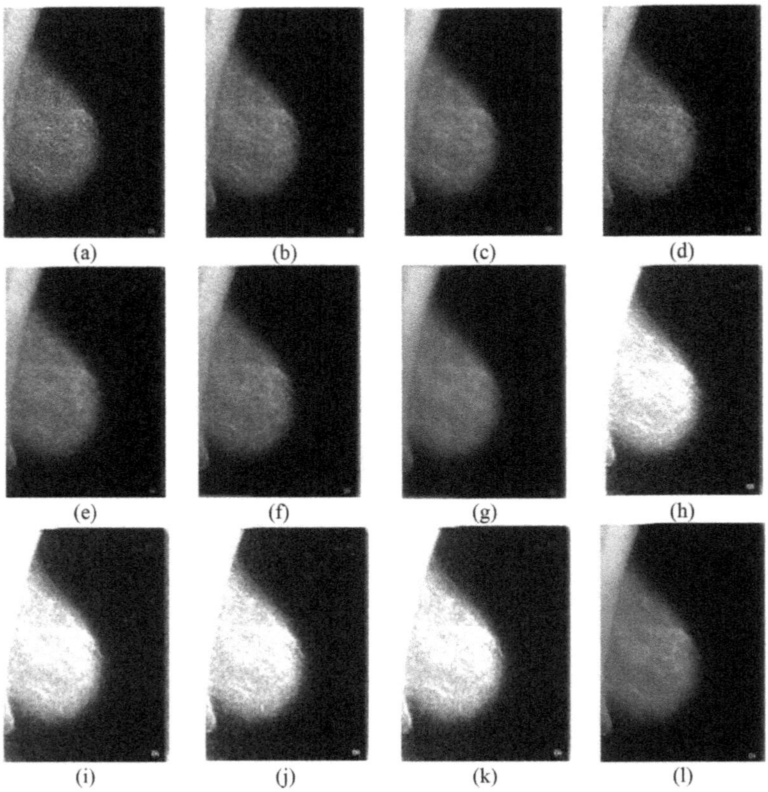

Figure 10.12. (a) Image with Gaussian noise, (b) 3 × 3 averaging filter output, (c) 5 × 5 averaging filter output, (d) 3 × 3 median filter output, (e) 5 × 5 median filter output, (f) Gaussian, (g) Butterworth, (h) wavelet-HL, (i) wavelet-LH, (j) wavelet-HH, (k) wavelet-LH-HH, (l) CNN.

Table 10.2. Performance evaluation for Gaussian noise.

		MSE	SNR	PSNR	Mean	Variance
Mean Filter	3 × 3	65.961	−0.0532	10.217	55.4081	15.829
	5 × 5	64.536	0.0415	10.3106	55.0900	15.389
Median	3 × 3	0.0078	58.9497	69.2261	0.2055	0.0235
	5 × 5	0.0089	58.3976	68.6582	0.2021	0.0225
Gaussian		65.803	−0.1113	10.158	55.8923	15.617
Butterworth		63.604	0.0290	10.3136	55.7716	14.509
Wavelet	HL	0.1015	47.6403	58.0667	−0.0107	0.0096
	LH	0.1012	47.6519	58.0783	−0.0112	0.0074
	HH	0.0106	47.6370	58.0034	−0.0117	0.0086
	LH-HH	0.1008	47.6687	58.0951	−0.0112	0.0055
CNN		0.0026	63.5801	74.0101	0.2191	1.1413

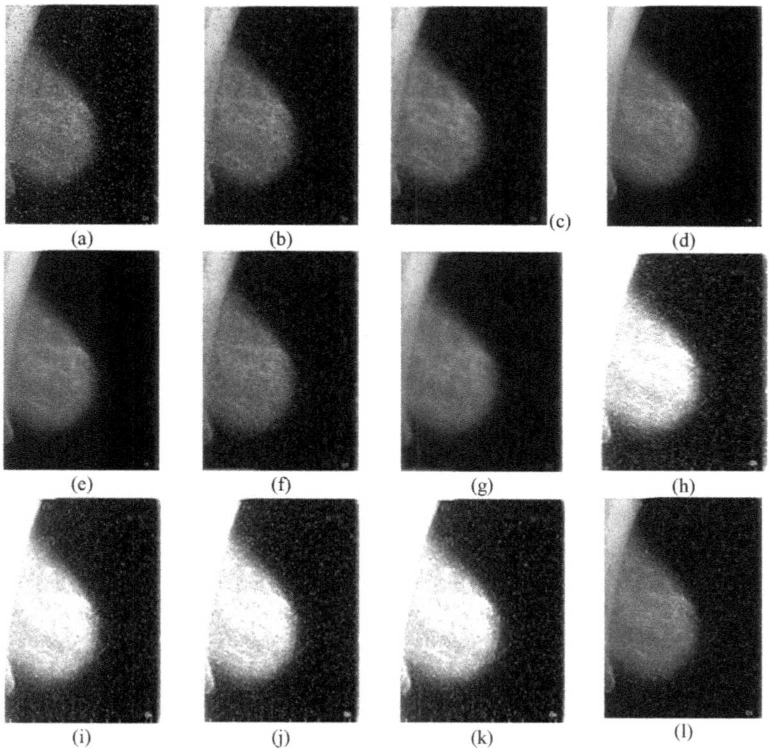

Figure 10.13. (a) Image with impulse noise, (b) 3 × 3 averaging filter output, (c) 5 × 5 averaging filter output, (d) 3 × 3 median filter output, (e) 5 × 5 median filter output, (f) Gaussian, (g) Butterworth, (h) wavelet-HL, (i) wavelet-LH, (j) wavelet-HH, (k) wavelet-LH-HH, (l) CNN.

that indicates that the median filter, wavelet, and CNN have low MSE, and high SNR and PSNR. Subjective analysis of different filtering techniques in figure 10.13 shows that median filtering is the best option for impulse noise reduction, but we have also seen that median filter also causes image smoothing when we increase the window size.

10.7 Conclusion

In this chapter, we have discussed image enhancement techniques both in the spatial domain and frequency domain. In spatial domain techniques, we have used the point processing techniques like histogram, histogram equalization, and histogram matching and some masking techniques like median filtering, mean filtering, Gaussian filtering, etc and in the frequency domain, ideal and Butterworth low pass filter, Gaussian filters, homomorphic filters, etc and observed that low pass filtering causes ringing effect in the output of the image. In the case of the Butterworth filter, it reduces the ringing effect but for higher-order, it also causes a ringing effect. However, a Gaussian filter does not cause any ringing effect. The homomorphic filter can enhance the image with very low illumination.

Table 10.3. Performance evaluation for impulse (salt and pepper) noise.

		MSE	SNR	PSNR	Mean	Variance
Mean Filter	3 × 3	63.961	−0.0565	10.4326	50.6045	15.725
	5 × 5	65.954	0.5104	10.2862	54.6008	16.189
Median	3 × 3	0.0206	55.2174	64.9820	0.2007	0.0225
	5 × 5	0.0214	55.0598	64.8287	0.1993	0.0221
Gaussian		67.502	0.3170	10.1007	55.5180	16.925
Butterworth		63.708	0.5178	10.2909	55.5329	13.917
Wavelet	HL	0.1098	47.5402	57.7268	−0.0108	0.0157
	LH	0.1096	47.5469	57.7329	−0.0113	0.0134
	HH	0.1102	47.5222	57.7083	−0.0118	0.0140
	LH-HH	0.1086	47.5876	57.7736	−0.0113	0.0084
CNN		0.1020	55.0312	65.2191	0.2190	0.0236

This chapter also discussed the recent developments in image denoising methods and showed their merits and demerits. Many times, noise in the image makes its analysis very difficult for researchers. A breast mammogram enhancement by removal of Gaussian, salt pepper, and speckle noise based on spatial domain filtering, frequency domain filtering, wavelet transform, and a CNN-based approach is developed. The proposed method is effective in image noise reduction and gives better enhancement for diagnosis. It is also shown that the performance of different filters depends upon the types of noises. The experimental result shows that the CNN-based filtering approach has been proven to be the best technique when the image is corrupted with Speckle, Gaussian, and impulse noise. The wavelet-based approach has been analyzed and results show that it is a good alternative for de-noising images corrupted with Gaussian and impulsive noise, but it also causes over enhancement and an image that appears brighter than the original mammographic image, so it becomes very difficult to identify the microcalcification. It is observed that low pass filtering can remove the noise, but it causes blurring and image smoothing. It can be concluded that the selection of image enhancement techniques either in the spatial domain or in the frequency domain is application-specific. It is also shown that the performance of different filters is varied and depends upon the types of noises.

References

[1] World Health Organization 2020 WHO report on cancer: setting priorities, investing wisely and providing care for all (February 2020) pp 17–36

[2] https://breastcancer.org/ (accessed on 10, January 2021)

[3] Knutzen A M and Gisvold J J 1993 Likelihood of malignant disease for various categories of mammographically detected, nonpalpable breast lesions *Mayo Clin. Proc.* **68** 454–60

[4] Weigelt B, Geyer F C and Reis-Filho J S 2010 Histological types of breast cancer: How special are they? *Mol. Oncol.* **4** 192–208

[5] www.cancer.gov/cancertopics/factsheet/Detection/screening-mammograms

[6] Armstrong K, Eisen A and Barbara W 2000 Assessing the risk of breast cancer *New Engl. J. Med.* **342** 564–71

[7] Shepherd J A, Malkov S, Fan B, Laidevant A, Novotny R and Maskarinec G 2008 Breast density assessment in adolescent girls using dual energy x-ray absorptiometry a feasibility study *Cancer Epidemiol. Biomarkers Prev.* **17** 1709–13

[8] Salzmann P, Kerlikowske K and Philips K 1997 Cost effectiveness of extending screening mammography guidelines to include women 40 to 49 years of age *Ann. Intern. Med.* **127** 955–65

[9] Wolfe J N 1967 Mammography: ducts as a sole indicator of breast carcinoma *Radiology* **89** 206–10

[10] boyd N F, Rommens J M, Vogt K, Lee V, Hopper J L, Yaffe M J and Paterson A D 2005 Mammographic breast density as an intermediate phenotype for breast cancer *Lancet Oncol.* **6** 798–808

[11] Byrne C, Schairer C, Brinton L A, Wolfe J, Parekh N, Salane M, Carter C and Hoover R 2001 Effects of mammographic density and benign breast disease on breast cancer risk (United States) *Cancer Causes Control* **12** 103–10

[12] Martin L and Boyd N 2008 Mammographic density potential mechanisms of breast cancer risk associated with mammographic density: hypotheses based on epidemiological evidence *Breast Cancer Res.* **10** 1–14

[13] Park J M, Franken E A Jr, Garg M, Fajardo L L and Niklason L T 2007 Breast tomosynthesis: present considerations and future applications *Radiographics* **27** 231–40

[14] Moy L, Elias K, Patel V, Lee J, Babb J, Toth H and Mercado C 2009 Is breast MRI helpful in the evaluation of inconclusive mammographic findings? *Am. J. Roentgenol.* **193** 986–93

[15] Gelderen V 2004 *Understanding X-Rays: A Synopsis of Radiology* 1st edn (Berlin: Springer)

[16] Benson C C, Rajamani K and Lajish V L 2015 A review on automatic marker identification methods in watershed algorithms used for medical image segmentation *Int. J. Innov. Sci. Eng. Technol.* **2** 829–39

[17] Kumar N and Arora S 2012 Medical evaluation of marker controlled watershed technique for detecting brain tumors *Int. J. Comput. App.* **54** 975–8887

[18] Chan R H, Chung-Wa C W and Nikolova M 2005 Salt and pepper noise removal by median type noise detectors and detail preserving regularization *IEEE Trans. Image Process.* **14** 1479–85

[19] Jagya P 2015 Comparison of two segmentation methods for mammographic image *Int. J. Comput. App.* **126** 31–43

[20] Amendolia S R, Bisogni M G, Bottigli U, Ceccopieri A, Delogu P, Fantacci M E, Marchi A, Marzulli V M, Palmiero R and Stumbo S 2001 The CALMA project: a CAD tool in breast radiography *Nucl. Instrum. Methods Phys. Res., Sect.* A **460** 107–12

[21] Tang J, Rangayyan R M, El-Naqa J, Xu I and Yang Y 2009 Computer-aided detection and diagnosis of breast cancer with mammography: recent advances *IEEE Trans. Inf. Technol. Biomed.* **13** 236–51

[22] Nema M K, Rakshit S and Chaudhuri S 2009 Image denoising using edge model-based representation of Laplacian subbands *7th Int. Conf. on Advances in Pattern Recognition (Kolkata, February 2009)* pp 329–32

[23] Shukla A K, Pandey R, Yadav S and Pachori R B 2019 Generalized fractional filter-based algorithm for image denoising *Circuits Syst. Signal Process.* **39** 363–90

[24] Adam D, Beilin-Nissan S, Friedman Z and Behar V 2006 The combined effect of spatial compounding and nonlinear filtering on the speckle reduction in ultrasound images *Ultrasonics* **44** 166–81
[25] Chen Y, Yin R M, Flynn R and Broschat S 2003 Aggressive region growing for speckle reduction in ultrasound images *Pattern Recognit. Lett.* **24** 677–69
[26] Djurovic I 2016 BM3D filter in salt-and-pepper noise removal *EURASIP J. Image Video Process.* **13** 1–11
[27] Michailovich O V and Tannenbaum A 2006 Despeckling of medical ultrasound images *IEEE Trans. Ultrason. Ferroelectr. Freq. Control* **53** 64–78
[28] Papadopoulos A, Fotiadis D and Costaridou L 2008 Improvement of microcalcification cluster detection in mammography utilizing image enhancement techniques *Comput. Biol. Med.* **38** 1045–55
[29] Cheng H D, Cai X, Chen X, Hu L and Lou X 2003 Computer-aided detection and classification of microcalcifications in mammograms: a survey *Pattern Recognit.* **36** 2967–91
[30] Chen Z K, Tao Y and Chen X 2001 Multi-resolution local contrast enhancement of x-ray images for poultry meat inspection *Appl. Opt.* **40** 1195–200
[31] Cheng H D, Xue M and Shi X J 2003 Contrast enhancement based on a novel homogeneity measurement *Pattern Recognit.* **36** 2687–97
[32] Stark J A 2000 Adaptive image contrast enhancement using generalizations of histogram equalization *IEEE Trans. Image Process.* **9** 889–96
[33] Kim J Y, Kim L S and Hwang S H 2001 An advanced contrast enhancement using partially overlapped sub-block histogram equalization *IEEE Trans. Circuits Syst. Video Technol.* **11** 475–84
[34] Dong W, Zhang L, Shi G and Li X 2012 Nonlocally centralized sparse representation for image restoration *IEEE Trans. Image Process.* **22** 1620–30
[35] Xie J, Xu L and Chen E 2012 Image denoising and inpainting with deep neural networks *25th Int. Conf. on Neural Information Processing Systems* vol 1 *(Red Hook, NY)* pp 341–9
[36] Lyu S and Simoncelli E P 2006 Statistical modeling of images with fields of Gaussian scale mixtures *Adv. Neural Inform. Process. Syst.* **31** 945–52
[37] Gonzales R and Woods R 2008 *Digital Image Processing* 3rd edn (Hoboken, NJ: Pearson Education Prentice Hall) pp 144–72
[38] Jayaraman S, Veerakumar T and Esakkirajan S 2010 *Digital Image Processing* 3rd edn (New Delhi: Tata McGraw-Hill Education)
[39] Mohideen S K, Perumal S A and Sathik M M 2008 Image de-noising using discrete wavelet transform *IJCSNS Int. J. Comput. Sci. Netw. Sec.* **8** 213–6
[40] Kimlyk M and Umnyashkin S 2018 Image denoising using discrete wavelet transform and edge information *2018 IEEE Conf. of Russian Young Researchers in Electrical and Electronic Engineering (EIConRus) (Moscow and St. Petersburg, February 2018)* pp 1823–5
[41] Zhai J H, Zhang S F and Liu L J 2008 Image recognition based on wavelet transform and artificial neural networks *Int. Conf. on Machine Learning and Cybernetics (Kunming, July 2008)* 789–93
[42] Hiremath P, Akkasaligar P T and Badiger S 2011 Performance comparison of wavelet transform and contourlet transform based methods for despeckling medical ultrasound images *Int. J. Comput. App.* **26** 34–41
[43] Thakur R S, Yadav R N and Gupta L 2019 State-of-art analysis of image denoising methods using convolutional neural networks *IET Image Proc.* **13** 2367–80

[44] Alpaydin E 2004 *Introduction to Machine Learning* 2nd edn (Cambridge, MA: MIT Press)
[45] Cheng H D, Shan J, Ju W, Guo Y and Zhang L 2010 Automated breast cancer detection and classification using ultrasound images: a survey *Pattern Recognit.* **43** 299–317
[46] Liu Z, Yan W Q and Yang M L 2018 Image denoising based on a CNN model *Int. Conf. on Control, Automation and Robotics (ICCAR) (Auckland, April 2018)* pp 389–93
[47] Hossain B, Chai H Y, Faisal A, Pingguan-Murphy B and Lai K W 2014 Speckle noise reduction of ultrasound knee biomarker with edge and detail preservation using improved diffusivity function *IEEE Conf. on Biomedical Engineering and Science (Kuala Lumpur, December 2014)* pp 639–43
[48] Pal S K, Bhandari D and Kundu M K 1994 Genetic algorithms, for optimal image enhancement *Pattern Recognit. Lett.* **15** 261–71
[49] Padmasini N, Abbirame K S, Mohamed Yacin S and Umamaheswari R 2014 Speckle noise reduction in spectral domain optical coherence tomography retinal images using anisotropic diffusion filtering *Int. Conf. on Science, Engineering and Management Research (Chennai, February 2014)* pp 1–5
[50] Santhos K A, Kumar A and Bajaj V *et al* 2020 McCulloch's algorithm inspired cuckoo search optimizer based mammographic image segmentation *Multimedia Tools App.* **79** 30453–88

IOP Publishing

High Performance Computing for Intelligent Medical Systems

Varun Bajaj and Irshad Ahmad Ansari

Chapter 11

Computational intelligence for eye disease detection

Amit Kumar Verma

High performance computing has an important role to play as the medical field depends on fast sensing, proper examination and analysis. Computational intelligence thus has a greater role to act in the detection of eye diseases, especially related to the retina. Changes in the retina may be the indicator of various eye diseases along with diseases or disorder related to the central nervous system and cardiovascular circulation. The retina is a membranous layer of tissue which is thin and provides central vision. Many eye diseases manifested through the retina are retinal tear, glaucoma, optic nerve disorder, diabetic macular edema, diabetic retinopathy, detachment of retina, hole in macula, degeneration of macula and other cardiovascular disorders like myocardial infarction and atherosclerosis. The retina is vulnerable to various organ specific as well as many systemic diseases, while retina imaging helps in the diagnosis of proper eye disease along with complications of diabetes retinopathy, hypertension, myocardial infarction etc. Retina analysis is a non-intrusive diagnosis technology. Through the use of computational intelligence via image processing techniques, the various eye diseases can be detected at a very early age of their initiation. This chapter focuses on the anatomy of the eye, physiology of the various eye diseases, retinal imaging methods-2D fundus imaging and 3D optical coherence tomography (OCT) and their comparative analysis. The chapter actually deals with retinal imaging and its clinical implications in the diagnosis or detection of eye diseases. In addition to this, the chapter also discusses different methods which are used for detection of glaucoma.

11.1 Introduction

Globally, the problem of loss of vision due to various eye diseases has attracted various researchers from medical, pharmaceutical and computer science backgrounds. As per the first world vision report compiled by WHO on October 8, 2019—2.2 billion

doi:10.1088/978-0-7503-3815-8ch11

people have a problem with vision impairment, out of which 1 billion people could have been prevented from vision loss. It also points out that elderly people are the most affected in terms of vision impairment or vision loss. Presbyopia affects 1.3 billion people in which there is difficulty seeing nearby objects. Myopia disturbs 2.6 billion people with 312 million under 19 years of age. Similarly, diabetic retinopathy affects 3 million, glaucoma affects 6.9 million, age related macular degeneration affects 10.4 million of the population. The report explains that accessibility for eye care and the high costs involved, particularly in rural areas, were the main contributor of vision loss and impairment. Retinal imaging is the technique of taking digital pictures of the back of the eye using computational intelligence. It depicts the retina, the disk that holds the main optic nerve and blood vessels involved; thus doctors find various retinal diseases and examine the status of the eye, however, an opthalmoscope is used to examine the eye but retinal imaging provides an opportunity for the ophthalmologist to get a much wider digital view of the retina, thus adding extra precision to the regular eye examination.

11.2 Anatomy of the eye

The sight organ of the human body is the eye, which is a slightly symmetrical globe measuring an inch in diameter, approximately 25 mm (figure 11.1). The remarkability of the eye is that it can detect a single light photon. The perception of the colour, depth, motion, distance, speed, lightning etc, makes it the primary sense organ of the human body. When you see yourself in the mirror, the front part of the eye includes:

1. Iris: this is the coloured portion;
2. Cornea: this is clear domed shaped over iris;
3. Pupil: this is circular opening black in colour in the iris for incoming light;

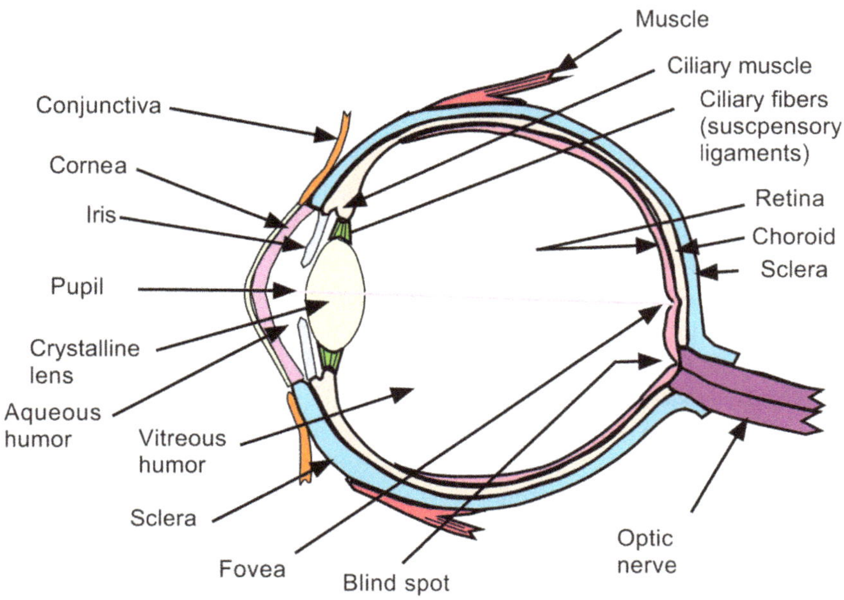

Figure 11.1. Anatomy of human eye.

4. Sclera: this is white part of the eye;
5. Conjunctiva: leaving the cornea, this is the tissue layer that covers the entire front of the eye.

11.2.1 The cornea

In the front of the iris and pupil lies the most anterior part of the body called the cornea. It is considered to be a highly dense innervated tissue of the body. The average dimension of the cornea of the adult human eye covers 11.5 mm horizontal diameter and 10.5 mm of the vertical diameter with constant curvature [1]. The trigeminal nerve has the ophthalmic entity which is the source of the corneal nerve [2]. Four millimetre is the size of pre-pupillary cornea, also termed the optic zone and situated in the middle of the cornea in a photopic condition. There is a difference in the physiology and pathological condition of both the central and the other type of cornea, that is, peripheral [3].

The human eye consists of five layers:

I. The epithelium;
II. The Bowman's membrane;
III. The lamellar stoma;
IV. The Descemet's membrane;
V. The endothelium.

I. **The corneal epithelium**

Its surface is covered by the tear film which has the vital role of protecting the corneal surface from microbes, toxic chemicals or any xeno substances. The tear film has an outer lipid layer and inner water mucus layer. The tear film gets spread with each eyelid blink due to interaction between the epithelial cells and the outer lipid layer. The corneal epithelium consists of:

(a) 2–3 layers of superficial cells;
(b) 2–3 layers of the wings cells;
(c) one layer of basal cells.

The folding of microplicae contribute irregularity to the surface of the superficial cells of the epithelium and shows interaction with the overlying tear film. Around seven to ten days is the renewal time of the cells of the corneal epithelium. The presence of the cell junction provides impermeability, stability and anchoring to the corneal epithelium [4].

II. **The Bowman's layer**

It separates the epithelium from the corneal lamellar stroma. It is a cellular zone of 10-15 micronmeters.

III. **The corneal lamellar stroma**

It provides structural anchoring to the cornea of the eye. The transparency and the hydration state of the cornea is maintained by the stroma keratocytes (stellar shaped cells) which release collagen and proteoglycans, collagen fibres in parallel arrangement ($n = 200$–250) running from limbus to limbus [5] constitute the bulk of the stromal extracellular matrix. Collagen fibres' regular organisation contributes to the corneal transparency and also provides mechanical strength to the cornea. Due to the compact packaging of the fibril more in the pre-pupillary cornea than the peripheral cornea, the cornea has mechanical strength and dioptric stability [6]. Proteoglycans, which surrounds the stromal collagen fibrils consists of keratin sulfate or chondroitin sulphate/dermatan sulphate side chain, thus regulating hydration of the eye.

IV. **The corneal endothelium**

It is 5–7 sided cuboidal cells in a single layer. They secrete Descemet's elastic membrane which causes separation between stroma and the endothelium. The endothelium has an osmotic transport system where the osmotic gradient generates a constant percentage of the water in the stroma maintaining clarity and transparency of the cornea (hypoosmotic stroma to hypertonic aqueous); this whole process is called deturgescence, and its disturbance results in corneal edema.

Note: in a normal transparent cornea, visible light neither gets absorbed nor scattered. The condition of corneal scattering occurs due to:

- corneal edema;
- restoration of the collagen fibrels;
- hazes;
- surgical irregularities.

11.2.2 The human retina

The inner surface of the eye is lined by the inner tissues surrounding the vitrous cavity and held by the surrounding sclera and cornea. The neural retina is inside of the optical wall encircling the vitrous cavity, whereas the outside of the wall is surrounded by pigment epithelium (sclera and choroid) [7, 8]. Mullerian glia is the backbone of the neural retina and the light is captured by neural retina, having six main class of neuron—ganglion cells, bipolar cells, horizontal cells and amacrine cells. The outer nuclear consists of a nuclear of the photoreceptor cells, and in the inner nuclear of the retinal lies the cells of bipolar, horizontal, amacrine and Maglia. The inner nuclear further has the layer of the outer plexiform composed of photoreceptors joined with horizontal and bipolar cells. On the other hand, a layer of the inner plexiform has amacrine and bipolar cells which have synapses with the cells of the ganglion. Mullerian glia processes extend to the retina. In a human there are two types of photoreceptor—rods and cones. Cones consist of the pigment with the absorption signal in various spectral ranges of colour of yellow, blue, and green. Rods having pigment show absorption in the colour region of green and blue. Rods are not involved in colour vision, they are active in low light levels [9].

Foveola is the thin, avascular bottom of fovea containing densely packed cone cells resulting in highest visual acuity. Henle's Fibres are the elongation fibres. RPE is a monolayer adjacent layer of the choroid. Light enters the eye and is captured by the photoreceptor at the back of the retina. After passing the lens, visual images are inverted, the right half image is projected onto the nasal retina of the right eye, and the left half of the image is projected onto the temporal retina of the right eye and the nasal retina of the left eye. The neural retina's neuron passes the visual information into the nerve impulse which travels through the optic nerve to the brain.

11.3 Retinal diseases

The various existing diseases related to the retina are:

1. Detachment of retina/tear problem;
2. Retinopathy caused by diabetes;
3. Hole in the macula;
4. Degeneration of macula;
5. Disorders of optic nerve;
6. Glaucoma;
7. Diabetic macular edema (DME);
8. Retinopathy of prematurity (ROP).

11.3.1 Retinal tear

In retinal detachment, there is separation of retina from the pigment epithelium. This may be due to an injury or tumour or inflammation to the eye or inflammation of the underlying choroid. The characteristic feature is the development of a hole as well as a tear. The tear is formed due to the forces applied on attachments between the retina and the vitreous humour that fills the interior of the eye. Vitreous pulling of the retina can be due to injury or changes due to age factor or sudden movement of the eye which further causes fluid to enter the small hole and causing striping. Retinal detachment is common to myopic (near-sighted) eyes. The pull of the vitreous on part of the retina creates a retinal tear. There is observation of brief light flashes observed by the affected person during eye ball rotation. The perception of coming shadow in the front of the eye indicates the beginning of a tear in the retina.

11.3.2 Diabetic retinopathy

Diabetic retinopathy is an eye illness that results due to the metabolic disorder of diabetes. In this alarming disorder a high level of glucose damages the retina of the eye. There is ceasation of blood through the blood capillaries, hence abnormal dilation is possible. There is additional development of blood capillaries on the retina. This all leads to the development of blurring then blindness. Swelling of the capillaries can result in the creation of edema of the macula. The disease progression signs include two-fold vision, eye ache, macular hole, floaters.

11.3.3 Macula hole

One important part, the macula, plays a vital role in the various activities related to vision such as book reading, vehicle driving and perception of things, thus causing promotion of fine proper vision. The drawing of the eye fluid vitreous humour is responsible for the creation of a gap in the macula. The gap is responsible for the softening of the macula. Extreme short sightedness, advancement of epiretinal membranes, separation of the retina and diabetic retinopathy all contribute to the creation of macular gap.

11.3.4 Degeneration of the macula

The degeneration of the macula can be inherited or can be from age related factors. It is an uncommon class of retinal degenerative diseases collectively called retinitis, pigmentosa of retina and similar disorders. The preliminary sign is night blindness, observed in childhood because of a change in the function of the rods. The thinning of vessels and the dispersion of pigment clumps progresses to 'tunnel vision'. Retinitis pigmentosa is due to malfunctioning in genes coding of amino acids sequences engaged in light sensitivity. Age-related macular degeneration (ARMD) is possible in patients over fifty and affects central vision and spares peripheral vision. This is a major contributor of vision loss. Age-related macular degeneration disease is categorised as

(a) Dry type macular degeneration

There is development of colour filler, that is, drusen slightly yellow; the other incorporation is epithelium percentage, all collectively leading to the dry type of degeneration.

(b) Wet macular degeneration (containing abnormal blood vessels)

In this, there is bleeding, and detachment of vessels filled with blood in the gap that exists between two anatomical features of sensory retina part and pigment epithelium part. This is noticed in someone suffering from a high blood glucose problem and high blood pressure. Degeneration of the macula affects central visual acuity, however, it does not cause total blindness but makes reading or fine detail work difficult or impossible.

11.3.5 Disorders of the optic nerve

The optic nerve is responsible for the signal transmission from the eye to brain and from brain to eye, therefore, proper nerve transmission is important for the good health of the eye. Due to the development of the various pressures inside the skull the eye may face problems which in due course of time lead to the development of various eye diseases. When this pressure remains persistent for continuous time it inflammes the nerve and hence swelling can occur. This starts to damage the fibres of the optic nerve resulting in various disorders of the optic nerve like low vision. Young adults are the main sufferers. Optic neuritis may be a manifestation of multiple sclerosis where the sheaths of the optic nerves have changed and interfere with the transmission of nervous impulses.

11.3.6 Glaucoma

This is caused when drainage of the aqueous humour is blocked due to blockage of specialized drainage channels at the base of the iris. This intraocular pressure may cause atrophy of retinal nerve fibres and causes blurred vision, so enhanced strain on human eye pressure is a risk contributor for the development of glaucoma, which is combination of problems that result in the development of nerve damage. Glaucoma is a strain sensitive disease depending mainly on the optimum strain of the eye. In normal conditions the human eye can withstand strain in the range of ten to twenty mm of Hg. So, the calculation of the strain is considered an appropriate marker for the detection of this disease, however, there are many clinical cases reported where there is glaucoma in spite of normal strain values. Two main categories of this disease are open angle type, common in older patients and angle closure glaucoma, caused due to blockage of the outflow of aqueous humour through the trabecular meshwork.

11.3.7 Diabetic macular edema

Fluid accumulation in the macula, or central portion of the eye, caused by the complication of diabetes results in swelling of the macula. Filling of the macula with cells causes blurred vision that plays a vital role for sharp, straight ahead vision that helps in reading and driving.

11.3.8 Retinopathy of prematurity

Retinopathy of prematurity is a disease which widely affects children or infants and is the main cause of vision loss. Basically, there is a problem occurring in the retina of babies having non-appropriate weight.

11.4 History of retinal imaging

In order to get the visual photo of inner retina, various special techniques are needed. For various analyses there was publication of a method that applied fluorescein angiography for image analysis based on mathematical morphology, primarily focused on vessel segmentation [9], done by Matsui *et al.* The French physician Jean Mery successfully depicted that on immersing a live cat in water, the cat's retinal vessels would become visible from the outside and this idea inspired Jan Evangelista Purkyně, who was a researcher, to invent the principles of the ophthalmoscope in 1823, then Charles Babbage reinvented it in 1845 [10, 11]. Lastly, the same attempt was made in 1851 by researcher von Helmholtz [12]. In the year 1853 the Dutch ophthalmologist van Trigt [13] published the first image of the retina. In 1891 Gerloff, a doctor from Germany, showed very important photographs of the eye retina depicting the blood vessels [14].

The fundus camera was developed by Gullstrand in 1910 and used in modern times to image the retina and for this he received the Nobel prize for his contribution [15]. The invention of fluorescein angiographic imaging was the next major development where the functional state of the retina was known by the help of a fundus camera with narrow filters [16]. Due to safety concerns this was replaced by tomographic imaging methods. In 1964 Allen described stereo fundus photography to represent 3D shape of the retina, further there occurred the development of confocal scanning laser ophthalmoscopy where at different confocal depths multiple images of the retina are obtained. The development of the super luminescent diodes and femtosecond lasers make tomographic imaging of the retina possible and popular. In addition to this, 3D sectioning of the retina gives reality to retinal imaging [17] by the various newer methods.

11.5 Current status of retinal analysis

The last 160 years saw the progression of imaging of the retina, which is now the backbone of clinical care of the eye patient having various retinal and systemic diseases. These techniques are used successfully for the diagnosis of diseases and disorders of high blood sugar, high blood pressure, dementia, atherosclerosis and other related cardiovascular diseases, which are detected by fundus photography. The popularly chosen methods are optical coherence tomography (OCT) and fluorescein angiography. In addition to this, OCT is also used in vireo-retinal surgery and its follow up.

11.5.1 Fundus imaging

In fundus imaging, there is a two-dimensional image projection of 3D retinal tissue. The intensity of the photo is directly proportional to the quantity of reflected light. The fundus imaging is cheap providing fine observation to the analyser.

The various categories of fundus imaging are fundus photography method, colour fundus photography method, stereo fundus photography method, hyperspectral imaging technique, scanning laser ophthalmoscopy technique, adaptive optics SLO, fluorescein angiography and indocyanine angiography methods.

(I) Fundus image analysis for the detection of diabetic retinopathy

The principle behind the detection of diabetic retinopathy from fundus images is based on the micro diagnosis of micro aneurysms, blood leakage and micro blood clots observed on the fundus, which reflects the inner parts of the retina.

(II) Image acquisition

This is the first step in the direction of detection of diabetic retinopathy. The acquisition of fundus colour image and its analysis helps us to observe abnormalities of the retina. Actually, in the process of fundus imaging there is projection of 3D half transparent tissues of the retina on the imaging plane. A special fundus camera is use to take the high-resolution image. The various manufacturers of cameras are Topcon, Canon, Kowa etc. The camera can be categorised into two types: mydriatic camera involving dilation of the pupil, and the other category of non-mydriatic camera. There are many databases available having numerous fundus images such as DRIVE, STARE, MESSIDOR, DIARETDBI, ARIA and ROC.

(III) Image pre-processing

Due to many limitations, the image quality of the image get deteriorated because of many factors such as low focus, unwanted motion of the patient, non-uniformity of light and improper calibration. The unusual features can only be detected if the quality of fundus images is up to standard. It is therefore suggested to apply image pre-processing techniques. Various algorithms are designed to remove the background abnormalities of the image. Three of the best known methods are histogram specification, histogram equalization and grey word normalization.

There are multiple features that indicate the damage caused due to retinopathy:

1. There is bright appearance of the exudates;
2. Dark appearance of vessels of blood as well as fovea (grey border);
3. Appearance of the optic disk as orange or pink in colour with diameter of 1.5 millimetre;
4. Micro-aneurysms are characteristic anatomical features that are dark circle shaped regions;
5. Haemorrhages are considered a major hallmark for determining the background of retinopathy caused by high glucose level;
6. Appearance of 'dot and blot' pattern and the colour is the same as that of vessels.

11.5.2 Optical coherence tomography

The theory behind the working of OCT is to estimate the 'depth at which a specific backscatter arises by calculating its time of flight'. Backscatters arises due to the differences in refractive index in transitions from one tissue to another tissue. The deeper tissues backscatter can be differentiated from backscatter arising in more superficial tissue due to longer time for the light to arrive at the sensor. Interferometry is used to measure the differences in 'time of flight' [17]. There are three major OCT theories:

I. Time-domain OCT, also called time-of-flight;
II. Swept-source or time encoded frequency domain OCT;
III. Spectral-domain OCT [18].

11.6 Disease specific analysis of retinal images

In order to increase the precision of eye patient management, to increase the eye clinician productivity and to reduce the cost, the requirement of reliable computerized methods or approaches for the retinal image analysis is the need of the time.

11.6.1 Early detection of retinal disease from fundus photography

Retinal disease detection is the most obvious example of a retinal screening application, in which the person suffering from eye disease is photographed in a distanced teleconsultation. This approach involves the utilization of cheap cameras for fundus photography which test the retinal images, and then focus on the preparation of the final output. it is considered the best example of telemedicine [19]. The preliminary diagnosis of retinopathy in a patient suffering from high blood glucose level through this technology is the hot spot nowadays but a screening program is available for the diagnosis of hypertension, dementia, disorder of optic nerve and various cardiovascular disorders. It has been observed that problems in the retinal vision can be prevented by the early diagnosis or detection of diabetic retinopathy [20, 21]. The work can be done successfully by applying the aforementioned sophisticated technology.

11.6.2 Early detection of systemic disease from fundus photography

Apart from the prior diagnosis of diseases of retina, early diagnosis of diseases of systemic circulation such as cardiovascular diseases or disorders can also be determined using fundus photography. Such determination is based on the calculation of retinal vessel characteristics, for heart stroke, hypertension or myocardial infarction [22, 23].

11.6.3 3-Dimensional OCT and retinal diseases—image guided therapy

3D OCT imaging, explains about the retinal morphology which helps in the close monitoring of a retinal disease like retinopathy caused due to high blood glucose level, glaucoma, tear, optic neuritis etc. The application of image guided treatment technology is proved to be beneficial in the treatment of retinopathy, macular edema in patient suffering from diabetes where the central part of the retina, the macula, is filled with leakage fluid causing visual loss or blindness. According to the research, the Early Treatment in Diabetic Retinopathy Study [24–26] shows that therapy taken for a diabetic macular edema (DME) with a focal laser, can prevent deterioration in the situation. The use of novel anti-vascular endothelial growth factor drugs, for example—ranibizumab combined with focal laser depicts better results in the treatment of DME. Recently, OCT imaging has shown the extent and amount of thickening in the retina, which helps with further treatment.

Neo-vascularization of the choroid is another form of vision loss category disease that has shown good results from image guided therapy. With the introduction of the anti-vascular endothelial growth factor agents like ranibizumab and bevacizumab, case improvements related to vision have been noticed [28, 29]. 3D representation of the optic nerve can be applied for early diagnosis and precise treatment to reduce the risk of blindness due to glaucoma [30].

11.7 Fundus image analysis

The most reliable means of fundus imaging is retinal imaging. Until recently, fundus image analysis was the only source of quantitative indices reflecting retinal morphological features. Subjects that lend themselves for fundus image analysis include: quantification of image quality (verification of image quality); detection, imaging of artifact; iatrogenic lesion detection (laser scars, etc); retinal structure's location and segmentation (retinal vessels, vessel diameter; artery and vein classification; vessel occlusion detection, fovea, optic disc-cup and rim; cupping); abnormalities segmentation (blood vessel related abnormalities/hemorrhages; microaneurysms; neovascularizations; nerve fiber infarcts—cottonwool spots); pigment epithelium related abnormalities (drusen hyper and hypopigmentation); choroid related abnormalities (nevus and melanoma detection; uveitis related choroidal lesions).

11.7.1 Glaucoma detection using retinal imaging

The thickness of the retinal nerve fiber layer (RNFL) [31] is the major hallmark for the diagnosis of this disease. In the case of glaucoma, fundus imaging is one of the most reliable techniques and photos can be easily accessed. After the analysis is done the results obtained can be interpreted to detect the disease [32–34].

The process of glaucoma diagnosis is depicted in the diagram in figure 11.2 hence the sequence involved in the process is as follows:

(i) There is observation and analysis of the provided image;
(ii) Pre-processing of analysed entity mainly depends on sampling process, region of interest, extraction and selection of channel;
(iii) Segmentation of provided photo image;
(iv) There is reorganization of analysis pattern by applying the technique of segmentation;
(v) There is the extraction of characters and then their selection;
(vi) Now the role of the classifiers comes into the play.

The detection and diagnosis of glaucoma is done by different classifiers, such as

I. **SVM classifier-based technique** Vapnik was the first to propose the support vector machine (SVM), which has sparked a lot of interest in the machine learning community. Several recent studies have shown that SVMs are typically capable of delivering higher classification accuracy than other data classification algorithms [35–38].
II. **Thresholding-based techniques** If the image intensity is less than a constant, the simplest thresholding methods replace each pixel in an image with a black pixel, and if the image intensity is greater than that constant, each

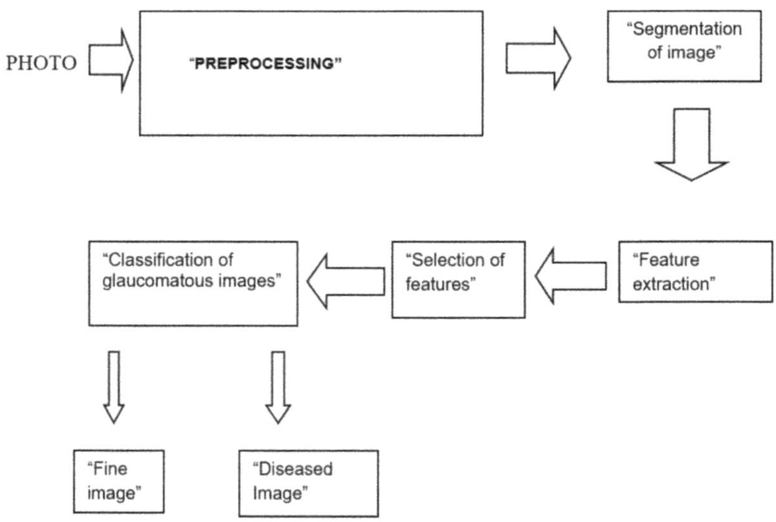

Figure 11.2. The diagram representing the diagnosis of the disease glaucoma using the technology retinal fundus imaging.

pixel is replaced with a white pixel. The dark tree becomes completely black, and the white snow becomes completely white, as seen in the example picture on the right [39].

III. **ANN classifier-based techniques** Artificial neuronal networks (ANNs) have been successfully used in a variety of fields, including geotechnics, civil engineering, mechanics, industrial surveillance, defense, automation, and transportation. ANN's image management processes include image pre-processing, data reduction, segmentation, and identification. An image can be represented as a matrix, with each pixel's colour information stored in each unit of the matrix. In the neuronal network, the matrix is used as input data. The size of the vector and the number of input vectors are determined by the images' small dimensions, which make learning easier and faster. A sigmoidal transfer function was used [40].

IV. **NB classifier-based techniques** Based on statistical knowledge learned from a training set, this transforms a color image to a binary (labeled) image. The probability density function (PDF) for the random variables plant (P) and background (B), each of which contains the random variables hue (H), saturation (S), and value (V), is calculated from the training set (colour channels). Using Bayes theorem and the naive assumption that the random variables are independent, we calculate the joint probability that a pixel is from random variable P or B given these PDFs (for convenience). If P(pixel = plant) > P(pixel = background), output pixels are classified as plant (255) or background (0) [41].

11.7.2 Dementia detection using retinal imaging

The basic principle behind the detection of dementia is that the neuronal retinal cells share similar properties to those of the central nervous system neurons, similarly that arterioles venules of retina pattern are the same as cerebral vessels of blood, so it is considered that degradative changes in retinal features can be extrapolated for neuro-degenerative changes and these degenerative changes are an early indicator of dementia.

11.7.3 Heart diseases detection using retinal imaging

The fundamental concept that lies in the detection of heart diseases is analysis of microvasculature and the appropriate vascular design. For maintaining the proper and healthy functioning of the heart correct vascular design is very important for proper flow of blood and its efficient diffusion. On the other hand, if there is a problem in the geometry of microvasculature then it gets mirrored in the retinal vasculature, which is the hallmark for the early detection of cardiovascular diseases. It is observed that in hypertensive condition there is thinning of the arterioles of the retina, similarly the parameter of arteriolar tortuosity is a marker of blood pressure so increased pressure of the blood causes increase in the tortuosity of anatomical features of the retina. Stiffness of the arterioles is another parameter to define the normal functioning of the CVS System. QUARTZ-Quantitative Analysis of Retinal Vessel Topology and Size is the automatic software for performing the retinal imaging.

11.7.4 Choroidal melanoma detection using retinal imaging

This melanoma of the eye can be detected on recognising its characteristic feature of orange coloured pigment on the surface of the tumour; the tumour is touched within the optic disc up to three millimetres.

11.7.5 Advantages of retinal imaging

1. Retina image template file size is small, therefore, the time consumed in the process is very small and can be saved for future use.
2. It is a painless and safe technique.
3. It is superior to overdilation because overdilation allows the doctor to see only 16% of the eye, while in retinal imaging this percentage is 80%.
4. There is no temporary light sensitivity or blurring of eye vision.

11.8 Comparative analysis between various retinal imaging methods

In the field of ophthalmology, eye examination was initially done with indirect operating ophthalmoscopy, direct operating ophthalmoscopy, then by slit lamps involving various lenses, through angiography technique of fluorescein, photography of fundus, 3D photography, laser techniques and OCT to novel techniques of multimodal imaging. Photography of the retina based on film is now no longer in use so we can say that the conventional system has been overtaken by a digital system. In telemedicine mode various cameras of different resolution are used, many non-mydriatic cameras are now used. The assessment of high blood pressure, various types of cancers and bacterial infection can be done with colour fundus photography of the retina, providing the correct scenario of health of eye.

The technique of fundus autofluorescence is useful for detecting the physiological changes that happened in the retina during autofluorescence. Angiography technique is now commonly used where there is I.V. injection of dye which is fluorescent in Nature. OCT due to its high resolution and low coherence is widely used for obtaining the cross-sectional ocular tissues photos. Fast scanning and repeatability of calculations makes it a front runner of the race. OCT angiography is the novel technique of eye retinal imaging based on motion contrast, which does not require dye injection and is much preferred. Many research projects are being started using the novel concepts of multimodal imaging providing high speed and fine resolution imaging with increased illumination penetration.

11.9 Conclusion

Retina imaging helps in the diagnosis of proper eye disease along with complication of diabetes retinopathy, hypertension, myocardial infarction etc. Retina analysis is a non-intrusive diagnosis technology. Through the use of image processing techniques, the various eye diseases can be detected at a very early age of their initiation. Rapid development in techniques of retinal imaging focuse on enhanced resolution, non-invasiveness and rapid speed.

There will be efforts to establish the relationship between retina and metabolic-cellular level through fluorescence lifetime imaging technology. It is predicted that the image acquisition and subsequent image analysis works to establish the integrity of analysis, some imaging concepts or techniques are still in the research and developmental phase which may provide in-depth knowledge about the various pathological processes. The modification of images for better understanding has changed the concepts of image modalities, novel OCT platforms are front runners for better judging of the retina, similarly, further advances in laser and optical technologies are providing wings to the future of telemedicine.

Within the next decade, the retinal imaging techniques utilization will creep up beyond the direct requirements of eye disease management. The advancement in the retinal examination helps in the assessment of various systemic disease both for patient health care and for population case studies. In future, diseases like multiple sclerosis, Huntington's disease, psychiatric diseases and neuropathies can be soft targets of retinal eye imaging.

References

[1] Rüfer F, Schröder A and Erb C 2005 White-to-white corneal diameter: normal values in healthy humans obtained with the Orbscan II topography system *Cornea* **24** 259–61

[2] Müller L J, Marfurt C F, Kruse F and Tervo T M T 2003 Corneal nerves: structure, contents and function *Exp. Eye Res.* **76** 521–42

[3] Van Buskirk E M 1989 The anatomy of the limbus *Eye (Lond)* **3** 101–8

[4] Farjo A A, McDermott M L and Soong H K 2009 Corneal anatomy, physiology, and wound healing 3rd edn ed M Yanoff and J S Duker *Ophthalmology* (Edinburgh: Mosby Elsevier) pp 203–8

[5] Maurice D M 1970 The transparency of the corneal stroma *Vision Res.* **10** 107–8

[6] Boote C, Dennis S, Newton R H, Puri H and Meek K M 2003 Collagen fibrils appear more closely packed in the prepupillary cornea: optical and biomechanical implications *Invest. Ophthalmol. Vis. Sci.* **44** 2941–8

[7] Miller N R and Newman N J 2005 Embryology, anatomy, and physiology of the afferent visual pathway *Walsh and Hoyt's Clinical Neuro-Ophthalmology* vol 1 6th edn (Philadelphia, PA: Lippincott Williams & Wilkins) pp 3–82

[8] Schubert H D 2009 Structure and function of the neural retina. Retinal pigment epithelium. Retinal and choroidal circulation 3rd edn ed M Yanoff and J S Duker *Ophthalmology* (Edinburgh: Mosby Elsevier) pp 511–21

[9] Matsui M, Tashiro T, Matsumoto K and Yamamoto S 1973 A study on automatic and quantitative diagnosis of fundus photographs. I. Detection of contour line of retinal blood vessel images on color fundus photographs (author's transl.) *Nippon Ganka Gakkai Zasshi* **77** 907–18

[10] Flick C S 1947 Centenary of Babbage's ophthalmoscope *Optician.* **113** 246

[11] Keeler C R 1997 150 years since Babbage's ophthalmoscope *Arch. Ophthalmol* **115** 1456–7

[12] von Helmholtz H L F 1851 Beschreibungeines Augen-Spiegels *A Farstnerische Verlagsbuchhandlung*

[13] Van Trigt A C 1853 Trajectiad Rhenum *Dissertatio ophthalmologica inauguralis de speculo oculi*

[14] Gerloff O 1891 Uber die Photographie des Augenhintergrundes *Klin Monatsblätter Augenheilkunde* **29** 397–403

[15] Gullstrand A 1910 Neue methoden der reflexlosen ophthalmoskopie *Berichte Deutsche Ophthalmologische Gesellschaft* 36

[16] Novotny H R and Alvis D L 1961 A method of photographing fluorescence in circulating blood in the human retina *Circulation.* **24** 82–6

[17] Huang D *et al* 1991 Optical coherence tomography *Science* **254** 1178–81

[18] Choma M, Sarunic M, Yang C and Izatt J 2003 Sensitivity advantage of swept source and fourier domain optical coherence tomography *Opt. Express* **11** 2183–9

[19] 2004 [Online]. Available http://www.atmeda.org/ICOT/diabeticretionpathy.FINAL.pdf

[20] Bresnick G H, Mukamel D B, Dickinson J C and Cole D R 2000 A screening approach to the surveillance of patients with diabetes for the presence of vision-threatening retinopathy *Ophthalmology.* **107** 19–24

[21] Kinyoun J L, Martin D C, Fujimoto W Y and Leonetti D L 1992 Ophthalmoscopy versus fundus photographs for detecting and grading diabetic retinopathy *Invest. Ophthalmol. Vis. Sci.* **33** 1888–93

[22] Cheung N, Liew G, Lindley R I, Liu E Y, Wang J J, Hand P, Baker M, Mitchell P and Wong T Y 2010 Retinal fractals and acute lacunar stroke *Ann. Neurol* **68** 107–11 [Online]. Available http://www.biomedsearch.com/nih/Retinal-fractals-acute-lacunar-stroke/20582985.html

[23] Wong T Y, Cheung N, Islam F M, Klein R, Criqui M H, Cotch M F, Carr J J, Klein B E and Sharrett A R 2008 Relation of retinopathy to coronary artery calcification: the multi-ethnic study of atherosclerosis *Am. J. Epidemiol* **167** 51–8

[24] Early Treatment Diabetic Retinopathy Study Research Group 1991 Early photocoagulation for diabetic retinopathy. ETDRS Rep. 9 *Ophthalmology.* **98** 766–85

[25] Early Treatment Diabetic Retinopathy Study Research Group 1985 Photocoagulation for diabetic macular edema. Early treatment diabetic retinopathy study report number 1 *Arch. Ophthalmol* **103** 1796–806

[26] Early Treatment Diabetic Retinopathy Study Research Group 1991 Fundus photographic risk factors for progression of diabetic retinopathy. ETDRS Rep. 12 *Ophthalmology* **98** 823–33

[27] Rosenfeld P J, Brown D M, Heier J S, Boyer D S, Kaiser P K, Chung C Y and Kim R Y 2006 Ranibizumab for neovascular age-related macular degeneration *New Engl. J. Med* **355** 1419–31

[28] Boyer D S, Antoszyk A N, Awh c c, Bhisitkul R B, Shapiro H and Acharya N R 2007 MARINA study group. Subgroup analysis of the marina study of ranibizumab in neovascular age-related macular degeneration *Ophthalmology.* **114** 246–52

[29] Lalwani G A, Rosenfeld P J, Fung A E, Dubovy S R, Michels S, Feuer W, Davis J L, Flynn H W Jr and Esquiabro M 2009 A variable-dosing regimen with intravitreal ranibizumab for neovascular age-related macular degeneration: Year 2 of the pronto study *Am. J. Ophthalmol* **148** 43–58

[30] Heijl A, Leske M C, Bengtsson B, Hyman L, Bengtsson B and Hussein M 2002 Early manifest glaucoma trial group. Reduction of intraocular pressure and glaucoma progression: results from the early manifest glaucoma trial *Arch. Ophthalmol* **120** 1268–79

[31] Bedke G C, Manza R R, Patil D D and Rajput Y M 2015 Secondary glaucoma diagnosis technique using retinal nerve fiber layer arteries *Proc. Int. Conf. on Pervasive Computing, Pune* pp 1–4

[32] Schacknow P N and Samples J R 2010 *Practical, Evidence-Based Approach to Patient Care, the Glaucoma Book* (Berlin: Springer)

[33] Poshtyar A, Shanbehzadeh J and Ahmadieh H 2010 Automatic measurement of cup to disc ratio for diagnosis of glaucoma on retinal fundus images *Med. Biometrics.* 64–72

[34] Vlachokosta A A, Asvestas P A, Matsopoulos G K, Uzunoglu N and Zeyen T G 2007 Preliminary study on the association of vessel diameter variation and glaucoma *Proc. 29th Annual Int. Conf. on IEEE Engineering in Medicine and Biology Society, Lyon* pp 888–91

[35] Narasimhan K and Vijayarekha K 2011 An efficient automated system for glaucoma detection using fundus image *Theor. Appl. Inf. Technol.* **33** 104–10

[36] Hussain S A and Holambe A N 2015 Automated detection and classification of glaucoma from eye fundus images: a survey *Comput. Sci. Inf. Technol.* **6** 1217–24

[37] Zhang Z, Lee B H, Liu J, Wong D W K, Tan N M, Lim J H, Yin F, Huang W, Li H and Wong T Y 2010 Optic disc region of interest localization in fundus image for glaucoma detection in ARGALI *Proc. Int. Conf. on Industrial Electronics and Applications, Taichung* pp 1686–9

[38] Mittapalli P S and Kande G B 2016 Segmentation of optic disc and optic cup from digital fundus images for the assessment of glaucoma *Biomed. Signal Process. Control* **24** 34–46

[39] Ho C Y, Pai T W, Chang H T and Chen H Y 2011 An automatic fundus image analysis system for clinical diagnosis of glaucoma *Proc. Int. Conf. on Complex, Intelligent, and Software Intensive Systems, Seoul* pp 559–64

[40] Zhang Z, Kwoh C K, Liu J, Cheung C Y L, Aung T and Wong T Y 2012 Automatic glaucoma diagnosis with mRMR-based feature selection *Biometrics Biostat.* 2155–6180

[41] Noronha K P, Acharya U R, Prabhakar Nayak K, Martis R J and Bhandary S V 2014 Automated classification of glaucoma stages using higher order cumulant features *Biomed. Signal Process. Control* **10** 174–83

IOP Publishing

High Performance Computing for Intelligent Medical Systems

Varun Bajaj and Irshad Ahmad Ansari

Chapter 12

Recent trends in medical image segmentation with special focus on brain tumours and retinal images

Mithlesh Prasad Singh, Aheibam Dinamani Singh, Rajesh Kumar, Kishorjit Nongmeikapam and Wahengbam Kanan Kumar

In a variety of areas from diagnosis and prediction to treatment based on the course of a disease, medical imaging plays a pivotal role. Image segmentation is a process that extracts the area of interest automatically or semi-automatically. Multimodality imaging is a concept used to capture an area of interest in the format used by various types, such as computer tomography (CT), magnetic resonance imaging (MRI), positron tomography (PET), etc. Various literatures demonstrated that their combination generates better classification of normal and abnormal tissues of brain, retina, lungs, kidney, etc. This chapter surveys state-of-the-art researches on biomedical image segmentation for brain tumours and retina segmentation, abnormality detection, advantages, disadvantages, and automated-learning techniques ranging from traditional machine learning to deep learning. The study also examines popular databases and contemporary approaches published so far. The chapter also provides a glimpse of key gaps and potential future scope for biomedical image segmentation of retina and brain tumours.

12.1 Introduction

One of the critical aspects of today's medical diagnosis process is biomedical imaging, as it is used in all fields of modern medicine [1]. Biomedical image examination is virtually always a complicated and prolonged task which specialists still struggle with [2, 3]. Biomedical image evaluation by medicinal specialists is an essential process for detection of pathologies. Analysis of different medical imaging modalities using computers has been in usage since as early as 1982 [4, 5]. Many techniques have been introduced since then, with each having an objective to increase accuracy/efficiency during computerized automated detection [6]. Today's technological progress could

doi:10.1088/978-0-7503-3815-8ch12

make it feasible to use new methods in the health domain. Throughout the practice with biomedical imaging, a medicinal practitioner relies upon subject reports and consequently makes specific and appropriate diagnosis about the subjects' status. Depending on the type of task there exist some forms of biomedical image examination techniques; some of them include segmentation based on organ and substructure, detection based on object, registration, prediction based on classification, classification based on objects, detection based on region and landmark, segmentation based on the item and others. A maximum number of researches focuses on segmentation based on organ and structure.

In patients' diagnosis and medication, imaging helps radiologists or clinicians make the diagnosis and prescription efficient. Currently, there is a wide variety of modalities for imaging soft and hard tissues/regions of the body. It has paved the way for more improved and early detection of abnormalities, and for possible early course of treatment. The foremost widely used modalities can be partitioned into two general categories: anatomical and functional. In this chapter, we only discuss the anatomical modality. These images can be represented in 2D, 3D and 4D systems. The elements of an image in 2D are referred to as pixels, while in 4D, they are referred to as voxels.

12.1.1 Types of biomedical imaging

A. X-ray. The most prevalent mode of screening that exists for identifying breaks and dislocation in bones is x-ray imaging. The image developed is 2D. One hundred thousand chest x-ray samples were provided by the National Institutes of Health (NIH) with relevant information and diagnostics to enhance imaging analysis techniques [7]. Similarly, a dataset comprising a sample of more than 350 000 body part x-rays for improving machine learning algorithms has been released by the Massachusetts Institute of Technology (MIT) to automatically diagnose specific disorders such as pneumonia or pinched lung, etc [8].
B. Computed tomography. It is also commonly referred to as a CT scan, and uses a computerised form or image acquisition in which 360 degrees of x-rays are aimed at the patient to create accurate cross-sectional representations of the body's inner organs, bones, soft tissue and blood vessels. Traditionally, the images are taken in the transverse plane or axial plane perpendicular to the body's long axis. However, it is possible to reformat these images, also known as slices, into multiple planes and create a three-dimensional image. By locating the presence of tumours and their scale, it is widely used to identify cancer and is among the most frequently addressed biomedical imaging issues. The National Institutes of Health (NIH) had given easy accessibility to 32 000 CT scan images with related information and diagnoses for enhancing lesion identification accuracy [9].
C. Magnetic resonance imaging. It is also commonly known by the term MRI scan, which uses intense magnetic fields to capture images of soft tissues within the region of interest of the human body. It is different from CT and

x-ray techniques which are rather used for capturing images of hard tissues of the body, such as bone fractures in different regions. Classification of grey matter, whiter matter and cerebrospinal fluid (CSF) using MRI scans has been carried out successfully. It has also led to the timely diagnosis of brain tumours, aneurysms, and haemmorhage. The OASIS project has collected neuro-imaging data sources for biomedical imaging studies comprising more than two thousand MRI sessions [10].

D. Ultrasound imaging (USI). It uses high-frequency vibration waves to give inside organ, tissue and bloodstream visual images. It is the most widely used technique in the reproduction process to track the foetus. It is mostly used for the stomach, vascular and thyroid filters and usually not used in the imaging of air-containing bones and tissues such as the lungs. The positive thing about using USI is that it is quick and free of radiation.

12.1.2 Biomedical image segmentation

Biomedical image segmentation (BIS) has been a comprehensive application since the 1990s. Segmentation is a process of partitioning an image picture into sub-images having similar grey scale intensities. The other elements can be colour, texture and brightness. The segmentation is used to subdivide the objects into detailed pictures used for depth analysis. Some of its crucial tasks are as follows: firstly, investigating the internal structure of human anatomy in detail; secondly, recognizing the precise location of abnormalities such as tumour or cancerous cell growth; thirdly, it helps in identification of multiple numbers of lesions, exudates, and other anomalies; and finally, it measures tissue volume to measure tumour expansion.

BIS approaches can be divided into three distinct classes depending on the extent of human involvement: manual segmentation, semi-automated segmentation, and fully automatic BIS [11, 12]. The following categories are described:

A. Manual segmentation of the biomedical image. Here, the region of interest (ROI) is specified by a well-qualified expert after which a contour is drawn around it [11, 13]. Prolonged and challenging work is manual segmentation. This process of manual segmentation is again composed of two different types, which are known as 'inter-rater', and intra-rater. In the case of the former, multiple experts segment the image in various ways, whereas in the latter, a single expert segments an image in a variety of ways [14]. Manual segmented images are utilized as ground truths in automated segmentation algorithms for teaching artificial intelligence (AI) on how a disease should look. High-resolution images can lead to images without sharp edges, which leads to small differences in the choice of ROI boundary pixels. The fact that the approach relies on knowledge and experience is another issue of manual segmentation and thus, therefore, experiences considerable heterogeneity between and within the experts [15]. Although manual segmentation is dependent upon the evaluator, it is used in clinical studies with non-significant time limitations [16, 17].

B. Semi-automatic segmentation. Semi-automatic segmentation strategies demand a restricted number of user encounters with automated algorithms in order to achieve precise segmentation outcomes [18]. The user interaction may include a set of estimated initial ROI, which is ultimately used to segment the whole picture. To reduce segmentation errors, manual testing and area boundary editing may be needed. The following are examples of semiautomatic segmentation strategies:
   (1) The Seeded Region Growth algorithm, which is based on a user's original seed point iteratively merges identical neighbourhood pixels [19].
   (2) A level-set active contour model that starts from an original boundary shapes with a specified ROI and updates them iteratively by shrinking or expansion process is not needed [20].
   (3) Localised region active contour methods that use region boundary conditions to use tiny local sections to define the image's foreground and background and have the benefit of managing heterogeneous textures [21].

C. Fully automatic segmentation. There is no interference from the customer. However, many of these systems concentrate on supervised methods of learning and training data, such as atlas segmentation methods, support vector machines (SVMs) and deep neural networks (DNNs). In unsupervised learning both training samples and the sample validation require ground truth images. With a completely intelligent segmentation in biomedical images, significant variations in form, size, texture and in some cases ROI colour between patients and low contrast between section are obvious challenges [22].

Noise may also lead to substantial deviations during data capture, as is often the case with modern devices. As a result, most emerging methods based on clustering and machine learning are confronted with the lack of global deployment that restricts their use to a limited range of applications. In addition, the feature extraction techniques used by SVM or neural networks takes a while and does not process natural data in its raw state and may not necessarily adapt to changing data. However, deep learning approaches can examine data without extracting features manually [23]. For semantic segmentation they are most favoured for BIS [24].

12.1.3 Segmentation evaluation

A. **Accuracy**

Manual accuracy represents the percentage of correct biomedical image pixels as described in equation (12.1). It is also recognised as a complete pixel precision. This is the most fundamental assessment method, but in the case of class imbalance it restricts the error of representation of biomedical image segmentation results. The other class inequality arises when one segmentation category dominates. In such a situation, a higher accuracy will overwhelm the lower accuracy of the other class and thus a skewed result for the dominant class. Per class accuracy analysing and then estimating the proportion of pixels correctly labelled for each group is an alternative to this concept of accuracy [25]. This test can be used in the case of a class imbalance for sample data set. A decline in the confidence measurement of specific classes is the downside of average class precision. Fewer cases of a given class can lead to a substantial variance in the reliability of the results in comparative analyses.

$$\text{Accuracy} = \frac{\text{TP} + \text{TN}}{\text{TP} + \text{FP} + \text{FN} + \text{TN}} \tag{12.1}$$

where TP stands for true positives, FN for false negatives, TN are the number of true negatives, and FN is the number of false negatives.

B. **Precision**

As specified in equation (12.2), precision is reflecting the relation of disease pixels in automatic segmentation results measures that corresponds to the pixels of the ground reality disease. Precision is a valuable measure of performance segmentation as it reacts to over-segmentation. The over-segmentation leads to low accuracy values.

$$\text{Precision} = \frac{\text{TP}}{\text{TP} + \text{FP}} \tag{12.2}$$

C. **Sensitivity**

This value reflects the true positive rates reported in test data. It indicates the number of times the test provided a positive outcome when the sample did indeed have a condition [26]. Defined in equation (12.3)

$$\text{Sensitivity} = \frac{\text{TP}}{\text{TP} + \text{FN}} \tag{12.3}$$

D. **Specificity**

This specificity value indicates the true negative rates reported by the test data. It refers to the proportion of negative samples identified by the test that are actually negative [26]. The specificity is described in equation (12.4):

$$\text{Specificity} = \frac{\text{TN}}{\text{TN} + \text{FP}} \tag{12.4}$$

E. **F1 measure**

The measure F1 specifically states the harmonic mean of precision and recall and is suitable for contour matching the predicted segmentation with ground truth segmentation.

$$\text{F}_1 = \frac{2\text{TP}}{2\text{TP} + \text{FP} + \text{FN}} \tag{12.5}$$

F. **Hausdorff distance (*h*)**

This value is a measurement of distance among two test samples set. It is a set's maximal distance from the closest point in another set [27]. Hausdorff distance is shown in equation (12.6).

$$h(X, Y) = \max_{x \in X} \min_{y \in Y} ||x - y|| \tag{12.6}$$

where $X = \{x_1, x_2, x_3, \ldots, x_n\}$ and $Y = \{y_1, y_2, y_3, \ldots, y_n\}$ are sample sets.

12.2 Retinal images segmentation

12.2.1 Datasets

Several publicly accessible professional data sets containing blood vessel descriptions are available. The first step in the retinal database is to train and assess classifiers for segmenting blood vessels. Researchers have access to these databases—STARE and DRIVE etc, along with their ground truth files, which can be obtained freely. The performance and exactness of the classifier can be evaluated with the following data sets.

A. **Structured analysis of the retina (STARE)**

It contains 400 retinal images and possesses a 605 × 700 pixel 8 bit Color channel via TOPCON's TRV-50 fundus camera with 35-degree field of view (FOV). The average diameter of the FOV is 650 × 700. STARE consists of twenty samples of vessel ground truths files which can be used for training classifiers to segment blood vessel to demonstrate the presence of healthy and distinct types of ocular diseases. The very first specialist separated 10.4% of the blood vessel's pixels', whereas the second expert manually segmented the thinner retina vessel 14.9%. The ground truth obtained from these manual segmentations of the first professional is commonly used for evaluating a trained classifier's precision and efficiency

B. **Digital retinal images for vessel extraction (DRIVE)**

This dataset is a very widely used for studying segmentation of retinal blood vessels. It is made from 20 photographs of the retinals, each of which reveals mild retinopathy, with 33 healthy retinal fundus images and 7 images suffering from moderate diabetic retinopathy (DR). The Canon CR5 camera with 45 degrees FOV and then a color channel of 8 bit in JPEG format was used for taking photographs at 768 × 584 pixels. The circular field of view of each images has radius of 270 pixels. The DRIVE dataset was divided into 20 pictures each in a training and test package. In the training sets, 14 of 20 sample images were segmented by first specialists, while the second specialists segmented the six remaining sample images. The vessel was segmented twice in the test set for evaluation. During the first circumstance 13 and 7 sample pictures were segmented by first and second specialists, while the second scenario consisted of a segmentation procedure by a third specialist. 12.7% and 12.3% pixels were identified in both the circumstances.

C. **Child health and heart studies in England (CHASE_DB1)**
It contains different varieties of disorders prevailing in a retinal fundus image and their ground truth vessels [28]. The fundus images have been acquired with a TIF camera of 35 degree FOV and 1280 × 960. The picture has been captured with a complete exposure in the center of the optical disk. The database consists of 14 pairs of left and right eyes obtained from children. Two specialists were used for creating a ground truth mask of the vessel regions. However, diseases are not clearly registered. All videos are of high quality and well distinguishable.

D. **HRF**
Jan Odstrcilik and his group of researchers developed the high-resolution fundus (HRF) dataset to undertake an automated segmentation architectures critical review. 45 retinal fundus images are provided by the HRF database. It includes 15 samples for healthy eyes, 15 sample images for glaucoma and 15 sample images for DR. All images have a high resolution of 3504 × 2336 [29].

E. **Messidor**
For carrying out empirical studies on multiple segmentation algorithms for retinal fundus images the French Ministry of Science and Defense has established this dataset. It is a compilation of 1200 retinal images obtained by the non-mydriatic Topcon TRC NW6. Three of its ophthalmology divisions took part in the image acquisition process, which used 45-degree screen settings in TIFF format with a total colour-channel resolution of 8 bit, 2304 × 1536, 2240 × 1488, and 1440 × 936. 400 sample images does not have pupil dilation while others were taken with dilation. For each picture in the data set, the experts suggested two diagnoses of the potential macular oedema and retinopathy [30].

F. **Retinal vessel images for estimation of width (REVIEW)**
It consists of 16 mydriatic and 193 segmented retinal blood vessel images. It is an initiative of the University of Lincoln (United Kingdom), in the year 2008. In order to mark the divisions of blood vessels, three specialists used a special drawing technique. This set of data has been subdivided into four series consisting of 8 photographs with high definition, 2 with central light reflective pictures, 4 of images of vascular abnormalities and 2 pictures of kicks point [31].

G. **ImageRet**
The ImageRet project is FinnWell's technology project for diabetic retinopathy (DR), which began in 2008. This collection has 219 retinal images named as DIARETDB0 and DIARETDB1. iDIARETDB0 includes 130 fundus images where 110 healthier and 20 DR. And in DIARETDB, 84 images have DR and the remaining are healthy. The images were acquired in PNG format with a 50° fundus camera bearing 1500 × 1152 resolution [32].

H. **ROC micro-aneurysm**
The 2009 Microaneurysm Diagnosis Retinopathy Online Competition (ROC) took place at the University of Iowa. There are 100 retinal fundus

images, which comprise 50 training and test images each. The goal was to delineate micro-aneurysm sites in the given training images. The Images has resolutions of 1058×1061, 1389×1383 and 768×576 [33].

12.2.2 Fundus photography

A special fundus camera is used to record the principal anatomical structures of the eye, including the optical disc, fovea, blood and macula. A laser or a flash camera with a low power microscope is usually used. The fundus camera, which has specific dyes and filters to represent various intrinsic characteristics, captures various joint structures of the eye. Fundus photography has different shapes, including a colour fundus photography, red-free fluorescent angiography and concurrent stereo fundus photography. The retina has white light and full colour photographs. Special filters having spectral wavelength equal to 540–570 nm that can retain green chromaticity while removing red colour capture superficial lesions. A fluorescent colored dye is imparted in the blood circulation of the patient to record the images during the course of fluorescein angiography. The angiography of sodium fluorescein uses 490 nm blue light, and 530 nm yellow light fluoresces. For studying DR, it is a highly standardized photography technique. The choroidal vessels are observed using indocyanine green angiography using an 805 nm infrared diode

12.2.3 Challenges in retinal vessel segmentation

The performance of the retinal vessel segmentation methods recorded in the reports in the test sets and evaluation criteria [6, 34, 35] is usually nearer to that of human observers. Both documents and the latter in particular, a restriction which usually controls medical imaging techniques, are not consistent. The debate on the validation of algorithms and the challenge of international design is increasing internationally [36–39]. Several image processing problems affect a coherent segmentation of the retinal fundus. The most important of them can be summed up here.

- Central light reflection produces a divide in the segmented vessel and two smaller versions are developed on the segmented image.
- Tiny vessels that lack segmentation have poor contrast.
- Split vessels at crossover/bifurcation points.
- Near, parallel blood vessels are segmented as a big one.
- Existence of unwanted imaging artefacts like blur, noise, and non-uniform lighting.
- Injuries like microaneurysms, bleeding, hard and soft exudates and neo-vascularization interrupts the blood vessel images, block and show false positive effects.

The challenges mentioned above are critical to ensure that the data obtained with a variety of different instruments, procedures, operators and patient specimens are secure, reproducible and extremely accurate and eventually allow for the efficient translation of research technologies to the healthcare sector. Recent methods of deep learning have been largely efficient in the case of vessels that have been evaluated in natural, public data sets, typically DRIVE or STARE, which consists of a few images that contain the ground truth [40–43]. We observe that such a restriction is changing progressively. For example, at MICCAI 2018, the REFUGE challenge created a dataset of 1200 images featuring annotations for optical disc/cup segmentation and detection of glaucoma [44].

12.2.4 Review of literature

Researchers use methods to assess representations of the retinal fundus based on profound learning algorithms. Various uses, including segmentation of the retinal blood vessel and images of the retinal fundus, are discussed.

A. **Retina image segmentation**

Global blindness is primarily caused by eye disorders, such as DR and diabetic maculopathy (DM). DM has a prolonged preclinical period in which eyesight is not impaired and visual loss will usually not be regained until the individual is in the eye clinic. Early diagnosis will avoid and protect the vision of the disease. Thus, retinal vessel research and analysis have become the basis for early diagnosis medical applications and successful monitoring of the retinal pathology, including blood vessels' diameter, angles and lengths of its branches. Retinal ophthalmology image assessment is a key step towards retinal pathology recognition. Retinal vessel segmentation is a critical element for the diagnosis of eye disease. For the identification of symptoms, the thick and thin vessels are essential.

One of the principal anatomical structures found in a retinal fundus image is retinal blood vessels. The structure and feature changes in it reflect the impact of cardiovascular diseases (CVDs) such as cataract, DR, and high blood pressure, etc. In the developed world, cataracts are by far the most common cause of blindness, contributing to over half of visual impairments. Effects like blindness can be avoided by early diagnosis and treatment. The region of the eye lens becomes thick and cloudy. It happens progressively as the eye's protein deposition expands and prevents the lens from transmitting clear images to the retina. Around 0.075 billion blind people are likely to be registered in 2020 [45, 46]. It is of three types depending on its location. Firstly, at the middle of the lens, the nuclear cataract imparts yellow colour and image-blur to the lens. Usually in elderly people, the cortical cataract features are found at the corner of the lens. The capsular cataract behind its lens is the seriously harmful form of cataract [47]. This index rises rapidly in the elderly over 40 years, particularly among older people. The increased incidence is a major problem in early detection and diagnosis for the WHO. Early intervention and treatment may reduce cataract patients' resilience and avoid vision problems. Retinal diseases can only be detected by segmentation, but experts for the detection and segmentation of manual vessels are required. It is typically divided into four groups that are average, mild, moderate and extreme as per the stage of the disease [48]. The stage depends on the optic disc's and vessels' sizes. The retinal fundus of the normal patient reveals the arteries (which can be large or small) and the optic disc very clearly. Less volume of blood vessels is seen in a patient whose eye is compromised by mild cataract, whereas, in the retinal fundus in patients with mild cataract, only large blood vessels are visible. Finally, absolutely nothing is found in the case of extreme cataract. These cataract classes differ between 0 and 3 with 0, 1, 2 and 3, respectively, meaning mild, medium, moderate and severe cataracts. Detection and classification of cataracts relies highly on the details of the blood stream and the optic disc. Segmentation of a blood vessel manually followed by its identification is a very time-consuming procedure. Consistent scientific attempts have been made in the field of retinal image processing [49]. A few statistical methods were designed to obtain the most powerful characteristics. Low levels such as morphology, colour, diameter of the vessel, shape, sharpness and thickness have indeed been incorporated inside the blood vessel, but some are equipped with advanced equipment and do not fit in remote clinics without specialist experts. Intermediate characteristics, such as the retinal fundus image saliency diagram, are used in retinal blood vessel extraction classifiers [50]. Vessel characteristics such as tortuosity, thickness, angle and width are extremely complicated to analyse for the early onset of retinal disease [51]. Manual segmentation is often very costly and time-consuming as an ophthalmologist needs to be employed [50]. Automatic extraction and differentiation of vessels through the use of the AI is also important for the early identification of the disease.

In the Kaggle diabetic retinopathy challenge held in 2015, Van Grinsven *et al* [52] released the first paper on retinal fundus images that focused on deep learning. According to our understanding, since then, only 17 deep learning scientific articles have been published. Out of this, 12 are connected to the segmentation of the retinal vessel, which is the current priority. Here, we provide a thorough review of these 12 approaches by examining and evaluating their advantages and weaknesses. Study results will encourage the precocious and reliable identification of retinal disease based on the latest machine learning study. The article gives recommendations for potential technology for significantly reducing the loss of vision, increasing the accuracy of early detection and significantly improving the quality of life of the patient. Flexible and accurate solutions are explored, which would automatically be able to detect blood vessel changes and anticipate future illness from the outset.

B. **Retinal vessel segmentation methods**

It can be further classified as unsupervised and supervised [6, 34, 35]. Classification techniques belonging to the supervised category train by using ground truth labels. Some of the most popular supervised ML techniques are —support vector machine (SVM), random forest, k-nearest neighbour (kNN), Neural Network (NN), bayes network, AdaBoost, and discriminant analysis [6, 34, 35]. On the other hand, Fuzzy C-means (FCM), Gaussian Mixture

Model (GMM), and k-means clustering algorithms are some popular unsupervised ML techniques. Another type of ML is Deep Learning that uses two-dimensional Convolutional Neural Networks (CNN) to learn attributes from images. Some of the noteworthy research works that apply these ML and DL techniques are discussed in the following subsections.

C. **Deep learning**

A desirable characteristic of DL models such as the CNN is the ability to measure description and categorisation representations. Vessel segmentation through CNN was implemented in [53, 54], and also jointly with random forest, and Conditional Random Field (CRF) [55–57]. Improved models that used more sophisticated deep learning layers has been implemented. An example that can be cited is the combined detection of blood vessels and optic disc highlighted in [53, 58, 59]. They used a pre-trained CNN with a large number of images which occur naturally. The use of Dense CRF as well reinforcement datasets aimed at reducing training time, which are a challenge to traditional techniques have been used effectively for thin vessel segmentation [60, 61]. In contrast to networks utilizing only fully-connected layers, a fully convolutional network (FCN) was also identified as improving results of segregation of vessels. [62–67] have also demonstrated techniques for integrating a multiple number of networks with an aim to reducing training volume. Such techniques also enable analysis in multiple scales for detecting blood vessels of specific lengths [43], or for implementing in a Hanning window-based wavelet transform [60]. The efficiency of segmentation in spite the presence of several types of lesions can be improved by using Generative Adversarial Networks (GANs), which can generate synthetic images from labelled images [68, 69].

D. **Supervised methods**

Neural Networks (NNs) which are based on backpropagation are used in combination with spatial textures to segment retinal vessels [70]. On similar lines, researchers have also made use of colours, pixel intensity, and moment independent features [71–73]. Vega *et al* [72] observed that lattice-based NN which has only one feed forward layer can provide improved convergence. In a different approach, researchers of [74] have demonstrated a wider and very deep NN that has cross-modality learning for segmenting vessels which is corrupted by noisy pathological aretefacts. Local Binary Patterns (LBPs), and different shape-based feature descriptors were implemented with NN for segmenting thin blood vessels [75]. In another blood vessel enhancement technique, features derived from GMM, wavelet, and Gabor features are mixed with intensity, and SIFT features to train NNs and LDA classifier [76].

A parameterized and curvilinear supported Gaussian filter known as SCIRD-TS was used for segmenting thin retinal vessels [77]. Researchers of [78] used pixel intensities, Gabor features and textures together with ensemble classifier to differentiate between vessel and background [78, 79]. The attributes observed through AdaBoost algorithm have been demonstrated to extract vessel data from normal and pathological retinal images by using various combinations of linear classifiers [73]. Directional, Gaussian, and multiple scale LBP feature descriptors have been used with fuzzy inference systems as well [80]. The use of divergence vector based ensemble learning, dictionary-based sparse classifier, and fusion of multiple classifiers have been able to impart resistance against clutter in lesion images [81–83]. In order to deal with poor segmentation issues related to weak priors, SVM has been combined with fully connected CRF. Each such pixel was perceived as a function of matched filter (MF), and gradient magnitude [84]. In [85] it is shown that features derived from the retinal vessel's shape and pixel intensities have a capacity to enhance retinal vessel segmentation that has lesions. Also, it is reported in [86] that a combination of hard k-means clustering and the SVM classifier can remove parallel retinal vessels that lie in proximity. Through the work of [86, 87], good image segmentation in lesion-affected hypertension and DR images have been achieved by using features such as Gabor, Binary Hausdorff symmetry measure, and multi-fractal features with the SVM classifier. In the random forest classifiers, visual attention modeling was used to deal with issues of near parallel vessels, CVR, slender vessels having low contrast, lesions and non-uniform illumination [88].

E. **Unsupervised techniques**

The main advantage of unsupervised segmentation techniques of blood vessels is that manual annotation is not necessary. The pixel is grouped into a vessel and non-vessel category by means of image features. Vessel segmentation has also utilized the GMM-expectation maximization (EM) technique. The EM algorithm was entrusted by the task to impart either a maximum or most like probability to pixels as belonging to the vessel or non-vessel category [89]. In this technique, the enhancement of blood vessels have been carried out with either top-hat transformation or high-pass filters. Here, optic disc and blood vessels have been processed by using a combination of GMM and gray voting. In another research work [90], the FCM soft clustering approach was implemented with multiple filters such as Frangi's, Gabor wavelets, and matched filter for eliminating blobs in retinal fundus image, and enhancing thin blood vessels in due course [90]. Natured inspired algorithms like bee colony optimization have also been used for identifying blood vessel specific cluster, and identifying background by evaluating texture and spatial dependence probabilities [91].

12.3 Brain tumour segmentation

Cell differentiation and irregular development in the brain tissue are brain tumours. Brain tumours can be classified according to their origin, as either primary or metastatic brain tumours. The primary cell's origin is cells with brain tissues, whereas metastatic cancer cells spread to the brain or some other part of the body. Gliomas are a form of glial cell brain tumour. It is the dominant brain tumour type and many of the research areas concentrate on the segmentation of brain tumours.

The expression glioma is being used to identify multiple kinds of gliomas, from low-grade gliomas like astrocytoma and oligodendrogliomas up to high-grade multiform glioblastoma and even the most damaging primary malignant brain tumour [92]. Radiotherapy, surgery and chemotherapy are procedures used, typically in tandem, for the treatment of gliomas [93].

Early glioma diagnosis plays a crucial role in enhancing treatment options. Imaging technologies including CT, PET, MRI have been employed in order to ensure valuable information about the structure, magnitude, location and metabolism of the brain tumour. While these methods could be used in conjunction with brain tumours to provide the best knowledge, the definitive soft-tissue contrast and wide adoption make MRI the base standard. MRI is a near-invasive *in vivo* imaging framework for implementing radio frequencies to influence target tissues to produce their internal images, under the effects of a very strong magnetic field. Images from various MRI sequences are created by altering the time when the image is recovered. Different MRI modalities provide different images of tissue contrast that provide useful structural information and allow the identification and segmenting of the tumour in conjunction with its sub-regions [94]. During the acquisition of MRI, although it can differ from device to device, almost a hundred slices of 2D pictures are generated to reflect the 3D brain volume. Moreover, when the fragments from the required normal modalities are fused for study, the data becomes densely populated and complex.

During a surgical procedure aimed at removing/depleting tumour cells, care must also be taken to preserve as much healthy tissue as possible. Brain tumour segmentation involves identification, delineation and differentiation of the tumour tissues of healthy brain tissues from necrotic cells or activated cells and edema. The strategy requires the manual annotation and segmentation of a large number of multimodal MRI images in a routine manner. However, since handcrafted segmentation is a pro-lengthy procedure, the development of robust automatic segmentation methods to provide effective and accurate segmentation has become an interesting and prominent scientific discipline in recent years [95]. Recently, high segmentation results achieved by deep learning strategies make them good nominees to accomplish this task.

12.3.1 Brain tumour segmentation databases

A. **BrainWeb**

The McConnell Brain Imaging Centre developed the BrainWeb dataset; an anatomical representation of normal and dysfunctional brains is provided by an MRI simulator. The BrainWeb's strength scale consists of 0, 20 and 40 non-uniformity ranges, with each of the slices having thicknesses of 1 mm, 3 mm, 5 mm, 7 mm and 9 mm. The noise level remains 0 percent, 1 percent, 3 percent, 7 percent and 9 percent. The Centre for Morphometric Research has developed the Internet Brain Segmentation Repository (IBSR) (CMA). The brain tumours MRI dataset provides files of 16-bit integers formatted as 256×256 images.

B. **AANLIB database**

In the AANLIB repository released by the Harvard Medical School there are six major types of images, which are inflammatory, normal, degenerative, cerebrovascular, neuro-imaging and neoplastic anatomy. A computer-aided imaging analysis methods for diagnosis of brain disorders such as autism, Alzheimer's disease and dementias have been developed by the Section for Biomedical Image Analytics (SBIA) of the University of Pennsylvania. The Cancer Imaging Archive (TCIA) created the Reference Image Collection to Assess Therapy Response (RIDER) which includes imaging data collected from 19 patients. The neuroimaging initiative for Alzheimer's disorder (ADNI1) covers two types of Alzheimer's disorder which includes imaging reports from 400 patients. The Allen brain atlas includes a typical dataset of photographs containing imaging data from 20 patients.

12.3.2 Classification of brain tumour

A brain tumour is classified on the basis of the origin or cell involvement of the cancer cell. In the former, the cell genesis is found in the brain, and is not extended to other areas of the body, whereas, the latter develops in various parts of the body and is then subsequently transferred to the brain. Lung, colon, kidney and skin are among the most important organs that can spread cancer cells to the brain. They are also referred to as metastatic brain tumours.

Cell-based tumours are the least invasive category and are non-cancer cells of the brain tumour. Benign tumours normally grow low, and other neighbouring tissues do not penetrate. Malignant brain tumours range between non-invasive and highly invasive. Depending on growth rates, adjacent healthy brain tissues can invade various cancer cells. Probably the most widely-reported type of primary brain tumour in adults is glioblastomas, also called glioblastoma multiforme (GBM). Glioblastomas are a type of glial cell that develops rapidly. High-grade gliomas (HGGs) have a higher rate of proliferation than low-grade gliomas (LGGs), so they require intensive plans for therapeutic therapy. Most GBM patients die within less than one year, with almost no long-term chances of survival. The research community has drawn huge attention to these tumours; for the sufferer's early detection and therapeutic preparation. It will strengthen the patient's survival. In reality, because of the wide variety of appearances, configuration and orientation of the brain, the segmentation of multimodal MRI scans is one of the most critical tasks in bioimaging. The MRI offers detailed brain anatomy information across all three planes: axial, coronal and sagittal. It is beneficial for the diagnosis of a tumour, treatment plans, aid in operation and recovery.

12.3.3 Brain photography

Two kinds of MRIs exist: (1) fMRI (Functional MRI): it monitors brain activity through blood flow transition, (2) sMRI (Structural MRI): it captures brain structure and pathology. The emphasis of this chapter is focused on sMRI to deal with the pathology in the brain. Different modalities of sMRI capture responses of the brain tissues which lead to distinct biological information in the images. Different sMRI modalities are:

A. **Diffusion-weighted image (DWI) MRI**: It measures water molecules diffusion within the voxels of tissues. DWI is also used for hyperintensity visualisation.
B. **Flair MRI**: A sequence of MRI pulses that suppress the fluid and promotes edema in the image. The water molecule signal is essentially suppressed in FLAIR images, which can distinguish between cerebrospinal fluid (CSF) and edema.
C. **T1w MRI**: Standard MRI pulse sequence that captures tissue variations in longitudinal relaxation time. Time constant needed for exciting protons to revert to equilibrium. T1 images are typically used to differentiate between healthy tissues.
D. **T1Gd MRI:** Gadolinium is injected into the body as a contrast enhancement agent and then the T1 sequence is obtained. This contrast enhancement agent shortens the duration of T1, leading to the bright emergence of blood vessels and tumour-like pathologies. The tumour contours can be comfortably separated from the active cell of the tumour tissue by the bright signal of the accumulated contrast agent such as gadolinium ions. Necrotic cells do not intervene, which enable them to be accurately segmented from the active cell zone, by the hypo-intense portion of the tumorous central core.
E. **T2w MRI:** a simple MRI pulse sequence that catches tissue variations in transverse relationship time (T2). T2 imaging is being practised to identify the area of the edema which creates a bright image signal.

12.3.4 Challenges

Fully automated brain tumour segmentation is a highly challenging task. The tumour-bearing brain MRI metadata is 3D data that can vary greatly from patient to patient in its structure, size and location. In addition, with discontinuities, tumour borders are usually ambiguous and pose an important challenge for traditional borders. Brain tumour MRI knowledge from laboratory scanners or synthetic databases [96], by contrast, is highly complex. For each individual picture frame in the datasets, the MRI devices and protocols used for the acquisition vary greatly from scan to scan, which leads to intensity distortions and other variations.

There are some additional difficulties in implementing deep learning methods and algorithms to process brain-tumor images. The shortage of extensive data sets is a severe obstacle for deep learning methods. MRI and CT mechanisms that accumulates loads of medical images were implemented in different installations over the past decade. In several other disciplines, image data are used for a specific purpose. CT instruments are not commonly used in other fields of medicine, such as pathology and ophthalmology.

In addition to prolonging the labelling of the tumour sample, a high level of awareness that is problematic in research on brain tumours is also essential.

Teaching systems based on deep learning algorithms, which are almost always carried out in 3D networks, require a slice-by-slice specification which is not only complicated but time-consuming. Another major disadvantage of deep learning algorithms lies in their inefficiency to learn from a limited amount of image data. 3D segmentation models proposed by several researchers used 2D segmentation [97]. BraTS datasets are extensively used for the tumour analysis algorithms and to estimate a tumour condition in brain MRIs.

Another issue with the data set is the class imbalance. For example, data increase strategies are employed by applying rotation and scaling technologies to produce additional brain tumour samples. This may cause class disequilibrium problems. Pereira [98] explores data augmentation techniques to overcome class imbalance for brain tumour segmentation.

Another problem is the implementation of the same or fixed kernel size, which can mask useful information that may occur in areas outside the kernel.

12.3.5 Image pre-processing

Medical image pre-processing plays a very important role in the appropriate inputs to computer-assisted research techniques. Preprocessed images help to even get accurate outputs since these images demonstrate proper voxel relationships. The repository has images of various diagnostic practice and scanners, the variability is simplified and put all the scans on the same scale. Apart from the image registration and skull stripping, additionally, there are other improved pre-processing methods like:

A. **Noise reduction (NR)**

   The distortion in the MRI at the time of acquisition is caused by a radio wave or a magnetic field. Various noise amplification methods are suitable for noise elimination.

B. **Histogram matching (HM)**

   Based on a different configuration of the MRI devices the intensity level of the images acquired may differ. Intensity ratios are to be adjusted to the same scale using the corresponding histogram process.

C. **Intensity normalization (IN)**

   Different modality images possess a different intensity range. They must map to the equivalent range. Zero mean and unit variance are considered by standardisation of all scans.

12.3.6 Image post-processing

Due to inappropriate or incorrect feature selection, the segmentation output formed by computer-assisted procedures could include false segmentation in the image. The use of post-processing approaches, for example, can improve the segmentation.

A. **Connected component analysis (CCA):**

   CCA clubs the voxels depending on the connectivity depending on the similar voxel intensities values. The consecutive components which are extremely small are excluded from the decision as such components are considered to be false positives due to spurious segmentation outcomes.

B. **Conditional random field (CRF):**

The voxel class is predicted by the classifier based on the characteristics associated with that voxel, and does not depend on the voxel's adjacent interaction with other nearby voxels. In order to enforce the dependencies between the predictions, CRF takes this correlation into account and constructs a graphical model.

12.3.7 Traditional machine learning in tumor segmentation

In a technique proposed in [99], the researchers applied morphological erosion and dilation operators with global thresholding on a binary tumour masking for segmenting tumour afflicted regions. An overall accuracy of 97% was achieved on a test image dataset which had about 100 MRI images derived from different individuals. In another research work [100], the SRC technique has used K-SVD dictionary-based learning for segmenting MRI brain images. The segmentation result was further refined by applying Active Contours Without Edges (ACWE). The data collection consisted of 80 T2 brainMRI images, 50 and 30 of which, respectively, were used for training and validation. Researchers of [101] proposed an MRI image brain tumour segmentation technique by using multiple fractal dimension, intensity, and texton features with AdaBoost classifier. Some improved versions of Fuzzy C-Means (FCM) algorithms named as Particle Swarm Optimization with FCM (PSOFCM) [102], Genetically Improved Fuzzy Markovian Relational Clustering Matrix (GIFMRCM) [103], Fast and Automatically Adjustable GRBF Kernel FCM (FAAGKFCM) [104], and Enhanced Possibilistic FCM (EPFCM) [105], have been used for segmenting MRI brain images. A Computer Aided Design (CAD) based segmenting technique that used pre-processing, segmentation or Region of Interest (ROI) development, feature extraction, and machine learning phases has been described in [106]. In this work, histogram equalization was the pre-processing method, which was followed by morphological dilation and erosion segmentation. They investigated using a wide variety of machine learning techniques like Particle Swarm Optimization (PSO), Support Vector Machines (SVMs), Artificial Neural Network (ANN), and K-Nearest Neighbour (KNN). An accuracy of 100% was achieved while using kNN and PSO techniques. Local independent projection-based classification (LIPC) has been used together with connected component analysis and morphological operator for segmenting MRI images [107]. In another different approach for segmenting brain tumour, Jiang *et al* [108] proposed and demonstrated the usage of a learning process that used a graph constructed from population and patient-centric Gabor and image modality feature descriptors. A 3D PCNN was used with morphological erosion and dilation operators for segmenting brain images of rodents. A spherical shaped mask was used for providing a smooth function [109]. A technique that is based on Markov Random Field (MRF) for segmenting MRI images that has multiple sclerosis (MS) lesions has been proposed in [110]. The MRF parameters were evaluated from the manually annotated images, and contextual information was included in the final stage. Their investigation was carried out on 24 axial T1, T2 and PD weighted images, where each has a resolution of 256 × 256. Another MS lesion identification technique for FLAIR brain MRI image that uses a combination of adaptive mixture model (AMM) and MRF has been proposed in [111]. In a unique approach, the content-based active contour model (CBAC) was used to initially demarcate tumour afflicted regions, after which a group of different feature descriptors were used for extracting features. The feature descriptors employed in their work are—directional Gabor, Laplacian of Gaussian (LoG), circular Gabor, rotation-invariant local binary patterns (RILBPs), GLCM and pixel intensity features. The final stage consisted of the PCA algorithm to reduce the feature vectors, after which the ANN was employed for training [112]. Brain tumour in MRI images has also been segmented by using kNN and CRF in [113]. The investigation was carried out using 40 MRI images, out of which 30 and 10 samples were derived from individuals having HG and LG tumours, respectively. Researchers of [114] used hard k-means with FCM clustering techniques initially, after which the level was set and adaptive thresholding techniques were applied. Before this final segmentation, the brain MRI images were filtered by median filter and brain surface extractor algorithm. Their experimentation on three data sets yielded accuracies of 90.5%, 100%, and 100% having 22, 152 and 81 images, respectively. In another research work, the GMM algorithm was used for extracting rich features from different tumour tissues, which were then combined with random forest and MRF for segmenting brain tumour images. They used a total of 520 brain images derived using multiple modalities—T1, T1C, FLAIR, and T2 [115]. The authors of [116] extracted features from T1 and FLAIR MRI brain images by using 80 different Histogram of Oriented Gradient (HOG) features, 20 GLRLM, 256 lBP, and 112 GLCM features. It resulted in the creation of a feature vector having 475 diverse descriptors. It was reduced to 20 dimensioned feature vectors by applying PCA. A hybrid technique that uses FCM clustering and Hopfield Neural Network has been investigated on the PDC and IBSR databases for image segmentation and visualisation capability [117]. Before training, they performed skull stripping by using morphological operation. The technique by [118] used global thresholding, morphological operation and watershed segmentation on brain MRI images. Another research work [119] also implemented Otsu's thresholding, hard k-means, and soft clustering for segmenting brain tumour images. An overall accuracy of 90.57% was attained.

12.3.8 Deep learning

Figure 12.1 below highlights the different constituents of a CNN-based brain tumour segmentation. The deep learning model (DL) of [120] uses 2D patches having different dimensions as inputs for two separate pathway CNN-layer stacks for performing convolution. The features liberated from the two CNNs were concatenated together. In a similar, yet improved version, the researchers of [121] investigated a two-pathway DL technique by having 3D patches as input. Their network used residual connection and produced multiple voxels as output. Another DL model that is used widely is the U-Net [122], which uses encoder-decoder model.

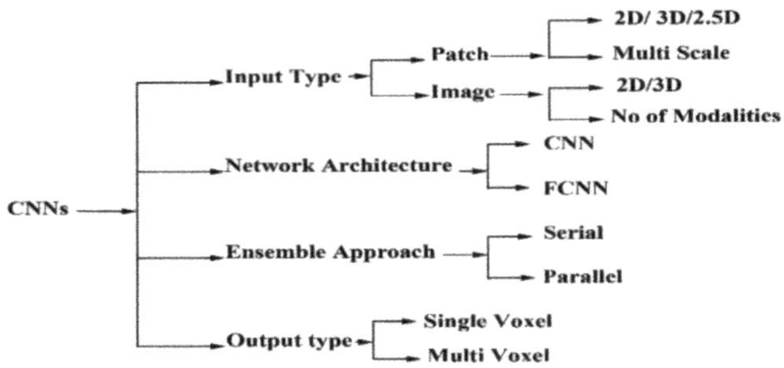

Figure 12.1. Design aspects of CNN architecture for brain tumor segmentation.

It consists of several skip connections between analysis layers and synthesis path layers. It is based on an approach to a serial ensemble. The very first system segments the entire tumour, then, the core of the tumour is segmented by the second system and, eventually, the output of the second stage is used in the third stage, which is the enhancing stage. The voxel-based image segmentation is initially performed by shallow CNN [123]. In [120] authors suggested the use of CNN multi-path architecture for voxel classification. One route uses a 32 × 32 2D patch and the other uses fully connected 5 × 5 patch-size input with a middle pixel similar to a 32 × 32 patch. There is a patch collection so that the labels are equiprobable. L1 and L2 regularizations overcome overfitting.

The depth of such a DL model increased. For instance, researchers of [124] made use of a DL model where FC layer has separate HGG and LGG layers. A cascaded CNN has been proposed in [125]. The model utilized a two-path deep CNN model initially, after which, the outputs are used with other 2D CNNs. Wang *et al* [123] also used residual connections with both pathways of a two-path deep CNN model, and trained using varying input image sizes. A dilated CNN type residual network has also been used for training with image patches in [126].

The authors in [127] implemented brain tumour segmentation using U-net architecture. The authors in [128] changed the 3D input U-net and reduced the network depth to three. In [129], the authors suggested new architectures of encoder-decoders that worked well on several problems with the biomedical image segmentation. For deep segmentation tasks, various CNN approaches using single-path have also been implemented in [130–134]. Ensemble CNNs are more efficient than single CNNs, as was the case in [135], where authors introduced a seven-network ensemble that uses DeepMedic, FCN, and U-net and variations in the three networks.

The authors in [136] had implemented the set of 10 architectures based on the encoder–decoder and the auto-encoder-stream for additional details and regularisation purposes. The authors' method suggested in [137] was expanded in [138]. They use U-net and Densenet combinations with an architecture like U-net that includes dense dilated convolution blocks. Three networks, which are WNet, TNet and ENet, were used by the authors in [123] to build a cascaded framework. These networks use axial, coronal, sagittal viewing angles to produce the final segmentation output.

In [139] there is a cascaded network that originally segmented the entire tumour and the tumour centre and reinforced the tumour segmentation.

A multi-scale 3D U-net mask was proposed by [140] authors with spatial pyramid pooling in which the first-network WT segmentation for the TC development was transferred to the second, in sequence to the end-net to establish ET output. Additional CNN approaches based on an ensemble have been defined in [141–145].

12.4 Discussion and conclusion

This chapter presents the work, i.e., pre-existing and current techniques, accomplished by other researchers related to biomedical images segmentation, especially retina vessel segmentation and brain tumour segmentation. Here every referenced paper is summarized. It presents numerous types of segmentation by using different methods. Each segmentation approach reviewed here has its leads and constraints, and setting a particular benchmark for comparison is inappropriate. The segmentation of biomedical images has been broadly categorized in this paper. The validation of segmentation outcomes is a quintessential subject in biomedical image analysis since it directly influences surgical judgments. Orthodox machine learning algorithms can be further improved. For example, the method of extraction is mostly performed using a series of pre-specified filters in most conventional machine learning algorithms. Thus it would greatly increase efficiency if data-driven extraction methods were devised for conventional learning algorithms. Recent research on the segmentation of biological images relies mostly on the paradigm of deep learning. Finding high-quality biomedical image data is always a challenge. Deep architectures like ResNet, VGGNet and GoogLeNet typically overfit the learning framework significantly in cases where there are not enough training images, even after including regularisation, dropouts, and model averaging. The accuracy of CNN in the classification task of biomedical image datasets with GoogLeNet architecture has been steadily increased due to an increase in training images. The current level of classification is too simple for practical biomedical imaging processing, such as segmentation, but a fundamental relationship between efficiency and consistency of the training data set has been identified. Researchers have trained 3D segmentation models with only 2D segmentation in brain tumours segmentation study. A further scientific difficulty in the segmentation of brain tumours is that researchers apply the same fixed size to a kernel, which may mask any helpful information from another area that the kernel does not know. The way to enlarge the data set is more manageable, by random translation, tossing and rotation, to transform the primary data set. In regular machine learning algorithms, this term known as data augmentation is used previously. A lot of hyperparameters are essential for modern and deep learning arrangements. Minute variations in hyperparameters can lead to excessively significant network performance changes. While background and optimization by stochastic gradient descent methods also automatically learn how to weigh the network, many hyperparameters are also involved empirically, such as layer numbers, regularity coefficients and dropout rates. Deep learning methods, however, have still not been adequately improved but related work has been examined to avoid problems arising with these heuristic choices. There are also conditions of health that must be tackled. As we move forward, it is necessary to consider the possible disadvantages of deep learning methodologies.

References

[1] Angell M, Kassirer J P and Relman A S 2000 Looking back on the millennium in medicine [editorial] *N. Engl. J. Med.* **342** 42–9

[2] Zhu W 2019 Deep Learning for Automated Medical Image Analysis. arXiv preprint arXiv:1903.04711

[3] Kumar E S and Bindu C S 2019 Medical image analysis using deep learning: a systematic literature review *Int. Conf. on Emerging Technologies in Computer Engineering* pp 81–97 (Berlin: Springer)

[4] Soomro T A, Gao J, Khan T, Hani A F M, Khan M A and Paul M 2017 Computerised approaches for the detection of diabetic retinopathy using retinal fundus images: a survey *Pattern Anal. Appl.* **20** 927–61

[5] Soomro S, Akram F, Kim J H, Soomro T A and Choi K N 2016 Active contours using additive local and global intensity fitting models for intensity inhomogeneous image segmentation *Comput. Math. Methods Med.* **2016** 9675249

[6] Fraz M M, Remagnino P, Hoppe A, Uyyanonvara B, Rudnicka A R, Owen C G and Barman S A 2012 Blood vessel segmentation methodologies in retinal images—a survey *Comput. Methods Programs Biomed.* **108** 407–33

[7] National Institutes of Health (NIH) chest X-ray NIHCC. 2017 [online] Nov. 2019, https://nihcc.app.box.com/v/ChestXray-NIHCC

[8] MIT Laboratory for Computational Physiology. Mimic-chest X-ray database (mimiccxr) [online] https://physionet.org/content/mimic-cxr/2.0.0/, Tech. Rep., Nov. 2019

[9] Yan K, Wang X, Lu L and Summers R M 2018 DeepLesion: automated mining of large-scale lesion annotations and universal lesion detection with deep learning *J. Med. Imag.* **5** 036501

[10] Fotenos A F, Snyder A Z, Girton L E, Morris J C and Buckner R L 2005 Normative estimates of cross-sectional and longitudinal brain volume decline in aging and AD *Neurology* **64** 1032–9

[11] Yao J 2006 Image processing in tumor imaging *New Techniques in Oncologic Imaging* (London: Taylor & Francis) pp 79–102

[12] Karsch K, He Q and Duan Y 2009 A fast, semi-automatic brain structure segmentation algorithm for magnetic resonance imaging *2009 IEEE Int. Conf. on Bioinformatics and Biomedicine* (Piscataway, NJ: IEEE) pp 297–302

[13] Ramkumar A *et al* 2016 User interaction in semi-automatic segmentation of organs at risk: a case study in radiotherapy *J. Digit. Imag.* **29** 264–77

[14] White D R, Houston A S, Sampson W F and Wilkins G P 1999 Intra-and interoperator variations in region-of-interest drawing and their effect on the measurement of glomerular filtration rates *Clin. Nuclear Med.* **24** 177–81

[15] Millioni R, Sbrignadello S, Tura A, Iori E, Murphy E and Tessari P 2010 The inter-and intra-operator variability in manual spot segmentation and its effect on spot quantitation in two-dimensional electrophoresis analysis *Electrophoresis* **31** 1739–42

[16] Bae K T, Shim H, Tao C, Chang S, Wang J H, Boudreau R and Kwoh C K 2009 Intra-and inter-observer reproducibility of volume measurement of knee cartilage segmented from the OAI MR image set using a novel semi-automated segmentation method *Osteoarthritis Cartilage* **17** 1589–97

[17] Gaonkar B *et al* 2015 Automated tumor volumetry using computer-aided image segmentation *Acad. Radiol.* **22** 653–61

[18] Iglesias J E 2017 Globally optimal coupled surfaces for semi-automatic segmentation of medical images *Int. Conf. on Information Processing in Medical Imaging* (Berlin: Springer) pp 610–21

[19] Fan M and Lee T C 2014 Variants of seeded region growing *IET Image Proc.* **9** 478–85

[20] Fan J, Wang R, Li S and Zhang C 2012 Automated cervical cell image segmentation using level set based active contour model *2012 12th Int. Conf. on Control Automation Robotics and Vision (ICARCV)* (Piscataway, NJ: IEEE) pp 877–82

[21] Kim Y J, Lee S H, Park C M and Kim K G 2016 Evaluation of semi-automatic segmentation methods for persistent ground glass nodules on thin-section CT scans *Healthcare Inform. Res.* **22** 305

[22] Roth H R, Shen C, Oda H, Oda M, Hayashi Y, Misawa K and Mori K 2018 Deep learning and its application to medical image segmentation *Med. Imag. Technol.* **36** 63–71

[23] Silva F H S D 2018 Deep learning for corpus callosum segmentation in brain magnetic resonance images *MSc Dissertation* COPPE/UFRJ

[24] Zhou X, Yamada K, Kojima T, Takayama R, Wang S, Zhou X, Hara T and Fujita H 2018 Performance evaluation of 2D and 3D deep learning approaches for automatic segmentation of multiple organs on CT images *Medical Imaging 2018: Computer-Aided Diagnosis* vol 10575 p 105752C (Bellingham, WA: SPIE)

[25] Csurka G, Larlus D, Perronnin F and Meylan F 2013 What is a good evaluation measure for semantic segmentation? *Proc. British Machine Vision Conf. 2013 (BMVC)* 27 *(Bristol, UK)* pp 10–5244

[26] Altman D G and Bland J M 1994 Diagnostic tests. 1: sensitivity and specificity *BMJ* **308** 1552

[27] Huttenlocher D P, Klanderman G A and Rucklidge W J 1993 Comparing images using the Hausdorff distance *IEEE Trans. Pattern Anal. Mach. Intell.* **15** 850–63

[28] Owen C G, Rudnicka A R, Mullen R, Barman S A, Monekosso D, Whincup P H, Ng J and Paterson C 2009 Measuring retinal vessel tortuosity in 10-year-old children: validation of the computer-assisted image analysis of the retina (CAIAR) program *Investigative Ophthalmol. Vis. Sci.* **50** 2004–10

[29] Köhler T, Budai A, Kraus M F, Odstrčilik J, Michelson G and Hornegger J 2013 Automatic no-reference quality assessment for retinal fundus images using vessel segmentation *Proc. 26th IEEE Int. Symp. on Computer-based Medical Systems* (Piscataway, NJ: IEEE) pp 95–100

[30] Decencière E *et al* 2014 Feedback on a publicly distributed image database: the Messidor database *Image Analy. Stereol.* **33** 231–4

[31] Al-Diri B, Hunter A, Steel D, Habib M, Hudaib T and Berry S 2008 A reference data set for retinal vessel profiles *2008 30th Annual Int. Conf. of the IEEE Engineering in Medicine and Biology Society* (Piscataway, NJ: IEEE) pp 2262–5

[32] Kauppi T, Kalesnykiene V, Kamarainen J K, Lensu L, Sorri I, Raninen A, Voutilainen R, Uusitalo H, Kälviäinen H and Pietilä J 2007 The diaretdb1 diabetic retinopathy database and evaluation protocol *Proc. British Machine Vision Conf. 2007 (BMVC)* **1** 1–10

[33] Niemeijer M *et al* 2009 Retinopathy online challenge: automatic detection of microaneurysms in digital color fundus photographs *IEEE Trans. Med. Imag.* **29** 185–95

[34] Srinidhi C L, Aparna P and Rajan J 2017 Recent advancements in retinal vessel segmentation *J. Med. Syst.* **41** 70

[35] Mookiah M R K, Acharya U R, Chua C K, Lim C M, Ng E Y K and Laude A 2013 Computer-aided diagnosis of diabetic retinopathy: A review *Comput. Biol. Med.* **43** 2136–55

[36] Galdran A, Costa P, Bria A, Araújo T, Mendonça A M and Campilho A 2018 A no-reference quality metric for retinal vessel tree segmentation *Int. Conf. on Medical Image Computing and Computer-Assisted Intervention* (Berlin: Springer) pp 82–90

[37] Zhao Y, Xie J, Su P, Zheng Y, Liu Y, Cheng J and Liu J 2018 Retinal artery and vein classification via dominant sets clustering-based vascular topology estimation *Int. Conf. on Medical Image Computing and Computer-Assisted Intervention* pp 56–64

[38] Zhang Y and Chung A C 2018 Deep supervision with additional labels for retinal vessel segmentation task *Int. Conf. on Medical Image Computing and Computer-Assisted Intervention* pp 83–91

[39] Wu Y, Xia Y, Song Y, Zhang Y and Cai W 2018 Multiscale network followed network model for retinal vessel segmentation *Int. Conf. on Medical Image Computing and Computer-Assisted Intervention* pp 119–26

[40] Fu H, Xu Y, Lin S, Wong D W K and Liu J 2016 Deepvessel: retinal vessel segmentation via deep learning and conditional random field *Int. Conf. on Medical Image Computing and Computer-Assisted Intervention* pp 132–9

[41] Zhou L, Yu Q, Xu X, Gu Y and Yang J 2017 Improving dense conditional random field for retinal vessel segmentation by discriminative feature learning and thin-vessel enhancement *Comput. Methods Programs Biomed.* **148** 13–25

[42] Liskowski P and Krawiec K 2016 Segmenting retinal blood vessels with deep neural networks *IEEE Trans. Med. Imaging* **35** 2369–80

[43] Yan Z, Yang X and Cheng K T 2018 A three-stage deep learning model for accurate retinal vessel segmentation *IEEE J. Biomed, Health Inform.* **23** 1427–36

[44] Orlando J I *et al* 2020 Refuge challenge: a unified framework for evaluating automated methods for glaucoma assessment from fundus photographs *Med. Image Anal.* **59** 101570

[45] Mitchell P, Cumming R G, Attebo K and Panchapakesan J 1997 Prevalence of cataract in Australia: the Blue Mountains eye study *Ophthalmology* **104** 581–8

[46] Congdon N, Vingerling J R, Klein B E, West S, Friedman D S, Kempen J, O'Colmain B, Wu S Y and Taylor H R 2004 Prevalence of cataract and pseudophakia/aphakia among adults in the United States *Arch. Ophthalmol.* **122** 487–94

[47] Tomlins P J and Shah S 2008 Clinical ophthalmology: a self-sssessment companion *Br. J. Ophthalmol.* **92** 441

[48] Yang J J, Li J, Shen R, Zeng Y, He J, Bi J, Li Y, Zhang Q, Peng L and Wang Q 2016 Exploiting ensemble learning for automatic cataract detection and grading *Comput. Methods Programs Biomed.* **124** 45–57

[49] Devi L M, Wahengbam K and Singh A D 2021 Dehazing buried tissues in retinal fundus images using a multiple radiance pre-processing with deep learning based multiple feature-fusion *Opt. Laser Technol.* **138** 106908

[50] Klein B E K, Klein R, Linton K L P, Magli Y L and Neider M W 1990 Assessment of cataracts from photographs in the Beaver Dam eye study *Ophthalmology* **97** 1428–33

[51] Mobley J A and Brueggemeier R W 2002 Increasing the DNA damage threshold in breast cancer cells *Toxicol. Appl. Pharmacol.* **180** 219–26

[52] Van Grinsven M J, van Ginneken B, Hoyng C B, Theelen T and Sánchez C I 2016 Fast convolutional neural network training using selective data sampling: application to hemorrhage detection in color fundus images *IEEE Trans. Med. Imag.* **35** 1273–84

[53] Maninis K K, Pont-Tuset J, Arbeláez P and Van Gool L 2016 Deep retinal image understanding *Int. Conf. on Medical Image Computing and Computer-Assisted Intervention* pp 140–8

[54] Guo Y, Budak Ü, Vespa L J, Khorasani E and Şengür A 2018 A retinal vessel detection approach using convolution neural network with reinforcement sample learning strategy *Measurement* **125** 586–91

[55] Wang S, Yin Y, Cao G, Wei B, Zheng Y and Yang G 2015 Hierarchical retinal blood vessel segmentation based on feature and ensemble learning *Neurocomputing* **149** 708–17

[56] Maji D, Santara A, Ghosh S, Sheet D and Mitra P 2015 Deep neural network and random forest hybrid architecture for learning to detect retinal vessels in fundus images *2015 37th Annual Int. Conf. of the IEEE Engineering in Medicine and Biology Society (EMBC)* (Piscataway, NJ: IEEE) pp 3029–32

[57] Fu H, Xu Y, Wong D W K and Liu J 2016 Retinal vessel segmentation via deep learning network and fully-connected conditional random fields *2016 IEEE 13th Int. Symp. on Biomedical Imaging (ISBI)* (Piscataway, NJ: IEEE) pp 698–701

[58] Tan J H, Acharya U R, Bhandary S V, Chua K C and Sivaprasad S 2017 Segmentation of optic disc, fovea and retinal vasculature using a single convolutional neural network *J. Comput. Sci.* **20** 70–9

[59] Jiang Z, Zhang H, Wang Y and Ko S B 2018 Retinal blood vessel segmentation using fully convolutional network with transfer learning *Comput. Med. Imag. Graph.* **68** 1–15

[60] Oliveira A, Pereira S and Silva C A 2018 Retinal vessel segmentation based on fully convolutional neural networks *Expert Syst. Appl.* **112** 229–42

[61] Dasgupta A and Singh S 2017 A fully convolutional neural network based structured prediction approach towards the retinal vessel segmentation *2017 IEEE 14th Int. Symp. on Biomedical Imaging (ISBI 2017)* (Piscataway, NJ: IEEE) pp 248–51

[62] Brancati N, Frucci M, Gragnaniello D and Riccio D 2017 Retinal vessels segmentation based on a convolutional neural network *Iberoamerican Congress on Pattern Recognition* (Cham: Springer) pp 119–26

[63] Meyer M I, Costa P, Galdran A, Mendonça A M and Campilho A 2017 A deep neural network for vessel segmentation of scanning laser ophthalmoscopy images *Int. Conf. on Image Analysis and Recognition* pp 507–15

[64] Yan Z, Yang X and Cheng K T 2018 Joint segment-level and pixel-wise losses for deep learning based retinal vessel segmentation *IEEE Trans. Biomed. Eng.* **65** 1912–23

[65] Hu K, Zhang Z, Niu X, Zhang Y, Cao C, Xiao F and Gao X 2018 Retinal vessel segmentation of color fundus images using multiscale convolutional neural network with an improved cross-entropy loss function *Neurocomputing* **309** 179–91

[66] Mo J and Zhang L 2017 Multi-level deep supervised networks for retinal vessel segmentation *Int. J. Comput. Assist. Radiol. Surg.* **12** 2181–93

[67] Xu X, Tan T and Xu F 2018 An improved U-net architecture for simultaneous arteriole and venule segmentation in fundus image *Annual Conf. on Medical Image Understanding and Analysis* pp 333–40

[68] Zhao H, Li H, Maurer-Stroh S and Cheng L 2018 Synthesizing retinal and neuronal images with generative adversarial nets *Med. Image Anal.* **49** 14–26

[69] Park K B, Choi S H and Lee J Y 2020 M-gan: retinal blood vessel segmentation by balancing losses through stacked deep fully convolutional networks *IEEE Access* **8** 146308–22

[70] Rahebi J and Hardalaç F 2014 Retinal blood vessel segmentation with neural network by using gray-level co-occurrence matrix-based features *J. Med. Syst.* **38** 1–12

[71] Franklin S W and Rajan S E 2014 Computerized screening of diabetic retinopathy employing blood vessel segmentation in retinal images *Biocybernet. Biomed. Eng.* **34** 117–24

[72] Vega R, Sanchez-Ante G, Falcon-Morales L E, Sossa H and Guevara E 2015 Retinal vessel extraction using lattice neural networks with dendritic processing *Comput. Biol. Med.* **58** 20–30

[73] Fraz M M, Rudnicka A R, Owen C G and Barman S A 2014 Delineation of blood vessels in pediatric retinal images using decision trees-based ensemble classification *Int. J. Compute. Assist. Radiol. Surg.* **9** 795–811

[74] Fathi A and Naghsh-Nilchi A R 2014 General rotation-invariant local binary patterns operator with application to blood vessel detection in retinal images *Pattern Anal. Appl.* **17** 69–81

[75] Kaur J and Mittal D 2017 A generalized method for the detection of vascular structure in pathological retinal images *Biocybern. Biomed. Eng.* **37** 184–200

[76] Shah S A A, Tang T B, Faye I and Laude A 2017 Blood vessel segmentation in color fundus images based on regional and Hessian features *Graefe's Arch. Clin. Exp. Ophthalmol.* **255** 1525–33

[77] Annunziata R and Trucco E 2016 Accelerating convolutional sparse coding for curvilinear structures segmentation by refining SCIRD-TS filter banks *IEEE Trans. Med. Imag.* **35** 2381–92

[78] Memari N, Ramli A R, Bin Saripan M I, Mashohor S and Moghbel M 2017 Supervised retinal vessel segmentation from color fundus images based on matched filtering and AdaBoost classifier *PLoS One* **12** e0188939

[79] GeethaRamani R and Balasubramanian L 2016 Retinal blood vessel segmentation employing image processing and data mining techniques for computerized retinal image analysis *Biocybern. Biomed. Eng.* **36** 102–18

[80] Sigurðsson E M, Valero S, Benediktsson J A, Chanussot J, Talbot H and Stefánsson E 2014 Automatic retinal vessel extraction based on directional mathematical morphology and fuzzy classification *Pattern Recognit. Lett.* **47** 164–71

[81] Javidi M, Pourreza H R and Harati A 2017 Vessel segmentation and microaneurysm detection using discriminative dictionary learning and sparse representation *Comput. Methods Programs Biomed.* **139** 93–108

[82] Zhu C, Zou B, Xiang Y, Cui J and Wu H 2016 An ensemble retinal vessel segmentation based on supervised learning in fundus images *Chin. J. Electron.* **25** 503–11

[83] Barkana B D, Saricicek I and Yildirim B 2017 Performance analysis of descriptive statistical features in retinal vessel segmentation via fuzzy logic, ANN, SVM, and classifier fusion *Knowl.-Based Syst.* **118** 165–76

[84] Orlando J I, Prokofyeva E and Blaschko M B 2016 A discriminatively trained fully connected conditional random field model for blood vessel segmentation in fundus images *IEEE Trans. Biomed. Eng.* **64** 16–27

[85] Tang Z, Zhang J and Gui W 2017 Selective search and intensity context based retina vessel image segmentation *J. Med. Syst.* **41** 1–12

[86] Panda R, Puhan N B and Panda G 2016 New binary Hausdorff symmetry measure based seeded region growing for retinal vessel segmentation *Biocybern. Biomed. Eng.* **36** 119–29

[87] Jebaseeli T J, Durai C A D and Peter J D 2019 Retinal blood vessel segmentation from diabetic retinopathy images using tandem PCNN model and deep learning based SVM *Optik* **199** 163328

[88] Srinidhi C L, Aparna P and Rajan J 2018 A visual attention guided unsupervised feature learning for robust vessel delineation in retinal images *Biomed. Signal Process. Control* **44** 110–26

[89] Roychowdhury S, Koozekanani D D and Parhi K K 2014 Blood vessel segmentation of fundus images by major vessel extraction and subimage classification *IEEE J. Biomed. Health Inform.* **19** 1118–28

[90] Oliveira W S, Teixeira J V, Ren T I, Cavalcanti G D and Sijbers J 2016 Unsupervised retinal vessel segmentation using combined filters *PLoS One* **11** e0149943

[91] Hassan G and Hassanien A E 2018 Retinal fundus vasculature multilevel segmentation using whale optimization algorithm *Signal, Image Video Process.* **12** 263–70

[92] von Deimling A 1999 Gliomas *JAMA* **282** 1096

[93] Stupp R and Roila F 2009 Malignant glioma: ESMO clinical recommendations for diagnosis, treatment and follow-up *Ann. Oncol.* **20** 126–8

[94] Drevelegas A and Papanikolaou N 2011 Imaging modalities in brain tumors *Imaging of Brain Tumors with Histological Correlations* (Berlin: Springer) pp 13–33

[95] Agravat R and Raval M S 2021 *A Survey and Analysis on Automated Glioma Brain Tumor Segmentation and Overall Patient Survival Prediction* arXiv preprint arXiv:2101.10599

[96] Prastawa M, Bullitt E and Gerig G 2009 Simulation of brain tumors in MR images for evaluation of segmentation efficacy *Med. Image Anal.* **13** 297–311

[97] Çiçek Ö, Abdulkadir A, Lienkamp S S, Brox T and Ronneberger O 2016 3D U-Net: learning dense volumetric segmentation from sparse annotation *Int. Conf. on Medical Image Computing and Computer-Assisted Intervention* pp 424–32

[98] Pereira S, Pinto A, Alves V and Silva C A 2016 Brain tumor segmentation using convolutional neural networks in MRI images *IEEE Trans. Med. Imag.* **35** 1240–51

[99] Akram M U and Usman A 2011 Computer aided system for brain tumor detection and segmentation *Int. Conf. on Computer Networks and Information Technology* (Piscataway, NJ: IEEE) pp 299–302

[100] Julazadeh A, Alirezaie J and Babyn P 2012 A novel automated approach for segmenting lateral ventricle in MR images of the brain using sparse representation classification and dictionary learning *2012 11th Int. Conf. on Information Science, Signal Processing and their Applications (ISSPA)* (Piscataway, NJ: IEEE) pp 888–93

[101] Islam A, Reza S M and Iftekharuddin K M 2013 Multifractal texture estimation for detection and segmentation of brain tumors *IEEE Trans. Biomed. Eng.* **60** 3204–15

[102] Laishram R, Kumar W K, Gupta A and Prakash K V 2014 A novel MRI brain edge detection using PSOFCM segmentation and canny algorithm *2014 Int. Conf. on Electronic Systems, Signal Processing and Computing Technologies* (Piscataway, NJ: IEEE) pp 398–401

[103] Nongmeikapam K, Kumar W K, Khumukcham R and Singh A D 2018 An unsupervised cluster-wise color segmentation of medical and camera images using genetically improved fuzzy-Markovian decision relational model *J. Intell. Fuzzy Syst.* **35** 1147–60

[104] Nongmeikapam K, Kumar W K and Singh A D 2017 Fast and automatically adjustable GRBF kernel based fuzzy C-means for cluster-wise coloured feature extraction and segmentation of MR images *IET Image Proc.* **12** 513–24

[105] Rajendran A and Dhanasekaran R 2013 Enhanced possibilistic fuzzy C-means algorithm for normal and pathological brain tissue segmentation on magnetic resonance brain image *Arab. J. Sci. Eng.* **38** 2375–88

[106] Ulku E E and Camurcu A Y 2013 Computer aided brain tumor detection with histogram equalization and morphological image processing techniques *2013 Int. Conf. on Electronics, Computer and Computation (ICECCO)* (Piscataway, NJ: IEEE) pp 48–51

[107] Huang M, Yang W, Wu Y, Jiang J, Chen W and Feng Q 2014 Brain tumor segmentation based on local independent projection-based classification *IEEE Trans. Biomed. Eng.* **61** 2633–45

[108] Jiang J, Wu Y, Huang M, Yang W, Chen W and Feng Q 2013 3D brain tumor segmentation in multimodal MR images based on learning population-and patient-specific feature sets *Comput. Med. Imaging Graph.* **37** 512–21

[109] Chou N, Wu J, Bingren J B, Qiu A and Chuang K H 2011 Robust automatic rodent brain extraction using 3-D pulse-coupled neural networks (PCNN) *IEEE Trans. Image Process.* **20** 2554–64

[110] Van Leemput K, Maes F, Bello F, Vandermeulen D, Colchester A and Suetens P 1999 Automated segmentation of MS lesions from multi-channel MR images *Int. Conf. on Medical Image Computing and Computer-Assisted Intervention* pp 11–21

[111] Khayati R, Vafadust M, Towhidkhah F and Nabavi S M 2008 A novel method for automatic determination of different stages of multiple sclerosis lesions in brain MR FLAIR images *Comput. Med. Imaging Graph.* **32** 124–33

[112] Sachdeva J, Kumar V, Gupta I, Khandelwal N and Ahuja C K 2013 Segmentation, feature extraction, and multiclass brain tumor classification *J. Digit. Imag.* **26** 1141–50

[113] Havaei M, Jodoin P M and Larochelle H 2014 Efficient interactive brain tumor segmentation as within-brain kNN classification *2014 22nd Int. Conf. on Pattern Recognition* (Piscataway, NJ: IEEE) pp 556–61

[114] Abdel-Maksoud E, Elmogy M and Al-Awadi R 2015 Brain tumor segmentation based on a hybrid clustering technique *Egypt. Inform. J.* **16** 71–81

[115] Tustison N J, Shrinidhi K L, Wintermark M, Durst C R, Kandel B M, Gee J C, Grossman M C and Avants B B 2015 Optimal symmetric multimodal templates and concatenated random forests for supervised brain tumor segmentation (simplified) with ANTsR *Neuroinformatics* **13** 209–25

[116] Nabizadeh N and Kubat M 2015 Brain tumors detection and segmentation in MR images: Gabor wavelet vs. statistical features *Comput. Electr. Eng.* **45** 286–301

[117] Megersa Y and Alemu G 2015 Brain tumor detection and segmentation using hybrid intelligent algorithms *AFRICON* 2015 (Piscataway, NJ: IEEE) pp 1–8

[118] Abdullah H N and Habtr M A 2015 Brain tumor extraction approach in MRI images based on soft computing techniques *2015 8th Int. Conf. on Intelligent Networks and Intelligent Systems (ICINIS)* (Piscataway, NJ: IEEE) pp 21–4

[119] Kaur A 2016 An automatic brain tumor extraction system using different segmentation methods *2016 Int. Conf. on Computational Intelligence and Communication Technology (CICT)* (Piscataway, NJ: IEEE) pp 187–91

[120] Havaei M, Davy A, Warde-Farley D, Biard A, Courville A, Bengio Y, Pal C, Jodoin P M and Larochelle H 2017 Brain tumor segmentation with deep neural networks *Med. Image Anal.* **35** 18–31

[121] Kamnitsas K, Ferrante E, Parisot S, Ledig C, Nori A V, Criminisi A, Rueckert D and Glocker B 2016 DeepMedic for brain tumor segmentation *International Workshop on Brainlesion: Glioma, Multiple Sclerosis, Stroke and Traumatic Brain Injuries* (Cham: Springer) pp 138–49

[122] Weng W and Zhu X 2021 INet: convolutional networks for biomedical image segmentation *IEEE Access* **9** 16591–603

[123] Wang G, Li W, Ourselin S and Vercauteren T 2017 Automatic brain tumor segmentation using cascaded anisotropic convolutional neural networks *International MICCAI Brainlesion Workshop* (Cham: Springer) pp 178–90

[124] Pereira S, Pinto A, Alves V and Silva C A 2015 Deep convolutional neural networks for the segmentation of gliomas in multi-sequence MRI *BrainLes* 2015 (Cham: Springer) pp 131–43

[125] Havaei M, Dutil F, Pal C, Larochelle H and Jodoin P M 2015 A convolutional neural network approach to brain tumor segmentation *BrainLes* 2015 (Cham: Springer) pp 195–208

[126] Lopez M M and Ventura J 2017 Dilated convolutions for brain tumor segmentation in MRI scans *International MICCAI Brainlesion Workshop* (Cham: Springer) pp 253–62

[127] Dong H, Yang G, Liu F, Mo Y and Guo Y 2017 Automatic brain tumor detection and segmentation using u-net based fully convolutional networks *Annual Conf. on Medical Image Understanding and Analysis* pp 506–17

[128] Feng X and Meyer C 2017 Patch-based 3D U-Net for brain tumor segmentation *Int. Conf. on Medical Image Computing and Computer-Assisted Intervention (MICCAI)* pp 67–72

[129] Chen L, Bentley P, Mori K, Misawa K, Fujiwara M and Rueckert D 2018 DRINet for medical image segmentation *IEEE Trans. Med. Imaging* **37** 2453–62

[130] Pawar K, Chen Z, Shah N J and Egan G 2017 Residual encoder and convolutional decoder neural network for glioma segmentation *International MICCAI Brainlesion Workshop* (Cham: Springer) pp 263–73

[131] Islam M and Ren H 2017 Multi-modal pixelnet for brain tumor segmentation *International MICCAI Brainlesion Workshop* (Cham: Springer) pp 298–308

[132] Kim G 2017 Brain tumor segmentation using deep fully convolutional neural networks *International MICCAI Brainlesion Workshop* (Cham: Springer) pp 344–57

[133] Pourreza R, Zhuge Y, Ning H and Miller R 2017 Brain tumor segmentation in MRI scans using deeply-supervised neural networks *International MICCAI Brainlesion Workshop* (Cham: Springer) pp 320–31

[134] Nuechterlein N and Mehta S 2018 3D-ESPNet with pyramidal refinement for volumetric brain tumor image segmentation *International MICCAI Brainlesion Workshop* (Cham: Springer) pp 245–53

[135] Kamnitsas K *et al* 2017 Ensembles of multiple models and architectures for robust brain tumour segmentation *International MICCAI Brainlesion Workshop* (Cham: Springer) pp 450–62

[136] Myronenko A 2018 3D MRI brain tumor segmentation using autoencoder regularization *International MICCAI Brainlesion Workshop* (Cham: Springer) pp 311–20

[137] McKinley R, Meier R and Wiest R 2019 Ensembles of densely-connected CNNs with label-uncertainty for brain tumor segmentation *International MICCAI Brainlesion Workshop* (Cham: Springer) pp 456–65

[138] Jungo A, McKinley R, Meier R, Knecht U, Vera L, Pérez-Beteta J, Molina-García D, Pérez-García V M, Wiest R and Reyes M 2017 Towards uncertainty-assisted brain tumor segmentation and survival prediction *International MICCAI Brainlesion Workshop* (Cham: Springer) pp 474–85

[139] Zhou C, Chen S, Ding C and Tao D 2018 Learning contextual and attentive information for brain tumor segmentation *International MICCAI Brainlesion Workshop* (Cham: Springer) pp 497–507

[140] Xu Y, Gong M, Fu H, Tao D, Zhang K and Batmanghelich K 2018 Multi-scale masked 3-D U-net for brain tumor segmentation *International MICCAI Brainlesion Workshop* (Cham: Springer) pp 222–33

[141] Hua R, Huo Q, Gao Y, Sun Y and Shi F 2018 Multimodal brain tumor segmentation using cascaded V-nets *International MICCAI Brainlesion Workshop* (Cham: Springer) pp 49–60

[142] Wang G, Li W, Ourselin S and Vercauteren T 2018 Automatic brain tumor segmentation using convolutional neural networks with test-time augmentation *International MICCAI Brainlesion Workshop* (Cham: Springer) pp 61–72

[143] Crimi A, Bakas S, Kuijf H, Keyvan F, Reyes M and van Walsum T (ed) 2019 Brainlesion: glioma, multiple sclerosis, stroke and traumatic brain injuries *4th Int. Workshop, BrainLes 2018, Held in Conjunction with MICCAI 2018, Granada, Spain, September 16, 2018, Revised Selected Papers, Part II* vol 11384 (Berlin: Springer)

[144] Chandra S, Vakalopoulou M, Fidon L, Battistella E, Estienne T, Sun R, Robert C, Deutsch E and Paragios N 2018 Context aware 3D CNNs for brain tumor segmentation *International MICCAI Brainlesion Workshop* (Cham: Springer) pp 299–310

[145] Yao H, Zhou X and Zhang X 2018 Automatic segmentation of brain tumor using 3D SE-inception networks with residual connections *International MICCAI Brainlesion Workshop* (Cham: Springer) pp 346–57

Chapter 13

Analysis of AI based PID controller for health care system

Vandana Dubey, Harsh Goud and Prakash Chandra Sharma

Ambiguity establishes one of the most difficult features in biomedical and control systems which aim to capture the physiology of a patient using mathematical modeling. In this chapter, we will elaborate a review of biomedical modeling and controller applied in a patient with chronic disease. A chronic disease is one that generally persists for three calendar months or longer and can become poorer with time. Some of the well-known chronic illnesses are cancer, heart disease, stroke, diabetes, and arthritis. Even so, one of the key conflicts to be taken into description is the huge intra-patient inconsistency, acknowledged using wide-reaching sensitivity examination using a conventional PID (Proportional Integral Derivative) controller of the biomedical system. Nowadays stakeholders of the health sector are putting emphasis on the point that Artificial Intelligence (AI) is going to gain greater importance in handling back-office activities in almost all the biomedical areas. To enhance the accuracy and stability of a biomedical system, the name of PID controller comes at the top of the list. In this chapter, we will discuss an AI based PID controller with various biomedical systems and also analyze how this study may be useful to enhance the stable state along with transient outcome of the biomedical system. A comparative study of all the primitive and novel control strategies for AI based PID controllers regarding the health care system will be address in this chapter. This study concludes with the superiority of the controller which copes with biomedical instruments effectively.

13.1 Introduction

Let us recall a famous quote: 'Prevention is better than cure'. This quote aptly applies to the transformation of the health care system in the United States (US). Earlier the focus was on treating the illness when it arose, rather than taking prior actions to prevent it. There are multiple changes in the processes which aim for the

doi:10.1088/978-0-7503-3815-8ch13

betterment of overall health of the patient. When compared to the health expenses of other countries, expenditure on health is persistently rising for the residents of the US [1–5]. Now the time has come to make a drastic change in this health system and use AI for its betterment. AI will help in the automation and proper information synthesis of the data of the patients and their family members. One thing must be kept in mind is that there should not be any misuse of data collected. In accordance with Oxford English Dictionary, AI is the ability of computers or additional devices to display or simulate intellectual performance. In accordance with Merriam-Webster dictionary, AI is a branch of computer science trading through the simulation of intellectual human actions in computers. Now the way we define AI has been changed from a collection of human-like abilities of computers to something big [6].

Diabetes, high blood pressure, cancer etc are some of the most common diseases today. These are also called non-communicable diseases (NCDs). NCDs are chronic in nature and are dependent on genetic, physiological and environmental factors. Today about 41 million people die every year due to NCDs and this figure is 71% of the total number of deaths every year. The World Health Organization (WHO) says this figure will rise to 55 million by 2030, if timely prompt actions are not taken. According to a recent report of WHO, one in four Indians has a risk of dying from an NCD before they reach the age of 70. The Indian Government, Ministry of Health and Family Welfare says that the NCDs' burden has increased from 30% in 1990 to 55% in 2016 and also the proportion of deaths has also increased from 37% to 61% [7].

An illness or state which generally survives for three months or longer and can grow worse by time is called a chronic disease (CD). CD tends to happen in older adults and may generally be handled but not cured. The foremost common categories of CD are cancer, heart disease, stroke, diabetes, and arthritis. The US spends about $5.3 trillion every year on its health care. Some of the common causes of CD are: tobacco use, nutrition deficiency, physical inactivity and alcohol addiction [8]. Extra care of the patient is essential for a healthcare center in today's lifestyle. Most of the electronic-healthcare systems have developed very well, however, some advanced research is required for the successful outcome from the entire health care unit (HCU). To know about a patient's history, present state of health etc, all are the part of an HCU. Nowadays, various controllers are presented and executed successfully. But, in the computer-controlled age, there is a chance to employ a novel controlling technique, which can comprise a large amount of information, beyond that of an ordinary controller. To fulfill the requirement of this computer controller era, there is a need to design and analyze a smart controller—a classical controller, with the help of AI techniques like genetic, neural networks and fuzzy etc, except with non-classical designing techniques, to design its parameters. The idea of the intelligent control scheme is unwrapped and simply designable. The effect of a conventional PID controller is not attractive for the requirements of complex and non-linear systems [9]. However, better results can be achieved by using smart PID controllers instead of conventional PID controllers.

For controlling and monitoring of biomedical systems, a well-known controller is used widely, i.e. a PID Controller, which performs very well in a variety of biomedical applications, for example arterial blood pressure (ABP), imbue/control, muscular rest in operation, combined slant control in unnaturally activated muscle, kidney transplant, glycemia control, control of unconsciousness etc. The wide-ranging applications of PID control are in industry and in the biomedical system, because it does continuous monitoring which is also essential in these fields. There should be a smart examination lab with smart doctor for respective labs. A lot of research has been done previously for the aforementioned workings [10–13]. Fast treatment and recovery of patients depend on the strong surroundings of the HCU such as drinking water, water used in toilets, nursing bed with commode facility. These constraints can be fulfilled by using an intelligent PID control system with fuzzy based tuning. A PID can be tuned in such a way that it can automatically control the input/output flow of supply water for wash out and clean-up purposes [14].

The Mamdani fuzzy deduction scheme has been investigated to manage a vapor engine and container amalgamation using a linguistic set of laws [15, 16]. Fuzzy based tuning is used to design PID controllers for several applications [17–19]. In [19], a relative comparison displays that fuzzy based tuning is better in comparison to Cohen–Coon, trial-error, and Ziegler–Nichols methods. A coupled tank's level can also be controlled by using PID [20, 21]. PID control is tempting for calculating blood glucose because it reproduces the reaction of initial and subsequent stages that are applied to conceal insulin through β-cells in the pancreas in contradiction of constantly examined glucose. For a patient's glucose control and maintainance, a switching technique based PID control algorithm is used [22]. Researchers studied Iletin Lente and internal secretion of a patient and used 'Meal Simulation model' and 'Havorka model' and show that the PID control technique achieves better results in several cases, for example Iletin Lente sensitivity.

In [23], researchers achieved success in systolic pressure controlling with the help of a nonlinear digital PID controller and by adding sodium nitroprusside into the drug. By this technique, high blood pressure can be controlled during open-heart surgery. Systolic pressure can also be controlled with the use of automatic control strategies [24] like PID control and variation in their parameter, best control, intelligent monitor, rule-based monitor counting fuzzy logic, and artificial neural system monitor. In [25] researchers applied automatically adjusting PID controlling technique for muscular rest in operation. A joint angle regulation scheme is also presented for the unnaturally activated muscle in [26]. A special PID system for a controlling and enhanced PID switching regulator for blood glucose control, a special PID and an advanced PID switching technique are presented in [27, 28]. PID technique is also used in liver transplantation, which models vecuronium pharma-co-kinetics and pharma-co-dynamics [29]. Use of anesthesia in children can also be controlled by using a smart PID control technique [30].

This chapter particularly focuses on CD and presents some literature review based on smart PID control techniques, by which diseases can be controlled at some level. The flow of work is as follows: In section 13.2 different types of CDs and their controlling techniques are discussed, section 13.3 discusses the types of different biomedical systems, and gives information about the classical PID controller and its operation, and section 13.4 represents mathematical modeling of the biomedical system.

13.2 Types of chronic disease

13.2.1 Cancer

Human cells normally divide and expand to produce fresh cells which are a requirement of the body. After cells grow and finally become old or damaged, they die and are substituted by fresh cells. In all forms of cancer, any of the body's cells start to split uncontrollably and spread into adjacent tissues. Cancer may begin in almost any part of the body.

Cancer cells versus normal cells: The key difference among normal cells and cancer cells is that cancer cells progressively divide without discontinuing. Normal cells develop to perform special functions while cancer cells do not.

Cancer classification:

(a) Common types of cancers: lung, breast, skin, prostate.
(b) Less common cancers: stomach, brain, ovarian, leukemia.
(c) Cancers occurring in children: osteosarcoma, neuroblastoma, acute lymphoblastic leukemia, childhood leukemia,

Carriers of cancer: The three main types of genes that are affected and contribute to cancer are tumor suppressor genes, DNA repair genes and proto-oncogenes. These variations are sometimes referred to as 'drivers of cancer'.

Tissue changes are sometimes misinterpreted as cancer: when cells within a tissue divide faster than normal pace then it is termed hyperplasia. This can be caused due to mere chronic irritation. When extra abnormal cells build up in an unusual manner, this is termed dysplasia, a more severe condition than hyperplasia. It has a greater chance of being converted into cancer.

Cancer controlling technique: An AI based PID controller is a tool to treat cancer in a better way. Cancer treatment is usually highly expensive. To curb the expenses and make it available to the everyone, a PID controller using Computed Torque Control (CTC) can be used that gives the best administration procedure for every patient. A feedback linearization-based controller has been created that is founded on the Hahnfeldt model [31]. The Hahnfeldt model uses a control engineering perspective for tumor regulation based on an optimal controller that decreases the dimensions of the tumor in the shortest way and also reduces the amount of medication, thus reducing the cost of treatment. It must be kept in mind that like any other medication, care should be taken to check any unforeseen result. This is a Robust Fixed-Point Transformation (RFPT) based control mechanism which decreases the total inhibitor concentration and at the same time increases the robustness of the controlled system. It is high time we should depart from the traditional model-based cancer chemotherapy practices. We can use a reinforcement learning-based (RL-based) method, a model-free method for the close control of cancer chemotherapy medicine dosing [32].

One of the important aspects of projected RL-based technique is that it requires less computational exertion and is less composite with respect to genetic algorithm-based approaches. In clinical pharmacology, progressive infusion of hormones and medicines can be optimized using RL. The use of RL-based monitoring was evaluated in the first closed-loop clinical trial for regulating propofol infusion in humans. Another RL-based technique is projected for the administration of anesthesia for ICU patients who require critical care. RL-based controllers are also used for the demonstration of robust control of propofol infusion and very good performance.

In [33–36] researchers used optimization technique with cancer chemotherapy control algorithms. In [35], an adaptive parameter controlling model of predictive control (MPC) is used for chemotherapy treatment. A cancer dynamics optical controlling problem as shown in figure 13.1 was investigated in [36]. Chemotherapy treatment can also be monitored and controlled by using genetic, computer controlled and evolutionary based methods [37, 38]. Diagnosis accuracy, speed and clinical managerial can be improved by the integration of AI techniques in cancer for improved health outputs.

13.2.2 Blood pressure

The heart pumps blood in arteries during beat time and the pressure experienced by the arteries is measured as BP. Further, blood pressure is of two types: one is systolic which is during beat time, and the other is diastolic which is during rest time between two beats. BP is measured in two numbers which shows systolic and diastolic pressures. The standard way to write the BP is to write systolic first than diastolic, e.g. 110/80 (110 is systolic and 80 is diastolic).

Much of the time high-BP (H-BP) does not show any symptoms. The only way to find the H-BP is with regular monitoring of BP. Commonly, H-BP has two types: primary and secondary. Primary H-BP is a very general type of BP and comes with age, while secondary H-BP occurs due to some other medical issues or medication. One may eliminate it by proper treatment or by stopping the medication that causes it. H-BP affects the heart function and that of other organs like the kidney. If H-BP stays for a long time, it may cause heart and kidney failure. For H-BP cure, it is necessary to change medicines and lifestyle related to the heart. Table 13.1 shows different categories of BP [39].

BP controlling technique: BP rises due to hypertension in a post-operative patient, particularly in a mature cardiac patient, and can be controlled by inserting an anti-

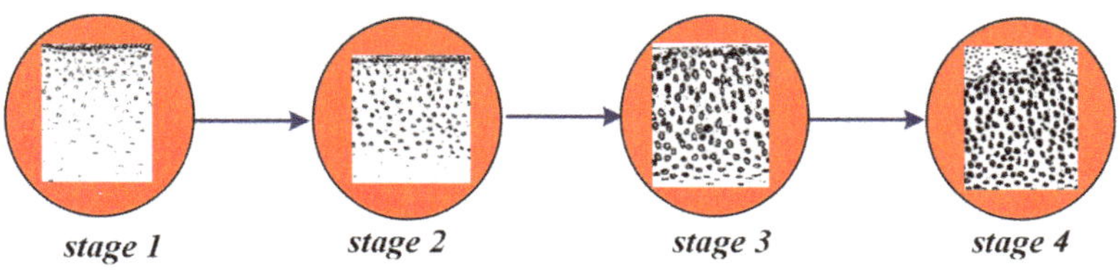

Figure 13.1. Cancer stages.

Table 13.1. BP categories.

Types of BP	Diastolic mm Hg (lower number)	Systolic mm Hg (upper number)
H-BP (Last stage)	>120	>180
H-BP (Second stage)	⩾90	⩾140
H-BP (First stage)	80–90	130–139
Low-BP	<80	120–129
Normal-BP	<80	<120

hypertension vasodilator medicine, sodium nitroprusside (SNP). By observation and control of the amount of medicine delivery to the patient one can reduce the BP to a recommended level, but proper medicine infusion is a very big problem in the biomedical-engineering field. Therefore, the accurate monitoring and controlling system of drug delivery is today's requirement so that a patient's recovery rate will be increased and their medical expenses also reduced. Table 13.2 shows that BP can be controlled and monitored very well with the help of various AI based PID techniques.

13.2.3 Diabetes

Diabetes is the common terminology for its medical name diabetes mellitus (DM). It is a metabolical disorder which affects the insulin production that causes uncontrolled blood glucose (BG) [45, 46]. There are various types of DM with different signs, and which affect the health undesirably such as: T(Type)1DM, T(Type)2DM, G(Gestational)DM, D(Double)DM, Gr (Genetic related) DM, and some extra forms of DM also occur by various types of disorder [47]. To regulate the glucose in the blood a system is used called Artificial Pancreas (AP). Insulin delivery in a diabetic body can also be managed by AP such as decreased insulin dose in a hyperglycemia patient and increased insulin dose in hypoglycemia.

T1DM: When the body is not able to make sufficient insulin to control blood sugar levels (BS-L). Insulin dependent and juvenile are other names for T1DM.

T2DM: Insulin independent and adult-onset are the name of T2DM. T2DM patients have the problem of high blood sugar and low insulin in the body, which causes repeated urine, mysterious weight loss and need for liquids.

Diabetes controlling technique or control algorithms for AP: Since DM is such a well-studied field of biomedical engineering, nearly every control method has been recorded. In [48] the researcher proposed an optimal technique to control blood glucose level (BGL) of a diabetic patient. However, without a general solution to the problem, there are highly valuable ways to concentrate upon the standard MPC, fuzzy logic centered, traditional PID control, or vigorous control methods [49–51]. Simply put, every control algorithm takes into account the same principles: the fulfilment of defined quality and quantity properties. PID control was the first attempt in this field, and it is even the best commonly utilized classical monitor

Table 13.2. AI based PID controller for BP monitoring system.

Year/type of the controller	First author	Type of work	Application	Key-idea	Summary	Ref.
2020/Embedded PID Controller (EPC)	Anna G C D Ribeiro	Designed an EPC for physical observation.	To control BP	An intelligent monitoring unit with the help of EPC to help in monitoring process and to mitigate the patient-care system.	A system has been designed around the PIC18F4520 micro-controller which gives auto configuration function. With the help of serial communication user can manipulate the parameters without changing the programmed code.	[40]
2019/Fractional-Order PID Control (FOPID)	Shabana Urooj	A BP controlling system (during surgery) using sodium nitroprusside was presented with the help of FOPID system.	Post-surgery Mean Arterial BP (MABP) controlling	The drug delivery rate to control the MABP is implemented using one Input one Output and FOPID system.	Stability of system enhanced using FOPID controller	[41]
2019/Robust IMC (Internal Model Control)-PID	Shahin Tasoujian	It estimates the efficiency of IMC PID in various hypotensive situations.	To control BP in serious hypotensive patient	To study the robust stability conditions the Small gain theorem is used for system uncertainty.	The explained controller is used for attenuation of overshoot and the oscillation reaction. It also produces a faster closed-loop system as well as keeping the bandwidth in a controlled range.	[42]

(Continued)

Table 13.2. (*Continued*)

Year/type of the controller	First author	Type of work	Application	Key-idea	Summary	Ref.
2018/PID, IMC (Internal Model Control) and MPC (Model Predictive Control) controller	A Alavudeen Basha	Review	Post-surgery BP monitoring and control of diabetic patients	The best insulin drug delivery can be achieved because of assistance of IMC—MPC controller.	The PID controller presents high response time in comparison to IMC and MPC regulator for patient while IMC and MPC present slow response time due to their nature.	[43]
2012/IMC Centered PI/ PID Controller	Sahaj Saxena	For constant, precise and relevant drug delivery with a broad variety of physiological deviations in patient, a new best IMC centered ODF (Single Degree of Freedom)-PI (Proportional-Integral) and TDF (Double Degree of Freedom)-PID controller are proposed.	To control Mean Arterial BP	Traditional PI-PID technique holds only single adjustable factor while IMC-PI-PID technique has a greater number of parameter variations, so this controlling technique is much better than PI-PID technique.	The SNP model has five constraints that differ from patient to patient and depend on medicine sensitivity while traditional PI-PID has only one tuning constraint, parameter. The IMC-PI-PID controller attains superior health performance for all types of patient such as normal, sensitive and non-sensitive patients.	[44]

procedure in the collection. However, the fundamental idea of PID control is simple, for the AP concept, advanced solutions such as robust PID [52, 53] or switching PID [54] have been used. In various carbohydrate ingestion and insulin sensitivity situations, the improved PID algorithm may work well. When compared to the standard PID algorithm, control efficiency is significantly improved, and hypoglycemia is avoided. With the use of PID, MPC and Fuzzy Logic a marvelous improvement has been noted of computerization rate of insulin mixture in AP [55, 56].

13.2.4 Arthritis

Joint pain is one of the most prevalent problems nowadays. In this there occurs swelling and stiffness in the joints. Osteoarthritis and rheumatoid arthritis are the most common types today. In osteoarthritis, there is breakdown of the tissue, while in rheumatoid arthritis, problem starts with the lining of joints. Arthritis is mostly seen in women and older people. Primary symptoms are problems in the motion of joints which can later lead to inability to do daily life activities. The worse case may be permanent joint changes [57].

Types of arthritis:

(i) Inflammatory arthritis: In this type the immune system attacks joints causing their decay. It may also lead to injury in internal organs. Rheumatoid arthritis is an example of inflammatory arthritis.

(ii) Degenerative arthritis: Excessive weight or hereditary traits may cause this type of arthritis. In this, the cushioning soft surface of the bone (cartilage) tears away, joints lose strength and may cause severe pain. Osteoarthritis is its example. Smoking, less frequent physical activity and some genetic factors are some of the possible reasons of osteoarthritis.

(iii) Metabolic arthritis: If the uric acid level in the body is not properly maintained by our glands, its excess causes the formation of some crystalline structure in the joints which causes pain. This arthritis may cause permanent disability in some part of the body.

Treatment: regular physical exercises, medicines, balancing of body mass index, the last option is surgery [58].

Arthritis controlling techniques: Proper care and control can avoid the symptoms of arthritis. Involvement of education and self-management by the patient can recover adherence and improve the efficiency of early treatment. The possibilities of involvement of new symptoms can be reduced by the combination of pharmacologic and rehabilitation management. Professional psychotherapy is a health environment that aims to enhance the daily routine activities by the patient. Multi-disciplinary follow up is essential for accurate management of the illness on different characteristics of life [59]. By the use of intelligent controlling techniques, the problem of arthritis may be controlled at some particular level. The problem of transferring secure and sufficient anesthesia during surgery can also be solved by using a strongly tuned PID controller [60].

13.3 Analysis of the biomedical system

Biomedical engineering (BME) is the well-known branch of engineering which is the combination of engineering ethics and methods used in the medicinal area. To improve the patient's health and life quality, it is necessary to use the engineer's skill with medicinal and natural discipline. Only conventional instruments were used previously, for disease identification and monitoring. There are numerous biomedical systems developed with new technology that modernize the health care system. Nowadays, hospice and health care centers use a variety of advanced and stylish instruments due to of technological improvement [61].

An apparatus that is used for a particular job is called an instrument. Most commonly used instruments are [62]:

1. Diagnostic instruments (DI): ECG (Electrocardiogram), EEG (Electroencephalogram);
2. Imaging instruments (II): e.g., MRI, CT Scan;
3. Therapeutic instruments (TI): e.g., Pace-makers (PMs).

ECG: It is used to measure the electrical signal generated by the heart muscles in cardiac functioning. It was invented by Wilhelm Einthoven. Electrocardiography is a technique to sense the electrical waveform generated by the heart. It is a specific arrangement of sensor (electrodes) in which two sensors are placed to receive the electric signals and another is for reference purposes. The electrical signals are of few millivolts, so they need to be amplified. After the proper conditioning of received signal they are ready to be saved or to display on screen. The ECG is an instrument which is used to measure the cardiac waveform to be stored, to display on screen or to print on paper. It indicates the functioning and condition of the heart, like heart beat cardiac output and myocardium etc. It gives information about the rate and rhythm of the heart and the condition of the heart muscles. Some diseases of the heart can be identified by it such as: heart attack, arrhythmia, cardiovascular etc.

EEG: A device that is used to measure the minute impulsive electrical movements of the brain by means of metal disc sensors positioned around the head. The technique of graphical representation of electrical waveforms generated by the brain is known as electroencephalography. 'Brain death' can be diagnosed with the help of EEG.

Imaging instruments (II): These are used to diagnose disease or any disorder of an organ in the very early phase, while the general or common diagnostic methods are not able to detect the same.

Magnetic resonance imaging: MRI gives images for organs or tissues of any layer of the body. This instrument was designed by Raymond Damadian and Bloch and Purcell. A computed tomography (CT) scan is a form of x-ray that is more advanced than a traditional x-ray. CT scan is an illustration technique which combines a computer to visualize the internals of the body with higher definition. A rotary arrangement of x-ray source and detector are used to imaging the body in a 360° angle.

Ultrasonography (USG): This works on the principle of Doppler effect in which a sound source with sound detectors is used to get an image of the internal body. The sound waves reflect from the internal organs are received by the detector to generate the two-dimensional image on the computer screen.

Therapeutic instruments (TI): An instrument that is used for therapy purposes. The PM is a small instrument which is used to keep the heart rhythm under control. It provides necessary electrical signals externally to the heart to maintain the proper heart beats.

13.3.1 Classical controller in a biomedical system

Feedback controllers are generally used in industry as well as in the biomedical field, known as PID. Elmer Sperry invented the first PID controller in 1911. PID has fast transient response and the ability to conquer steady state error. It has a quick momentary reaction and a lot of energy to beat steady state error. The PID has three controlling parameters: first is '*P*' that depends on present change in the error; the second is '*I*' that depends on past error; third is '*D*' that depends on future error. By adjusting these three parameters, researchers get the desired system outcome, as shown in table 13.3, according to need [63].

Error is the variation among the output (process variable) and the input (set point) of the controller. A PID controller uses a feedback phenomenon which can overcome the problem of error by adjusting the three parameters, i.e. *P*, *I* and *D*, as shown in figure 13.2 and in equation (13.1), according to system requirement.
Where: $u\ (t)$ = The PID controller's overall control function

K_p = Proportional benefit (present error)

K_i = Integral benefit (past error)

K_d = Derivative benefit (future error)

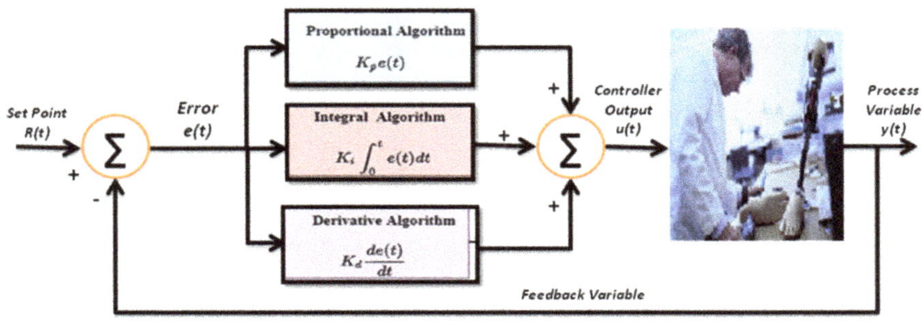

Figure 13.2. Biomedical system with PID controller.

Table 13.3. The effect of different gains of PID controlling parameters.

Controlling parameter	Overshoot	Steady-state error	Rise time	Settling time	Stability
K_p	Enlarge	Reduce	Reduce	Slight vary	Debase
K_i	Enlarge	Eradicate	Reduce	Enlarge	Debase
K_d	Reduce	No outcome	Slight vary	Reduce	Get better if K_d small

$$u(t) = K_p e(t) + K_i \int_0^t e(t)\mathrm{d}t + K_d \frac{d}{\mathrm{d}t} e(t) \tag{13.1}$$

13.4 Mathematical modeling of the biomedical system

13.4.1 MAP control

Mean arterial pressure (MAP) observation and controlling is necessary at the time of surgery. For same, researchers presented many controlling techniques, for example: PID control [64–66], model adaptive predictive control [67], fuzzy logic control [68], PI-PID control tuned with traditional technique [69] and PID tuning with PSO technique [70]. Figure 13.3 shows controlling of MAP using PID optimization techniques. Patient blood pressure can be represented by [71]:

$$G_{p1}(s) = \frac{Y(s)}{U(s)} = \frac{K(1 + \tau_3 s)e^{-Ls}}{[(1 + \tau_3 s)(1 + \tau_2 s) - \alpha](1 + \tau_1 s)} \tag{13.2}$$

$$P = p_0 - Y \tag{13.3}$$

where: G_{p1} = MAP Laplace based model

Y = decrease in the main burden because of the medicine effect;

p_0 = preliminary trunk pressure, P the subsequent pressure;

P = resulting pressure;

U = percentage of medicine infusion;

K = system gain;

L = time delay of system.

13.4.2 Intracranial tumor's temperature control

The primary aim is to automatically control the minimum temperature of brain tissues of a tumor patient who received interstitial hyperthermia treatment (IHT) [72]. In IHT, a catheters array is embedded in the tumor tissue during neurosurgery. The catheters work as temperature sensors as well as actuators. Tumor's temperature control using PID optimization techniques is shown in figure 13.4. The model for tumor tissues temperature control was established in [72] and can be represented by:

$$G_p(s) = \frac{Y(s)}{U(s)} = \frac{Ke^{-sL}}{1 + sT} \tag{13.4}$$

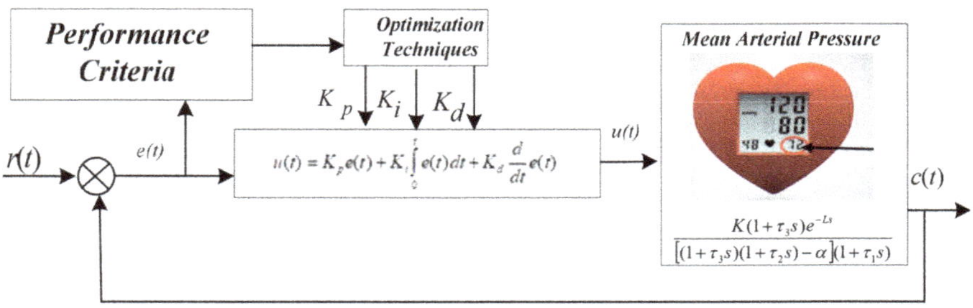

Figure 13.3. MAP control using PID.

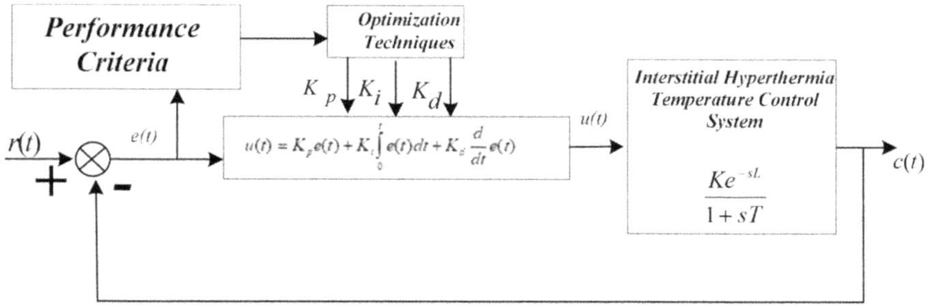

Figure 13.4. Tumor's temperature control using PID.

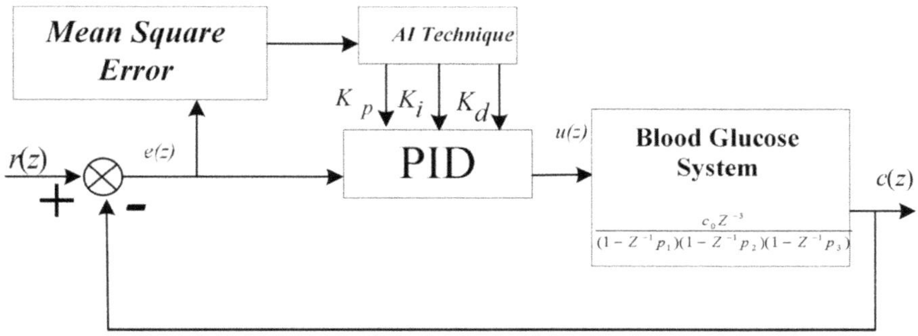

Figure 13.5. BP control using PID.

where Y = the least tissues heat;
U = the energy utilized to the pipe;
K = the system benefit (°CW-1);
T = system time constant;
L = the system time delay correlated by the conveyance moment among the source temperature and the expected calculating goals.

13.4.3 Blood glucose

To control the three special glucose dilutions 90, 120 and 150 mg dl^{-1}, a low order model with Black box technique is known widely, by which three linear models can be obtained for each diabetic patient [73]. Basal insulin (Ib) is considered for meticulous glucose level at steady state level, later than Ib added with sinusoidal insulin. After that, glucose deviation is recorded by locating the sampling time at 10 min A third order system used with Subspace identification method, for controlling the variation of BG, as shown in figure 13.5.

$$X_O(Z) = \frac{c_0 Z^{-3}}{(1 - Z^{-1}p_1)(1 - Z^{-1}p_2)(1 - Z^{-1}p_3)} \tag{13.5}$$

where $p_1 = 0.965$, $p_2 = 0.95$, $p_3 = 0.93$ are the poles of the system; and $c_0 = 0.932$ is a constant.

13.4.4 BP control after surgery in a diabetic patient

To control BP is a big challenge after surgery of a diabetic patient since diabetes and hypertension are related with each other, so constant observation and control are required. This problem can be overcome by obtaining automatic drug infusion technique. Generally, BP can be controlled in such cases by using SNP at an advised level, as shown in figure 13.6. The SNP performance for BP control can be represented as [43]:

$$G_{BP}(s) = \frac{\Delta Pd(s)}{I_i(s)} = \frac{ke^{-T_i s}(1 + \alpha e^{-T_C S})}{\tau s + 1} \tag{13.6}$$

where $\Delta Pd(s)$ = pressure difference (mmHg);
$I_i\ (s)$ = rate of infusion of SNP (ml h^{-1});
k = sensitivity of the patient (high value of k will show sensitive patient);
α = Index for recirculation;
τ = time constant;
T_i = opening transportation delay;
T_c = time for recirculation.

Generally, there are three types of modeling: standard, sensitive, and non-sensitive. Table 13.4 illustrates the different values of model parameter for all three types of modeling, which will vary patient-to-patient.

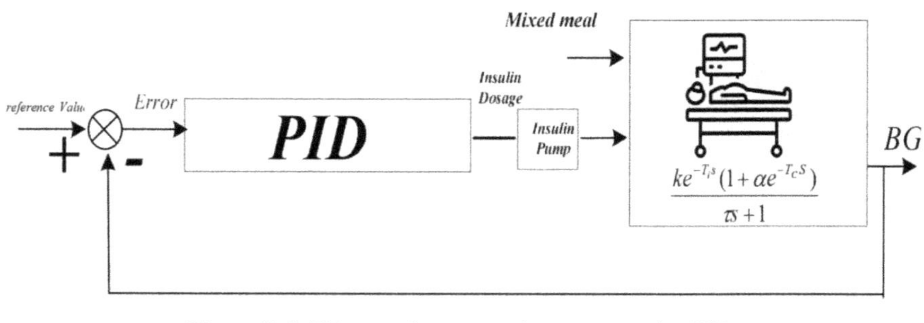

Figure 13.6. BP control strategy after surgery using PID.

Table 13.4. Model parameter.

Parameter	Non-sensitive	Sensitive	Standard
K	−0.179	−9	−0.714
A	0.4	0	0.4
τ	60	20	30
T_i	75	30	45
T_c	60	30	40

13.4.5 Heart modeling using PM

For heart-rate stabilization, the transfer functions of PM, heart and controller are all required, as shown in figure 13.7. PM is an I-order linear time variant system that may be modeled as [74]:

$$G_p(s) = \frac{k}{1 + s\tau} \tag{13.7}$$

$$Ms^2X(s) + BsX(s) + KX(s) = F(s)$$

$$G_h^c = \frac{X(s)}{F(s)} = \frac{1}{Ms^2 + Bs + K} \tag{13.8}$$

where: K = steady state gain;
M = volume of cardiac muscle;
B = constants of proportionality for sticky drag of myocardial unit;
K = constants of proportionality for torsional drag myocardial unit;
$F(s)$ = force utilized by the cardiac muscle sample then this force is produced through electrical and electrochemical action;
$X(s)$ = movement of the cardiovascular structure;
$Gc\ h(s)$ = heart's closed loop transfer function acknowledging unity feedback.

13.4.6 Tumor growth control

In today's life cancer is the most serious disease which increases death rates. Just about 1 373 500 people expired in 2017 due to cancer which is 3% extra compared to 2012 [75]. Due to this large number, cancer patient treatment is heavily dependent on the effectiveness of chemotherapy, as shown in figure 13.8. This problem can be overcome by using PID controller with the 'Hahnfeldt model' [76].

$$\dot{x}_1 = -\lambda x_1 \ln\left(\frac{x_1}{x_2}\right)$$

$$\dot{x}_2 = bx_1 - dx_1^{2/3}x_2 - ex_2g(t)$$

$$y = x_1$$

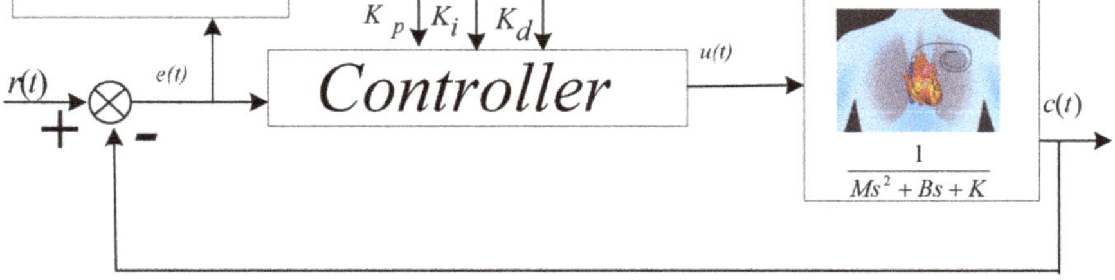

Figure 13.7. Heart disease control using PID.

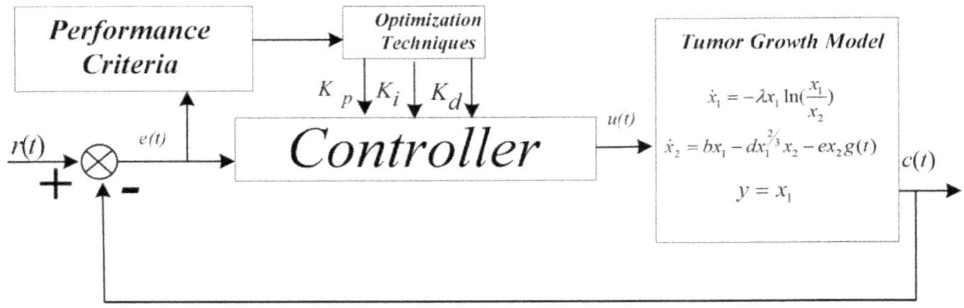

Figure 13.8. Tumor growth control using PID.

where x_1 = tumor size (mm^3);
x_2 = endothelial size (mm^3);
g = intensity of the controlled inhibitor (mg kg^{-1});
λ1 = tumor development speed (1/day);
b = stimulatory volume of tumor for vasculature (1/day);
d = endogenic inhibition of formerly created vasculature (1/day·mm^2);
e = anti-angiogenic impact of the controlled inhibitor on the tumor vasculature (kg/day·mg).

13.5 Conclusion

This work studied the application of a combination of AI and PID techniques in the medical diagnosis field. To get the most excellent and greatest response in the biomedical field, a PID controller is famous due to its simple design and intelligent tuning strategy. Non-noisy input provides more accuracy to the PID. The PID control systems are studied for controlling the different health issues such as, insulin delivery for diabetic patients, drug delivery control for H-BP during and post-surgery conditions, tumor growth monitoring, symptoms identification to control arthritis in preliminary stages etc. This work also studied the integration of AI based PID with different medical technologies to get better accuracy and enhanced diagnosis. The effectiveness of the AI based PID controller, mathematical modeling of various biomedical systems and drug infusion control systems are discussed. In this chapter the biomedical system based on a PID controller helps clinicians and control engineers to execute this progressive and harmless infusion method in actual time to automate the system delivery. The prototype models discussed are very effective in the field of medical health care systems.

References

[1] Alley D E 2016 Accountable health communities addressing social needs through Medicare and Medicaid *New Engl. J. Med.* **374** 8–11

[2] ASTHO (Association of State and Territorial Health Officials). Medicaid and Public Health Partnership Learning Series http://astho.org/Health-Systems-Transformation/Medicaid-and-Public-Health-Partnerships/Learning-Series/Managed-Care

[3] CMS (Centers for Medicare and Medicaid Services) 2019 Medicare and Medicaid Programs; Patient Protection and Affordable Care Act; Interoperability and Patient Access for Medicare Advantage Organization and Medicaid Managed Care Plans, State Medicaid Agencies, CHIP Agencies and CHIP Managed Care Entities, Issuers of Qualified Health Plans in the Federally Facilitated Exchanges, and Health Care Providers *Proposed Rule. Federal Register* 84 7610–80

[4] Kissam S M, Beil H, Cousart C, Greenwald L M and Lloyd J T 2019 States encouraging value-based payment: lessons from CMS's state innovation models initiative *Milbank Quart.* **97** 506–42

[5] Mendelson A, Kondo K, Damberg C, Low A, Motuapuaka M, Freeman M, O'Neil M, Relevo R and Kansagara D 2017 The effects of pay-for performance programs on health, healthcare use, and processes of care: a systematic review *Ann. Intern. Med.* **166** 341–55

[6] Israni S T and Verghese A 2019 Humanizing artificial intelligence *JAMA* **321** 29–30

[7] Patel V, Chatterji S, Chisholm D, Ebrahim S, Gopalakrishna G, Mathers C and Reddy K S 2011 Chronic diseases and injuries in India *Lancet* **377** 413–28

[8] Murray C J L, Inoue M and Lopez A D 1997 Alternative projections of mortality and disability by cause 1990–2020: global burden of disease study *Lancet* **349** 1498–504

[9] Govind K A and Sekhar R A 2014 Design of a novel PID controller for cardiac pacemaker *2014 Int. Conf. on Advances in Green Energy (ICAGE)* (Piscataway, NJ: IEEE) pp 82–7

[10] Sarangi L, Mohanty M N and Patnaik S 2017 Detection of abnormal cardiac condition using fuzzy inference system *Int. J. Autom. Control* **11** 372–83

[11] Sarangi L, Mohanty M N and Patnaik S 2016 Critical heart condition analysis through diagnostic agent of E-healthcare system using spectral domain transform *Indian J. Sci. Technol.* **9** 1–7

[12] Sarangi L, Mohanty M N and Patnaik S 2016 Design of ANFIS based E-health care system for cardio-vascular disease detection *Recent Developments in Intelligent Systems and Interactive Applications* (Berlin: Springer International Publishing) pp 445–53

[13] Sarangi L, Mohanty M N and Patnaik S 2015 An intelligent decision support system for cardiac disease cetion *Int. J. Control. Theory Appl.* **8** 2137–43

[14] Mohanty M D, Pattnaik D, Parida M, Mohanty S and Mohanty M N 2019 Design of intelligent PID controller for smart toilet of CCU/ICU patients in healthcare systems *Int. Conf. on Intelligent Computing and Applications* (Singapore: Springer) pp 97–107

[15] Yen J and Langari R 1999 *Fuzzy Logic. Intelligence, Control, Control, and information* (Englewood Cliffs, NJ: Prentice-Hall)

[16] Zhou Y S and Lai L Y 2000 Optimal design for fuzzy controllers by genetic algorithms *IEEE Trans. Ind. App.* **1** 93–7

[17] Vaishnav S R and Khan Z J 2007 Design and performance of PID and fuzzy logic controller with smaller rule set for higher order system *Proc. of the World Congress on Engineering and Computer Science* pp 24–6

[18] Venugopal P, Ganguly A and Singh P 2013 Design of tuning methods of PID controller using fuzzy logic *Int. J. Emerg. Trends Eng. Dev.* **5** 239–48

[19] Mallesham G and Rajani A 2006 Automatic tuning of PID controller using fuzzy logic *8th Int. Conf. on Development and Application Systems* pp 120–7

[20] Sharma S and Ma K K 2015 Analysis of liquid level control of coupled tank system by PI, PD, PID controller *Int. J. Sci. Res.* **4** 294–6

[21] Fellani M A and Gabaj A M 2015 PID controller design for two tanks liquid level control system using Matlab *Int. J. Elec. Comput. Eng.* **5** 436–42

[22] Kayani M H Q, Malik K N, Ahmad S, Khaqan A and Shuja S 2017 A switching based PID technique for blood glucose control *Biomed. Res.* **28** 8477–83

[23] Slate J B and Sheppard L C 1982 Automatic control of blood pressure by drug infusion *IEE Proc. A Phys. Sci. Meas. Instrum. Manag. Edu. Rev.* **129** 639–45

[24] Isaka S and Sebald A V 1993 Control strategies for arterial blood pressure regulation *IEEE Trans. Biomed. Eng.* **40** 353–63

[25] Denai M, Linkens D A, Asbury A J, MacLeod A D and Gray W M 1990 Self-tuning PID control of atracurium-induced muscle relaxation in surgical patients *IEE Proc. D: Control Theory Appl.* **137** 261–72

[26] Veltink P H, Chizeck H J, Crago P E and El-Bialy A 1992 Nonlinear joint angle control for artificially stimulated muscle *IEEE Trans. Biomed. Eng.* **39** 368–80

[27] Chee F, Fernando T L, Savkin A V and Van Heeden V 2003 Expert PID control system for blood glucose control in critically ill patients *IEEE Trans. Inf. Technol. Biomed.* **7** 419–25

[28] Marchetti G, Barolo M, Jovanovic L, Zisser H and Seborg D E 2008 An improved PID switching control strategy for type 1 diabetes *IEEE Trans. Biomed. Eng.* **55** 857–65

[29] O'Hara D A, Hexem J G, Derbyshire G J, Overdyk F J, Chen B, Henthorn T K and Li J K-J 1997 The use of a PID controller to model vecuronium pharmacokinetics and pharmacodynamics during liver transplantation *IEEE Trans. Biomed. Eng.* **44** 610–9

[30] Van Heusden K, Dumont G A, Soltesz K, Petersen C L, Umedaly A, West N and Mark Ansermino J 2013 Design and clinical evaluation of robust PID control of propofol anesthesia in children *IEEE Trans. Contr. Syst. Technol.* **22** 491–501

[31] Czakó B G, Sápi J and Kovács L 2018 Optimal PID based computed torque control of tumor growth models *IFAC-Papers Online* **51** 900–5

[32] Padmanabhan R, Meskin N and Haddad W M 2017 Reinforcement learning-based control of drug dosing for cancer chemotherapy treatment *Math. Biosci.* **293** 11–20

[33] Chen T, Kirkby N F and Jena R 2012 Optimal dosing of cancer chemotherapy using model predictive control and moving horizon state/parameter estimation *Comput. Methods Progr. Biomed.* **108** 973–83

[34] Kiran K L, Jayachandran D and Lakshminarayanan S 2009 Multi-objective optimization of cancer immunochemotherapy *Proc. 13th Int. Conf. on Biomedical Engineering* pp 1337–40

[35] Noble S L, Sherer E, Hannemann R E, Ramkrishna D, Vik T and Rundell A E 2010 Using adaptive model predictive control to customize maintenance therapy chemotherapeutic dosing for childhood acute lymphoblastic leukemia *J. Theor. Biol.* **264** 990–1002

[36] Engelhart M, Lebiedz D and Sager S 2011 Optimal control for selected cancer chemotherapy ODE models: a view on the potential of optimal schedules and choice of objective function *Math. Biosci.* **229** 123–34

[37] Tan K C, Khor E F, Cai J, Heng C and Lee T H 2002 Automating the drug scheduling of cancer chemotherapy via evolutionary computation *Artif. Intell. Med.* **25** 169–85

[38] Tse S-M, Liang Y, Leung K-S, Lee K-H and Mok T S-K 2007 A memetic algorithm for multiple-drug cancer chemotherapy schedule optimization *IEEE Trans. Syst. Man Cybern Part B (Cybern)* **37** 84–91

[39] American Heart Association 2014 Understanding blood pressure readings. Updated November 17

[40] Ribeiro A G, Maitelli A L, Valentim R A D M, Leite C R, Soares H B, de Almeida N C, Sizilio G R M A and Guerreiro A M 2011 Design of an embedded PID controller applied to blood pressure control *2011 Annual Int. Conf. of the IEEE Engineering in Medicine and Biology Society* (Piscataway, NJ: IEEE) pp 278–81

[41] Urooj S and Singh B 2019 Fractional-order PID control for postoperative mean arterial blood pressure control scheme *Procedia Comput. Sci.* **152** 380–89

[42] Tasoujian S, Salavati S, Franchek M and Grigoriadis K 2019 Robust IMC-PID and parameter-varying control strategies for automated blood pressure regulation *Int. J. Control Autom. Syst.* **17** 1803–13

[43] Basha A A, Vivekanandan S and Parthasarathy P 2018 Evolution of blood pressure control identification in lieu of post-surgery diabetic patients: a review *Health Inform. Sci. Syst.* **6** 17

[44] Saxena S and Hote Y V 2012 A simulation study on optimal IMC based PI/PID controller for mean arterial blood pressure *Biomed. Eng. Lett.* **2** 240–48

[45] Federation D 2013 *IDF Diabetes Atlas* 6th edn (Brussels: International Diabetes Federation)

[46] Fonyó A and Ligeti E 2008 *Physiology (in Hungarian)* 3rd edn (Budapest: Medicina) .

[47] American Diabetes Association 2011 Diagnosis and classification of diabetes mellitus *Diabetes Care* **34** S5–S10

[48] Mei Y 2017 Modeling and control to improve blood glucose concentration for people with diabetes. *Graduate Thesis* University of Iowa https://lib.dr.iastate.edu/etd/16102

[49] Chee F and Fernando T 2007 *Closed-Loop Control of Blood Glucose* 1st edn (Berlin: Springer)

[50] Cobelli C, Renard E and Kovatchev B 2011 Artificial pancreas: past, present, future *Diabetes* **60** 2672–82

[51] Shah V N, Shoskes A, Tawfik B and Garg S K 2014 Closed-loop system in the management of diabetes: past, present, and future *Diabetes Technol. Ther.* **16** 477–90

[52] Kamath S 2013 Model based simulation for type 1 diabetes patients *Asian Am. J. Chem.* **1** 11–9

[53] Ramprasad Y, Rangaiah G and Lakshminarayanan S 2004 Robust PID controller for blood glucose regulation in type I diabetics *Ind. Eng. Chem. Res.* **43** 8257–68

[54] Marchetti G, Barolo M, Jovanovic L, Zisser H and Seborg D E 2008 An improved PID switching control strategy for type 1 diabetes *IEEE Trans. Biomed. Eng.* **55** 857–65

[55] Bequette B W 2005 A critical assessment of algorithms and challenges in the development of a closed-loop artificial pancreas *Diabetes Technol. Therap.* **7** 28–47

[56] Peyser T, Dassau E, Breton M and Skyler J S 2014 The artificial pancreas: current status and future prospects in the management of diabetes *Ann. N.Y. Acad. Sci.* **1311** 102–23

[57] Stevens M A 2018 *Knee Osteoarthritis* Otterbein Iniversity, Nursing Student Class Projects (Formerly MSN) 300 https://digitalcommons.otterbein.edu/stu_msn/300

[58] Nkemdilim O C 2018 Differential diagnosis and tests of rheumatoid arthritis and its implication for physiotherapy *Int. J. Innov. Res. Adv. Stud. (IJIRAS)* **5** 18–22

[59] Almeida P H T Q D, Pontes T B, Matheus J P C, Muniz L F and Mota L M H D 2015 Occupational therapy in rheumatoid arthritis: what rheumatologists need to know? *Rev. Bras. Reumatol.* **55** 272–80

[60] Soltesz K, Van Heusden K, Dumont G A, Hägglund T, Petersen C L, West N and Ansermino J M 2012 Closed-loop anesthesia in children using a PID controller: a pilot study *IFAC Proc.* **45** 317–22

[61] Enderle J 2012 *Introduction to Biomedical Engineering* (New York: Academic)

[62] Singh M 2014 *Introduction to Biomedical Instrumentation* (New Delhi: PHI Learning Pvt. Ltd)

[63] Bequette B W 2012 Challenges and recent progress in the development of a closed-loop artificial pancreas *Annu. Rev. Control* **36** 255–66

[64] Guanzheng L, Wang L and Zhang Y 2009 A closed-loop feedback control method based on body sensor networks for mean arterial blood pressure regulation *Bull. Adv. Technol. Res.* **3** 12–6

[65] Enbiya S, Hossain A and Mahieddine F 2011 Neuro-PID adaptive control scheme for blood pressure regulation *5th Int. Conf. on Software, Knowledge Information, Industrial Management and Applications (SKIMA)* p 4

[66] Elamvazuthi I, Aymen O M, Salih Y and Tawfeig H 2013 An intelligent control of blood pressure system using PID and neural network *8th IEEE Conf. on Industrial Electronics and Applications (ICIEA)* pp 1049–53

[67] Clement Y, Roy R J and Bequette B W 1992 Multiple-model adaptive predictive control of mean arterial pressure and cardiac output *IEEE Trans. Biomed. Eng.* **39** 765–78

[68] Logesh K M, Harikumar R, Keerthi V A and Sudhaman V K 2009 Fuzzy controller for automatic drug infusion in cardiac patients *Proc. Int. Multi Conf. of Engineers and Computer Scientists* vol 1 *(Hong Kong)* p 5

[69] Jones R W and Tham M T 2005 An undergraduate CACSD project: the control of mean arterial blood pressure during surgery *Int. J. Eng. Ed.* **21** 1043–49

[70] Moura Oliveira P B, Vrančić D, Boaventura Cunha J and Solteiro Pires E J 2014 Teaching particle swarm optimization through an open-loop system identification project *Comput. Appl. Eng. Educ.* **22** 227–37

[71] Martin J F, Schneider A M and Smith N T 1987 Multiple-model adaptive control of blood pressure using sodium nitroprusside *IEEE Trans. Biomed. Eng.* **BME-34** 603–11

[72] DeFord J A, Babbs C F, Patel U H, Fearnot N E, Marchosky J A and Moran C J 1991 Design and evaluation of closed-loop feedback control of minimum temperatures in human intracranial tumours treated with interstitial hyperthermia *Med. Biol. Eng. Comput.* **29** 197–206

[73] Patricio C, Ricardo S, S´Anchez P, Ravi G, Eyal D and Francis J D III Reducing risks in type 1 diabetes using H 8 control *IEEE Trans. Biomed. Eng.* 201**461**

[74] Govind K A and Sekhar R A 2014 Design of a novel PID controller for cardiac pacemaker *2014 Int. Conf. on Advances in Green Energy (ICAGE)* (Piscataway, NJ: IEEE) pp 82–7

[75] Sápi J, Drexler D A and Kovács L 2013 Parameter optimization of H_∞ controller designed for tumor growth in the light of physiological aspects *2013 IEEE 14th Int. Symp. on Computational Intelligence and Informatics (CINTI)* (Piscataway, NJ: IEEE) pp 19–24

[76] Kovacs L, Szeles A, Drexler D, Sapi J and Harmati I 2013 Model-based angiogenic inhibition of tumor growth using modern robust control method *Comput. Methods Programs Biomed.* **114** 98–110

Lightning Source UK Ltd.
Milton Keynes UK
UKHW051627131021
392129UK00003B/82

9 780750 338134